Applications of FDG-PET in Central Nervous System Disorders

Editors

ANDREW B. NEWBERG
ERIC GUEDJ
ABASS ALAVI

PET CLINICS

www.pet.theclinics.com

Consulting Editor
ABASS ALAVI

October 2026 • Volume 21 • Number 4

ELSEVIER

1818 Market Street • Suite 3323 • Philadelphia, Pennsylvania, 19103-2899

http://www.pet.theclinics.com

PET CLINICS Volume 21, Number 4
October 2026 ISSN 1556-8598, ISBN-13: 978-0-443-52088-4

Editor: Stacy Eastman
Developmental Editor: Niharika Saxena

Publishing Office: *PET Clinics* (ISSN 1556-8598) is published quarterly by Elsevier Inc., 1818 Market Street, Philadelphia, PA 19103, United States. Periodicals postage paid at New York, NY and additional mailing offices. USA POSTMASTER: Send address changes to *PET Clinics*, Elsevier Customer Service Department, 3251 Riverport Lane, Maryland Heights, MO 63043, USA. Months of issue are January, April, July, and October. Subscription prices per year are $306.00 (US individuals), $100.00 (US students), $323.00 (Canadian individuals), $100.00 (Canadian students), $325.00 (foreign individuals), and $140.00 (foreign students). For institutional access pricing please contact Customer Service via the contact information below. To receive student and resident rate, orders must be accompanied by name of affiliated institution, date of term, and the signature of program/residency coordinator on institution letterhead. Orders will be billed at individual rate until proof of status is received. Foreign air speed delivery is included in all Clinics subscription prices. All prices are subject to change without notice. Orders, claims, and journal inquiries: Please visit our Support Hub page https://service.elsevier.com for assistance.

Reprints. For copies of 100 or more of articles in this publication, please contact the Commercial Reprints Department, Elsevier Inc., 360 Park Avenue South, New York, NY 10010-1710. Tel.: 212-633-3874; Fax: 212-633-3820; E-mail: reprints@elsevier.com.

PET Clinics is covered in MEDLINE/PubMed (Index Medicus).

Contributors

CONSULTING EDITOR

ABASS ALAVI, MD, MD (Hon), PhD (Hon), DSc (Hon)
Professor of Radiology, Division of Nuclear Medicine, Department of Radiology, Hospital of the University of Pennsylvania, University of Pennsylvania Perelman School of Medicine, Philadelphia, Pennsylvania, USA

EDITORS

ANDREW B. NEWBERG, MD
Professor, Departments of Integrative Medicine and Nutritional Sciences, and Radiology, Director, Research at the Marcus Institute of Integrative Health, Sidney Kimmel Medical College, Thomas Jefferson University, Philadelphia, Pennsylvania, USA

ERIC GUEDJ, MD, PhD
Professor of Biophysics and Nuclear Medicine, Aix-Marseille University (AMU), Head, Department of Nuclear Medicine, Timone Hospital, Research Leader, IMoTheP team, Institut Fresnel (AMU, CNRS, Ecole Centrale Marseille), Marseille, France

ABASS ALAVI, MD, MD (Hon), PhD (Hon), DSc (Hon)
Professor of Radiology, Division of Nuclear Medicine, Department of Radiology, Hospital of the University of Pennsylvania, University of Pennsylvania Perelman School of Medicine, Philadelphia, Pennsylvania, USA

AUTHORS

ABASS ALAVI, MD, MD (Hon), PhD (Hon), DSc (Hon)
Professor of Radiology, Division of Nuclear Medicine, Department of Radiology, Hospital of the University of Pennsylvania, University of Pennsylvania Perelman School of Medicine, Philadelphia, Pennsylvania, USA

CYRUS AYUBCHA, MD, PhD
Resident, Department of Neurosurgery, University of California San Diego, San Diego, California, and Department of Neurosurgery, Harvard Medical School, Boston, Massachusetts, USA

ARTUR MARTINS COUTINHO, MD, PhD
Assistant Physician, Clinical Research Coordinator, Nuclear Medicine Center (LIM-43), Institute of Radiology, Hospital das Clinicas, Faculdade de Medicina da Universidade de Sao Paulo (FMUSP), Sao Paulo, Brazil

ALEXANDER DRZEZGA, MD
Professor and Director (Chair), Department of Nuclear Medicine, University Hospital Cologne, University of Cologne, Cologne, Germany

RODOLFO FERRANDO, MD, MSc
Associate Professor, Academic Unit of Nuclear Medicine and Molecular Imaging, Hospital de Clínicas, Universidad de la República Head, Department of Functional Brain Imaging, Uruguayan Center for Molecular Imaging, Montevideo, Uruguay

ERIC GUEDJ, MD, PhD
Professor of Biophysics and Nuclear Medicine, Aix-Marseille University (AMU), Head, Department of Nuclear Medicine, Timone Hospital, Research Leader, IMoTheP team, Institut Fresnel (AMU, CNRS, Ecole Centrale Marseille), Marseille, France

YOUSR HASSAN, MD
Clinical Professional, Department of Radiology, Hospital of the University of Pennsylvania, Philadelphia, Pennsylvania, USA

JULIE HONG, MD
Assistant Professor, Department of Nuclear Medicine and Theranostics, David Geffen School of Medicine at UCLA, University of California, Los Angeles, USA

TATIANA HOROWITZ, MD, MSc
Associate Professor, CNRS, Biophysics and Nuclear Medicine, Aix Marseille University, Centrale Marseille, IMoTheP Team, Institut Fresnel, AP-HM, Timone Hospital, Nuclear Medicine Department, Service de Médecine Nucléaire, CHU Timone, CERIMED, Marseille, France

YINING HUA, MSc, PhD
PhD Candidate, Department of Epidemiology, Harvard T.H. Chan School of Public Health, Boston, Massachusetts, USA

ROLAND HUSTINX, MD, PhD
Full Professor, Faculty of Medicine, Head, Division of Nuclear Medicine and Oncological Imaging, University Hospital of Liège, Liège, Belgium

SATOSHI MINOSHIMA, MD, PhD
Professor, Anne G. Osborn Endowed Chair, Department of Radiology and Imaging Sciences, University of Utah, Salt Lake City, Utah, USA

MELIKA MIRBOD, MD
Researcher, Department of Radiology, Hospital of the University of Pennsylvania, Philadelphia, Pennsylvania, USA

SAHAR DARABI MONADI, MD
Neuroradiology Research Fellow, Department of Radiology, Thomas Jefferson University Hospital, Philadelphia, Pennsylvania, USA

DANIEL A. MONTI, MD
Chair and Professor, Department of Integrative Medicine and Nutritional Sciences, Marcus Institute of Integrative Health, Thomas Jefferson University, Philadelphia, Pennsylvania, USA

RIZWAN NASEER, MD
Internal Medicine Physician, Department of Medicine, Trinity Health System, Steubenville, Ohio, USA

ANDREW B. NEWBERG, MD
Professor, Departments of Integrative Medicine and Nutritional Sciences, and Radiology, Director, Research at the Marcus Institute of Integrative Health, Sidney Kimmel Medical College, Thomas Jefferson University, Philadelphia, Pennsylvania, USA

MONA-ELISABETH REVHEIM, MD, PhD, MHA
Professor II, Institute of Clinical Medicine, Faculty of Medicine, University of Oslo, Head of Department, The Intervention Center, Division for Technology and Innovation, Oslo University Hospital, Oslo, Norway

DANIEL H.S. SILVERMAN, MD, PhD
Professor, Department of Molecular and Medical Pharmacology, Head, Neuronuclear Imaging Section of the Ahmanson Translational Imaging Division, UCLA Medical Center, David Geffen School of Medicine at UCLA,University of California, Los Angeles, USA

CAMILLE STEENHOUT, MD
Medical Doctor, Division of Nuclear Medicine and Oncological Imaging, University Hospital of Liège, Liège, Belgium

THILO VAN EIMEREN, MD
Professor of Multimodal Brain Imaging, Departments of Nuclear Medicine and Neurology, University Hospital Cologne, University of Cologne, Cologne, Germany

ANTOINE VERGER, MD, PhD
Professor, Department of Nuclear Medicine, Nancyclotep Imaging Platform, IADI Laboratory, INSERM U1254, Université de Lorraine, Nancy, France

THOMAS J. WERNER, MSE
Clinical Research Assistant, Researcher, Department of Radiology, Hospital of the University of Pennsylvania, University of Pennsylvania Perelman School of Medicine, Philadelphia, Pennsylvania, USA

NADIA WITHOFS, MD, PhD
Professor, Faculty of Medicine, Physician, Division of Nuclear Medicine and Oncological Imaging, University Hospital of Liège, Liège, Belgium

Contents

PET CLINICS

FORTHCOMING ISSUES

January 2027
Applications of FDG-PET Imaging in the Management of Patients with Various Malignancies
Rakesh Kumar, *Editor*

April 2027
FDG-PET Applications in the Management of Patients with Infection and Inflammation
Rakesh Kumar, *Editor*

July 2027
FDG-PET in Theranostics and Therapeutic Decision Making
Sandip Basu, *Editor*

RECENT ISSUES

July 2026
Theranostics
Harshad Kulkarni and Abass Alavi, *Editors*

April 2026
PET/MRI and PET/CT in Pediatric Patients
Hongming Zhuang and Abass Alavi, *Editors*

January 2026
Computational and AI Methods in Theranostics and Nuclear Oncology
Arman Rahmim, Kuangyu Shi, and Babak Saboury, *Editors*

SERIES OF RELATED INTEREST

MRI Clinics of North America
Available at: MRI.theclinics.com
Neuroimaging Clinics of North America
Available at: Neuroimaging.theclinics.com
Radiologic Clinics of North America
Available at: Radiologic.theclinics.com

PROGRAM OBJECTIVE

The goal of the *PET Clinics* is to keep practicing radiologists and radiology residents up to date with current clinical practice in positron emission tomography by providing timely articles reviewing the state of the art in patient care.

TARGET AUDIENCE

Practicing radiologists, radiology residents, and other health care professionals who provide patient care utilizing radiologic findings.

LEARNING OBJECTIVES

Upon completion of this activity, participants will be able to:

1. Review the role of FDG PET as a diagnostic tool in integrative medicine and its use alongside clinical evaluation and complementary imaging modalities, including SPECT, CT, and MRI.
2. Discuss FDG PET as a powerful adjunct for the differential diagnosis of movement disorders, Parkinsonian Syndromes, traumatic brain injury (TBI), and evolving metabolic disturbances.
3. Recognize that neuroimaging plays a key role in the early and accurate assessment of diagnosis, prognosis, and treatment optimization for patients experiencing cognitive decline.

ACCREDITATION

The Elsevier Office of Continuing Medical Education (EOCME) is accredited by the Accreditation Council for Continuing Medical Education (ACCME) to provide continuing medical education for physicians.

The EOCME designates this journal-based CME activity for a maximum of 13 *AMA PRA Category 1 Credit*(s)™. Physicians should claim only the credit commensurate with the extent of their participation in the activity.

All other health care professionals requesting continuing education credit for this enduring material will be issued a certificate of participation.

DISCLOSURE OF RELEVANT FINANCIAL RELATIONSHIPS

The EOCME assesses conflict of interest with its instructors, faculty, planners, and other individuals who are in a position to control the content of CME activities. All relevant conflicts of interest that are identified are thoroughly vetted by EOCME for fair balance, scientific objectivity, and patient care recommendations. EOCME is committed to providing its learners with CME activities that promote improvements or quality in healthcare and not a specific proprietary business or a commercial interest.

The authors and editors listed below have identified no financial relationships or relationships to products or devices they have with ineligible companies related to the content of this CME activity:
Abass Alavi, MD, MD (Hon), PhD (Hon), DSc (Hon); Cyrus Ayubcha, MD, PhD; Rodolfo Ferrando, MD, MSc; Yousr Hasan, MD; Julie Hong, MD; Tatiana Horowitz, MD, MSc; Yining Hua, MSc, PhD; Roland Hustinx, MD, PhD; Satoshi Minoshima, MD, PhD; Melika Mirbod, MD; Sahar Darabi Monadi, MD; Daniel A. Monti, MD; Rizwan Naseer, MD; Andrew B. Newberg, MD; Mona-Elisabeth Revheim, MD, PhD, MHA; Daniel H. S. Silverman, MD, PhD; Camille Steenhout, MD; Antoine Verger, MD, PhD; Thomas J. Werner, MSE; Nadia Withofs, MD, PhD

The authors and editors listed below have identified financial relationships or relationships to products or devices they have with ineligible companies related to the content of this CME activity:
Artur Martins Coutinho, MD, PhD: *Advisor, Executive role, Ownership interest*: Masimo

Alexander Drzezga, MD: *Advisor/Speaker*: Siemens Healthineers, Sanofi, GE Healthcare, Biogen, Novo Nordisk, Invicro, Novartis/AAA, Bayer Vital, Lilly, Swiss Rockets; *Ownership Interest*: Siemens Healthineers, Lantheus Holding, Lilly, Bayer; *Patent Beneficiary*: 18F-JK-PSMA- 7 (PSMA PET imaging tracer), Patent No.: EP3765097A1; Date of patent: Jan. 20, 2021

Eric Guedj, MD, PhD: *Consultant*: GE Healthcare, Life Molecular Imaging, ABX-CRO

Thilo van Eimeren, MD: *Consultant*: Bial, ICON plc

The planners and staff listed below have identified no financial relationships or relationships to products or devices they have with ineligible companies related to the content of this CME activity:
Stacy Eastman; Prabhu Elangali; Michelle Littlejohn; Patrick J. Manley; Niharika Saxena

UNAPPROVED/OFF-LABEL USE DISCLOSURE

The EOCME requires CME faculty to disclose to the participants:

1. When products or procedures being discussed are off-label, unlabelled, experimental, and/or investigational (not US Food and Drug Administration [FDA] approved); and
2. Any limitations on the information presented, such as data that are preliminary or that represent ongoing research, interim analyses, and/or unsupported opinions. Faculty may discuss information about pharmaceutical agents that is outside of FDA-approved labelling. This information is intended solely for CME and is not intended to promote off-label use of these medications. If you have any questions, contact the medical affairs department of the manufacturer for the most recent prescribing information.

TO ENROLL

To enroll in the *PET Clinics* Continuing Medical Education program, call customer service at 1-800-654-2452 or sign up online at https://www.pet.theclinics.com/cme/home. The CME program is available to subscribers for an additional annual fee of USD 254.00.

METHOD OF PARTICIPATION

In order to claim credit, participants must complete the following:

1. Complete enrolment as indicated above.
2. Read the activity.
3. Complete the CME Test and Evaluation. Participants must achieve a score of 70% on the test. All CME Tests and Evaluations must be completed online.

CME INQUIRIES/SPECIAL NEEDS

For all CME inquiries or special needs, please contact elsevierCME@elsevier.com.

Introduction

Five Decades of Unparalleled Impact of Fluorodeoxyglucose-PET on Day-to-Day Practice of Medicine

The concept of synthesizing Fluorodeoxyglucose (FDG) was conceived by Abass Alavi, David Kuhl, and Martin Reivich in 1973, soon after the introduction of computed tomography (CT), which was considered a major threat to the standard practice of imaging with radiolabeled compounds in medicine. The main focus of radiotracer-based imaging at that time dealt with somewhat primitive single-gamma-emitting tracers by conventional planar scanners. This collaborative effort eventually led to the synthesis of 18F-FDG by chemists (Alfred Wolf and collaborators) at Brookhaven National Laboratory. In August 1976, this labeled compound was transported by a private aircraft to the University of Pennsylvania (Penn) for the first human studies. The first images of the brain were acquired by a Single-Photon Emission Computed Tomography instrument that was assembled at Penn for imaging conventional radiolabeled compounds. Determining brain glucose metabolism was achievable by this approach. Furthermore, the second subject was imaged by a conventional rectilinear scanner that was designed for tolerating high-energy single-gamma emitters. The latter image revealed total body distribution of FDG, which further demonstrated the ability of FDG to detect glucose metabolism in various organs of the human body. In parallel with this development, investigators at University of Washington, in St Louis, had designed early PET instruments that demonstrated the feasibility of imaging with such tracers. The early applications of FDG were carried out at Penn, Brookhaven National Laboratory, and UCLA. Such studies revealed the critical role of FDG-PET in assessing a variety of disorders with emphasis on brain diseases, malignancies, and cardiovascular disorders. During the past five decades, the impact of FDG-PET has been assessed extensively in other domains, including inflammation, infection, and many other benign disorders. The advancements that have been made in PET instrumentation along with novel quantitative techniques have truly revolutionized the day-to-day practice of medicine during the past decades. In particular, the introduction of PET/CT and PET/MR imaging has further expanded the applications of PET by convincing the medical community about the necessity of this modality in better management of patients in many settings. This has encouraged scientists around the world to synthesize numerous other compounds that have further expanded and enhanced the role of PET in medicine. In conclusion, the revolutionary impact of FDG-PET on research and clinical medicine is unparalleled by any other technique in decades. Therefore, at this juncture, it is very timely to celebrate the five decades since the introduction of FDG to the world and its enduring importance to the day-to-day practice of medicine.

Abass Alavi, MD, MD (Hon), PhD (Hon), DSc (Hon)
Division of Nuclear Medicine
Department of Radiology
Hospital of the University of Pennsylvania
University of Pennsylvania
Perelman School of Medicine
Philadelphia, PA, USA

E-mail address:
abass.alavi@pennmedicine.upenn.edu

PET Clin 21 (2026) xiii
https://doi.org/10.1016/j.cpet.2026.07.003
1556-8598/26/

Preface

Five Decades of [18F] Fluorodeoxyglucose–PET in Neuropsychiatric Disorders: From Brain Metabolism to Precision Functional Imaging

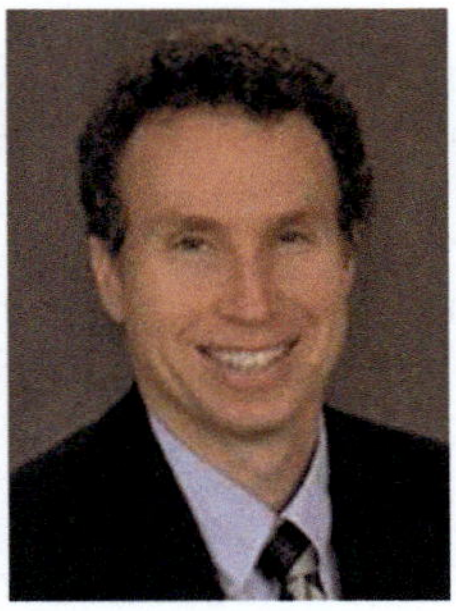
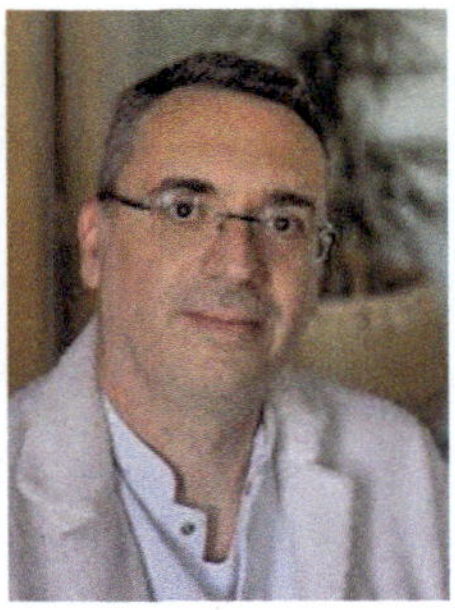
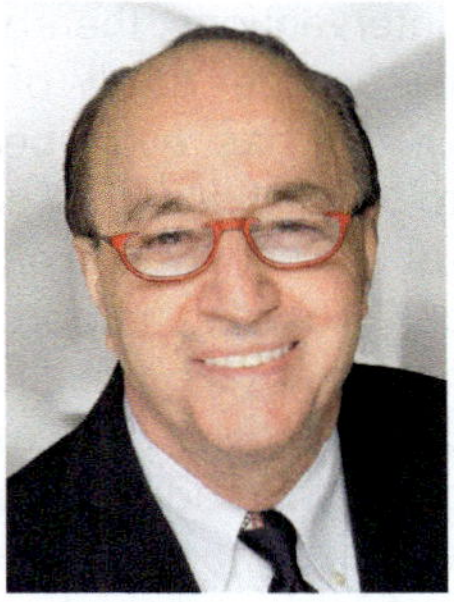

Andrew B. Newberg, MD Eric Guedj, MD, PhD Abass Alavi, MD, MD (Hon), PhD (Hon), DSc (Hon)
Editors

The development of fluorodeoxyglucose (FDG)-PET represents one of the most transformative advances in modern medical imaging. The concept of FDG-PET imaging originated in 1973 through the pioneering efforts of three investigators at the University of Pennsylvania—Abass Alavi, David Kuhl, and Martin Reivich. The first human FDG-PET study was subsequently performed at Penn in 1976. These early developments were deeply rooted in brain imaging and experimental neurophysiology, providing one of the first clinically interpretable in vivo maps of human cerebral glucose metabolism. Despite these groundbreaking achievements, the full clinical significance of PET imaging, and FDG in particular, was not widely appreciated until technical advances in its use for brain and oncologic imaging, particularly with the introduction of hybrid PET–computed tomography (CT) and, in selected settings, PET–MR imaging systems at the beginning of the twenty-first century. The integration of metabolic and anatomic imaging dramatically enhanced diagnostic accuracy and workflow, ultimately establishing PET-CT as an indispensable tool in both clinical medicine and biomedical research. Over the past two decades, FDG-PET has revolutionized patient care across numerous medical disciplines and has become firmly integrated into routine diagnostic algorithms worldwide.

FDG, as a radiolabeled glucose analogue, has played a central role in the success and expansion of PET imaging because of its ability to characterize tissue metabolism in vivo. This year marks the 50th anniversary of this landmark development in medicine, providing an opportunity to reflect on the extraordinary scientific and clinical impact of FDG-PET imaging. To commemorate this milestone, four issues of *PET Clinics* will be devoted to reviewing the major applications of FDG-PET in contemporary medicine. The present issue focuses on disorders of the central nervous system and the neuropsychiatric spectrum, including traumatic brain injury, aging, dementia, epilepsy, and neurodegenerative disorders. Additional focus will be placed on oncologic imaging, where FDG-PET has transformed cancer diagnosis, staging,

PET Clin 21 (2026) xv–xvi
https://doi.org/10.1016/j.cpet.2026.06.004
1556-8598/26/

treatment monitoring, and recurrence detection. The role of FDG-PET in infection and inflammation, including autoimmune and inflammatory disorders, will also be explored, as will emerging theranostic applications that combine molecular imaging with targeted therapy.

Beyond its conventional medical applications, FDG-PET has contributed substantially to advancing the understanding of human physiology, cognition, and behavior. FDG-PET has been used to investigate psychiatric disorders, stress responses, meditation practices, and integrative medicine interventions, thereby extending its impact into the broader study of brain-body interactions. FDG-PET has even been used in investigations exploring the neural correlates of consciousness, spirituality, and the nature of subjective experience, providing important insights into deep human philosophic questions. Across these domains, its distinctive value lies not simply in detecting abnormal metabolism, but in making the functional expression of disease visible, interpretable, quantifiable, and actionable within multidisciplinary care. Collectively, the history of FDG-PET reflects not only a remarkable technological achievement, but also the evolution of molecular imaging into a critical framework for understanding disease biology, therapeutic response, brain function, behavior, and patient-level clinical expression. As FDG-PET continues to evolve alongside advances in artificial intelligence, quantitative imaging, and precision medicine, we hope this issue will help readers appreciate both the historical importance of FDG-PET and its continuing potential to shape the next generation of clinical neuroscience.

Andrew B. Newberg, MD
Department of Integrative Medicine and Nutritional Sciences
Department of Radiology
Research at the Marcus Institute of Integrative Health
Thomas Jefferson University
Philadelphia, PA, USA

Eric Guedj, MD, PhD
Department of Nuclear Medicine
Aix-Marseille University
Timone Hospital (APHM)
ImoTheP research team
Fresnel Institute (AMU, CNRS
Ecole Centrale Marseille)
Marseille, France

Abass Alavi, MD, MD (Hon), PhD (Hon), DSc (Hon)
Division of Nuclear Medicine
Department of Radiology
Hospital of the University of Pennsylvania
University of Pennsylvania Perelman School of Medicine
Philadelphia, PA, USA

E-mail addresses:
Andrew.newberg@jefferson.edu (A.B. Newberg)
eric.guedj@univ-amu.fr (E. Guedj)
Abass.Alavi@pennmedicine.upenn.edu (A. Alavi)

18F-Fluorodeoxyglucose PET, the Brain, and Other Organs

From the First Human Studies (1976) to 2026

Abass Alavi, MD[a,*], Mona-Elisabeth Revheim, MD, PhD, MHA[b], Andrew B. Newberg, MD[c,d], Thomas J. Werner, MSE[e], Eric Guedj, MD, PhD[f]

KEYWORDS

• PET • FDG (18F-fluorodeoxyglucose) • Brain metabolism • Cancer imaging • Inflammation • Infection • Total body PET

KEY POINTS

- Following its introduction in 1976 by investigators at University of Pennsylvania, 18F-fluorodeoxyglucose (FDG)-PET was primarily used for brain imaging applications.
- While FDG was initially used for assessing central nervous system disorders and later cancer, its role substantially expanded over the years to include detection of inflammation and infection.
- Developments in PET instrumentation allowed imaging of the entire body, opening up new applications and eventually leading to long-axial field-of-view, Total Body PET/CT scanners.

Introduction of X-ray by Roentgen in 1895 led to a major revolution in practice of medicine that is still ongoing.[1] This invention allowed imaging of various anatomic sites and assessing many diseases and disorders of mankind over the years. While the original radiographic instruments were quite primitive and technically demanding, over the ensuing decades, its design and practical applications were optimized for routine clinical practice around the world. By the mid-20th century, conventional planar radiography with X-ray was employed as a major modality in patient care for a variety of indications.[2] The primary contrast agents used for planar X-ray imaging were barium and iodinated preparations administered through the GI tract or intravenously for a variety of indications.

The concept of tomography was born by David Kuhl and Roy Edwards at the University of Pennsylvania (Penn) in the 1960s. This approach was based on the back projection concept, which has formed the basis for reconstructed tomography as we know today. The validity of this innovative approach was validated by conventional single

[a] Division of Nuclear Medicine, Department of Radiology, Hospital of the University of Pennsylvania, Philadelphia, PA, USA; [b] Institute of Clinical Medicine, Faculty of Medicine, University of Oslo, The Intervention Center, Division for Technology and Innovation, Oslo University Hospital, Oslo, Norway; [c] Department of Integrative Medicine and Nutritional Sciences, Research at the Marcus Institute of Integrative Health, Thomas Jefferson University, Philadelphia, PA, USA; [d] Department of Radiology, Research at the Marcus Institute of Integrative Health, Thomas Jefferson University, Philadelphia, PA, USA; [e] Department of Radiology, Hospital of the University of Pennsylvania, Philadelphia, PA, USA; [f] Aix Marseille University, APHM, CNRS, Centrale Marseille, Institut Fresnel, Timone Hospital, CERIMED, Nuclear Medicine Department, Marseille, France

* Corresponding author. Laboratoire de Médecine Nucléaire, Hôpital de la Timone, 264 rue Saint Pierre, 13005 Marseille, France.

E-mail address: Abass.Alavi@pennmedicine.upenn.edu

PET Clin 21 (2026) 459–470
https://doi.org/10.1016/j.cpet.2026.05.001

Abbreviations

BNL	Brookhaven National Laboratory
CT	computed tomography
FDG	18F-Fluorodeoxyglucose
FUO	fever of unknown origin
NIH	National Institutes of Health
SPECT	single photon emission computed tomography
SUV	standardized uptake value
UCLA	University of California

photon emission computed tomography (SPECT), which was the only option at the time.[3] During the ensuing years, some primitive instruments were designed that further demonstrated the validity of the approach as a viable option for medical imaging during the 1970s. This early research was confined to brain diseases and disorders as the best option at the time.

By 1971, a relatively reliable instrument (Mark IV) was designed and assembled at Penn and became available for successful applications of tomography for both research and clinical purposes.[4] This research was confined to single gamma emitting radiotracers for assessing certain brain diseases and disorders.

Simultaneous with these developments at Penn, investigators at Washington University and Harvard were exploring the possibility of using positron emission tomography by developing instruments for this purpose.[2,5,6] However, it was not clear at that time whether this approach would eventually lead to practical applications in the future.

The introduction of X-ray-based computed tomography (CT) by Hounsfield in 1973 started another major revolution in medical imaging which truly transformed the role of this revolutionary concept in both patient care and research.[7] Over the past 5 decades with significant research at scientific institutions and investment by commercial companies, X-ray-based CT has become a very successful modality where its adoption as a standard technique has expanded its applications to include diseases and disorders of all organs and structures throughout the body.

The Department of Radiology at Penn was the first institution in the United States to install a commercial CT machine, which was designed primarily to assess structural abnormalities and blood-brain barrier breakdown by iodinated contrast agents. This instrument clearly demonstrated the success of X-ray tomography in detecting brain tumors, strokes, traumatic brain injuries, seizure sites, and several other central nervous diseases and disorders. However, investigators soon realized that the use of SPECT imaging for assessing only blood-brain barrier abnormalities would be seriously challenged by iodinated contrast enhanced CT scans, thereby limiting SPECT as a viable and competitive modality.

During the 1960s and early '70s, investigators at Penn and the National Institutes of Health (NIH) were conducting research with C14-labeled deoxglucose and a technique called *autoradiography* to assess regional glucose metabolism (therefore, brain function) in animals.[8] This technique involved administering this tracer at resting state and following various stimuli and demonstrating its ability as a unique probe for assessing regional brain function. In contrast to glucose, this radiolabeled tracer, after phosphorylation to C14-deoxyglucose phosphate, is not metabolized further and remains indefinitely in the cell as deoxyglucose-6-phosphate.

In December 1973, three investigators at Penn; Abass Alavi, David Kuhl and Martin Reivich, discussed the potential of labeling deoxyglucose with 18F and possibly other positron emitters for in vivo imaging of glucose metabolism in normal and disease states. They consulted investigators at Brookhaven National Laboratory (BNL) in Long Island, NY, about starting a joint research initiative for this purpose. Over the ensuing 3 years, 18F-Fluorodeoxyglucose (FDG) was synthesized and shown to mimic glucose metabolism in animal models, substantiating what had been accomplished by C14-deoxyglucose studies in the preceding animal models.[9,10] This development marked a critical transition from autoradiographic techniques to in vivo molecular imaging. Importantly, FDG should not be viewed as a tracer of a single biochemical pathway, but rather as an integrative marker of tissue metabolism. Its uptake reflects the combined effects of glucose transport, phosphorylation by hexokinase, and cellular metabolic demand. In the brain, this signal encompasses not only neuronal activity but also astrocytic and neurovascular contributions, thereby providing a systems-level representation of tissue function. This integrative property has been central to the robustness, reproducibility, and broad clinical applicability of FDG across both neurologic and systemic diseases.

In August 1976, a dose of FDG was flown from BNL to Philadelphia and administered to a volunteer human subject for the first time at Penn.[10] The first image with this tracer was generated by using the existing SPECT instrument (modified with heavy collimators to tolerate the high energy of gamma ray following annihilation of positron particles) (**Fig. 1**A).[9] This historical image demonstrated significant concentration of FDG in the brain with

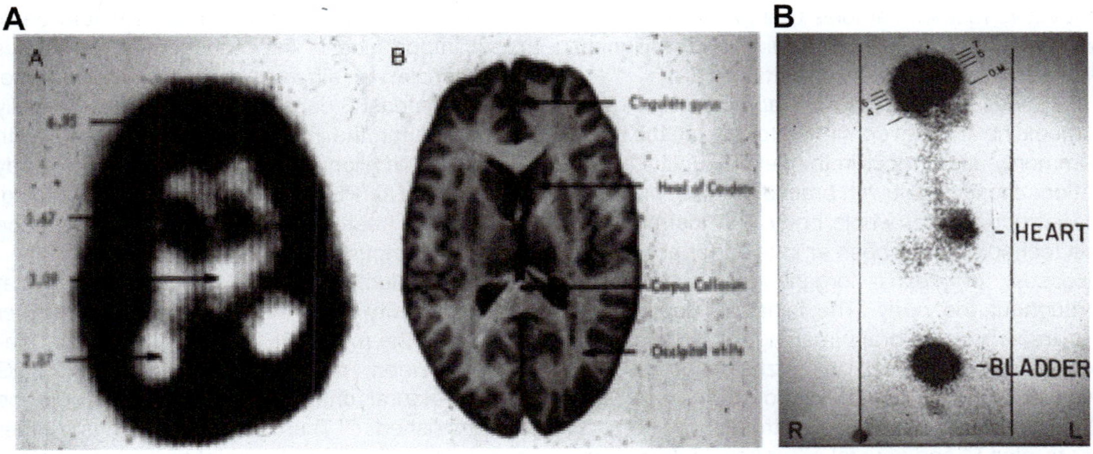

Fig. 1. (*A*) The first tomographic 18F-FDG images of the brain (*left*) acquired in 1976 at the University of Pennsylvania with a Mark IV scanner designed and built to examine central nervous system disorders with single-g-emitting radiopharmaceuticals. (*Right*), shows a corresponding slice of the brain and its comparable structures. (*B*) The first whole-body 18F-FDG images acquired with a dual-head Ohio Nuclear rectilinear scanner equipped with a set of high-energy collimators for performing strontium 85 (with an energy of 510 KeV) bone scans. The image revealed a significant concentration of 18F-FDG in the brain, heart, and bladder. (Abass Alavi, Martin Reivich, Guest editorial: The conception of FDG-PET imaging, Seminars in Nuclear Medicine, 32 (1), 2002, 2-5, https://doi.org/10.1053/snuc.2002.29269.[9])

higher uptake in the cortex and basal ganglia compared to the white matter. Soon after the acquisition of tomographic images of the brain, a whole body FDG scan was acquired using a conventional rectilinear scanner that was also equipped with high energy collimators. This image demonstrated the *in vivo* distribution of FDG throughout the body of a normal volunteer with pronounced uptake in the brain, heart, and kidneys, and excretion to the bladder (**Fig. 1**B).[10] This pilot observation was encouraging and eventually led to designing and building instruments that would allow successfully generating high-resolution PET images of the brain and other organs in the body.

Because of its complexity, it was challenging at the time to develop instruments that would allow imaging of the entire body within a reasonable period of time and determine applications of this novel and powerful technology in research and various clinical domains.

The original PET scanners could only image brain disorders and diseases due to design limitations and technical capabilities. However, because of the potential applications of PET for assessing the rest of the body, efforts were made to build whole body instruments during the ensuring decades. These early scanners were designed by modifying conventional planar imaging instruments (scintillation cameras) as coincident detectors, which made it possible to assess all the organs of the body.[11] However, the limited spatial resolution of the approach, along with other challenges, required a great deal of improvements and novel designs. By the mid to late 1980s, the potential applications of applying PET to the whole body enticed imaging companies to design specialized machines with an expanded field of view to achieve this goal.[12] By 2000, advanced PET instruments with longer axial field of view allowed faster imaging times and hence higher throughput for routine clinical and research.[11–13] The combination of rotating gantry PET technology with a spiral x-ray CT scanner led to the development of the first PET/CT system prototype.[14] This development marked the emergence of hybrid multimodal imaging, where the combination of metabolic and anatomic information resulted in a synergistic effect often described as *1 + 1= 3*. Beyond improved lesion localization, the integration of CT enabled accurate attenuation correction, significantly enhancing image quality and quantitative accuracy. This hybrid approach not only improved diagnostic performance but also fundamentally changed the way PET data are interpreted, by embedding metabolic information within a precise anatomic framework. Furthermore, improvements in reconstruction algorithms enabled the rapid processing of tomographic images, which were adopted from CT algorithms that had been refined throughout the later decades of the 20th century as well as the early 21st.

Soon after the introduction of FDG, investigators at Penn, University of California (UCLA) and BNL were funded by the NIH to conduct many innovative research studies to explore further applications of FDG in both benign and malignant diseases and in a variety of settings.

FDG was the initiator of the applications of PET in medicine and has continued to date as the most commonly used tracer in the field. Its initial applications mostly dealt with brain disorders, but after the introduction of whole body PET instruments, this technology has been employed for assessing diseases of many organs and structures throughout the body. The initial applications of this tracer was to brain imaging, which included normal aging (**Fig. 2**),[15,16] Alzheimer's Disease (AD) (**Fig. 3**),[17,18] brain tumors (**Figs. 4** and **5**),[19,20] seizures (**Fig. 6**),[21,22] strokes (**Fig. 7**)[17,23], depression,[24] and several other psychiatric disorders.[25] While these early applications primarily focused on regional abnormalities, it has become increasingly evident that FDG-PET captures distributed metabolic patterns reflecting large-scale functional organization of the brain.[26] Rather than isolated focal changes, many neurologic and psychiatric conditions are now understood as network-level disorders, and FDG provides a unique window into these integrated processes.

In particular, observations made in assessing brain tumors at various stages of the disease with FDG were of great value for adopting this PET tracer for assessing numerous malignancies throughout the body. For decades it was known that cancer cells are highly glycolytic, and therefore, an imaging technique that could detect glucose consumption in tumor cells would be of great importance in the management of various malignancies at different stages of the disease. During the past 3 decades, FDG has been heavily employed for the management of patients with numerous malignancies throughout the body (**Fig. 8**).[27] FDG-PET is used for diagnosis, staging, response to treatment and detection of recurrence following various interventions.[27]

The introduction of PET/CT by investigators at the University of Pittsburgh in 2000 further enhanced the role of PET imaging where correlation between metabolic imaging with FDG and structural changes seen on CT could be accomplished.[28] This development has further accelerated the importance of these modern imaging modalities by expanding its applications throughout modern medicine.

During the past decade, efforts have been to expand axial field of view of PET imaging beyond that provided by existing commercial instruments. This research initiative was started by Simon Cherry at University of California, Davis and eventually was marketed commercially by United Imaging (**Fig. 9**).[29] These total body PET instruments are able to image 1 to 2 m of a patient within a few minutes, allowing detection of disease activity simultaneously in every organ and structure.[30,31] This has allowed significant throughput of PET imaging and therefore increasing the volume of studies that can be performed in existing imaging facilities throughout the world. This novel approach has

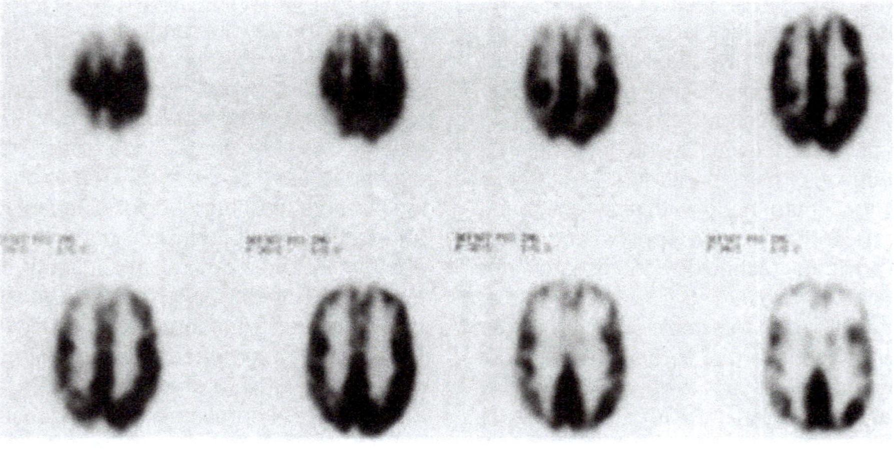

Fig. 2. Control subject PET image showing normal metabolism that is relatively evenly distributed throughout all brain regions. There is, however, minimal reduction in frontal lobe metabolism, which is consistent with normal aging. This research was originally published in *Journal of Nuclear Medicine (JNM)*. Alavi A, Newberg AB, Souder E, Berlin JA (1993) Quantitative analysis of PET and MR imaging data in normal aging and Alzheimer's disease: atrophy weighted total brain metabolism and absolute whole brain metabolism as reliable discriminators. (This research was originally published in JNM. Alavi A, Newberg AB, Souder E, Berlin JA (1993) Quantitative analysis of PET and MRI data in normal aging and Alzheimer's disease: atrophy weighted total brain metabolism and absolute whole brain metabolism as reliable discriminators. J Nucl Med 34, 1681-1687. © SNMMI.[16])

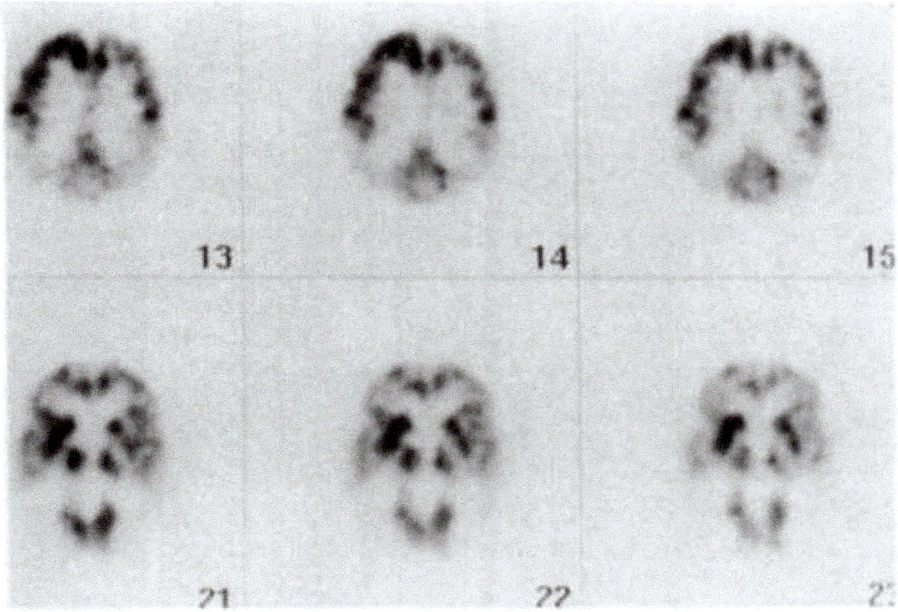

Fig. 3. Alzheimer's disease (AD) patient PET image shows marked hypometabolism, particularly in the parietal region. This research was originally published in *JNM*. Alavi A, Newberg AB, Souder E, Berlin JA (1993) Quantitative analysis of PET and MR imaging data in normal aging and Alzheimer's disease: atrophy weighted total brain metabolism and absolute whole brain metabolism as reliable discriminators. (This research was originally published in JNM. Alavi A, Newberg AB, Souder E, Berlin JA (1993) Quantitative analysis of PET and MRI data in normal aging and Alzheimer's disease: atrophy weighted total brain metabolism and absolute whole brain metabolism as reliable discriminators. J Nucl Med 34, 1681-1687. © SNMMI.[16])

great potential for expanding the role of PET in research and day-to-day practice of medicine.[32] Beyond improved sensitivity and throughput, total body PET enables simultaneous dynamic assessment of multiple organs, opening new perspectives for investigating systemic physiology. This includes the study of brain-body interactions, neuroimmune coupling, and multiorgan metabolic

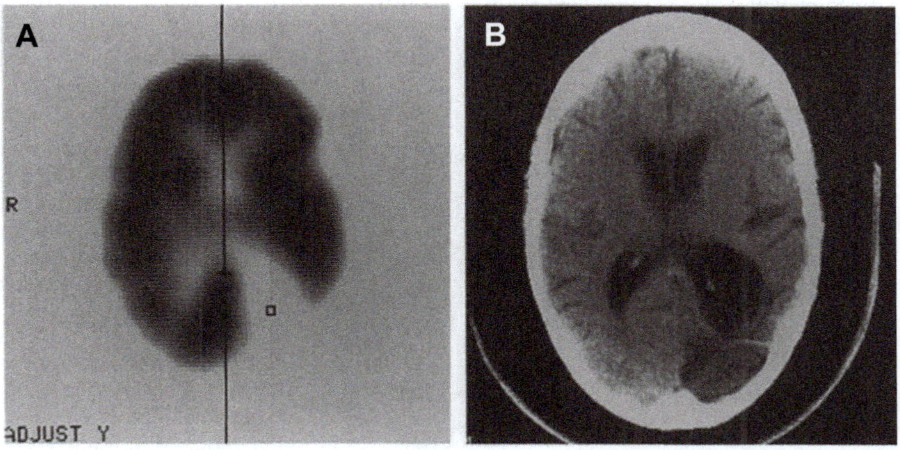

Fig. 4. (*A, B*) (*A*) PET scan of patient with low-grade tumor showing no metabolic activity in tumor. (*B*) Computed axial tomography (CAT) scans of the same patient. (Kim, C.K., Alavi, J.B., Alavi, A. et al. New grading system of cerebral gliomas using positron emisson tomography with F-18 fluorodeoxyglucose. J Neuro-Oncol 10, 85–91 (1991). https://doi.org/10.1007/BF00151249.[19])

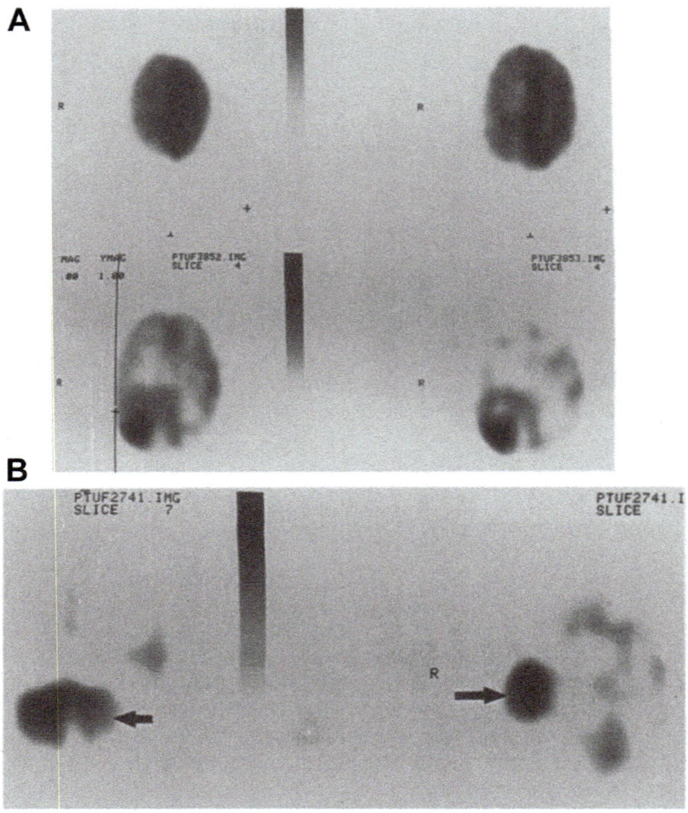

Fig. 5. (*A*) PET scan of patient with high grade glioma in right parietal area. There is decreased functional activity in ipsilateral hemisphere, and high metabolic activity in the tumor. (*B*) PET Scan of patient with high grade glioma in right temporoparietal area. There is high metabolic activity in the tumor (*arrow*), and reduced activity in the contralateral cerebellum (*arrow*). (Kim, C.K., Alavi, J.B., Alavi, A. et al. New grading system of cerebral gliomas using positron emisson tomography with F-18 fluorodeoxyglucose. J Neuro-Oncol 10, 85–91 (1991). https://doi.org/10.1007/BF00151249.[19])

responses, thereby extending the role of FDG from regional imaging to a tool for integrated whole-body functional assessment.

In recent years, the potential role of PET-MR imaging has been explored and discussed but its practical applications remain uncertain at this time.[33] The major issues relate to optimal attenuation correction and the feasibility of imaging the entire body within a short period of time.[33] In recent years, specialized instruments have been designed to image limited anatomic sites such as the brain[34] and breast.[35]

The major attribute of PET/CT imaging has been its ability to quantify the degree of disease activity in the affected sites as well throughout the body.[36,37] In this context, the introduction and widespread adoption of semiquantitative metrics such as the standardized uptake value (SUV)

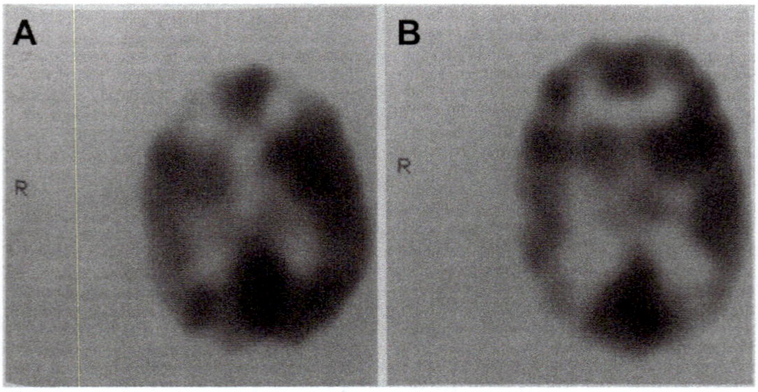

Fig. 6. (*A*) FDG-PET scan in epileptic patient shows diffuse right hemisphere cortical and basal ganglia hypometabolism excepting visual cortex. This patient had right hippocampal seizure onset defined with depth electrodes. (*B*) FDG-PET scan in another patient shows mainly right temporal and frontal hypometabolism in cortical regions. Right basal ganglia and thalamic hypometabolism is also evident. (Sperling, M.R., Gur, R.C., Alavi, A., Gur, R.E., Resnick, S., O'Connor, M.J. and Reivich, M. (1990), Subcortical Metabolic Alterations in Partial Epilepsy. Epilepsia, 31: 145-155. https://doi.org/10.1111/j.1528-1167.1990.tb06299.x.[22])

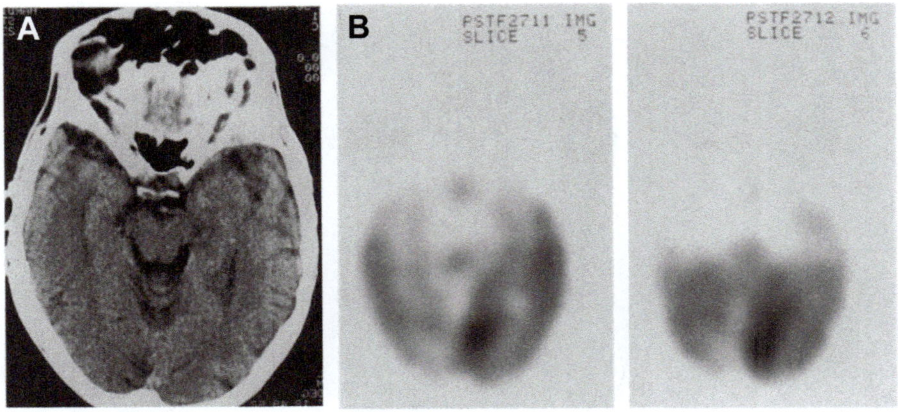

Fig. 7. Acute infarct. (*A*) X-ray computed tomography (XCT): an area of decreased density is seen in the left visual cortex. This area is poorly defined and primarily confined to the posterior calcarine cortex. (*B*) PET: a large area of metabolic abnormality is seen in the left visual cortex. This abnormality involves the entire left visual cortex and appears much larger than that seen on XCT. (Abass Alavi et al., Positron emission tomography imaging of regional cerebral glucose metabolism, Seminars in Nuclear Medicine, 16 (1), 1986, 2-34, https://doi.org/10.1016/S0001-2998(86)80002-2.[23])

have played a central role. SUV has provided a practical means to quantify tracer uptake in clinical routine, facilitating objective assessment of disease burden, treatment response, and longitudinal follow-up across a wide range of indications. Incorporating quantitative analysis into medical imaging has fundamentally changed the way disease activity is measured across various clinical scenarios and settings.[38,39]

While initially FDG was used for assessing central nervous system disorders and later on for examining patients with a variety of malignancies,

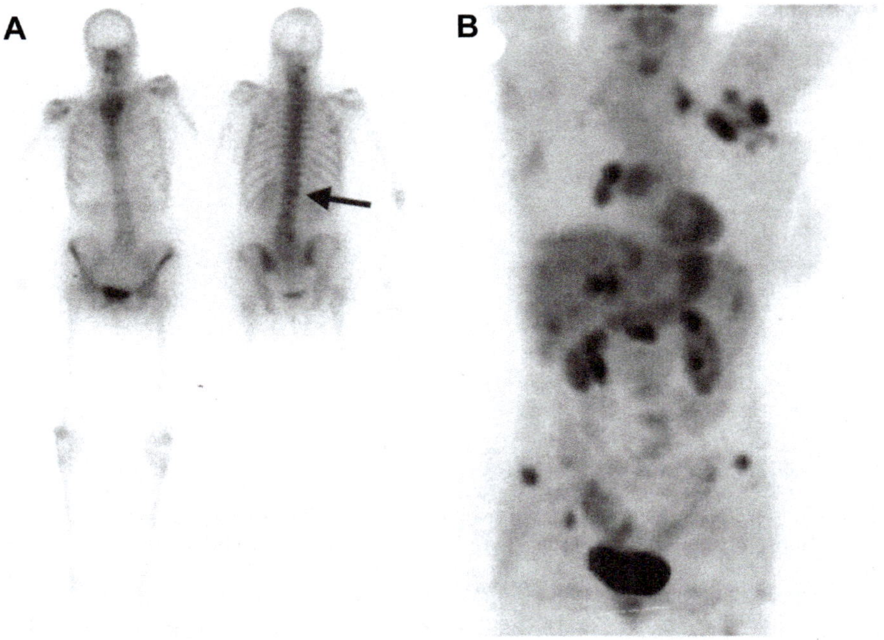

Fig. 8. FDG-PET imaging in a 62-year-old patient who was treated for breast cancer and presented with back pain. (*A*) A bone scan revealed a mild linear area of increased uptake (*straight arrow*), which was thought to represent a partial vertebral collapse. (*B*) Maximum intensity projection of FDG images revealed multiple bone and soft tissue metastases not seen on the bone scan, which influenced plans for treatment of this patient. (Roland Hustinx, François Bénard, Abass Alavi, Whole-body FDG-PET imaging in the management of patients with cancer, Seminars in Nuclear Medicine, 32 (1), 2002, 35-46, https://doi.org/10.1053/snuc.2002.29272.[27])

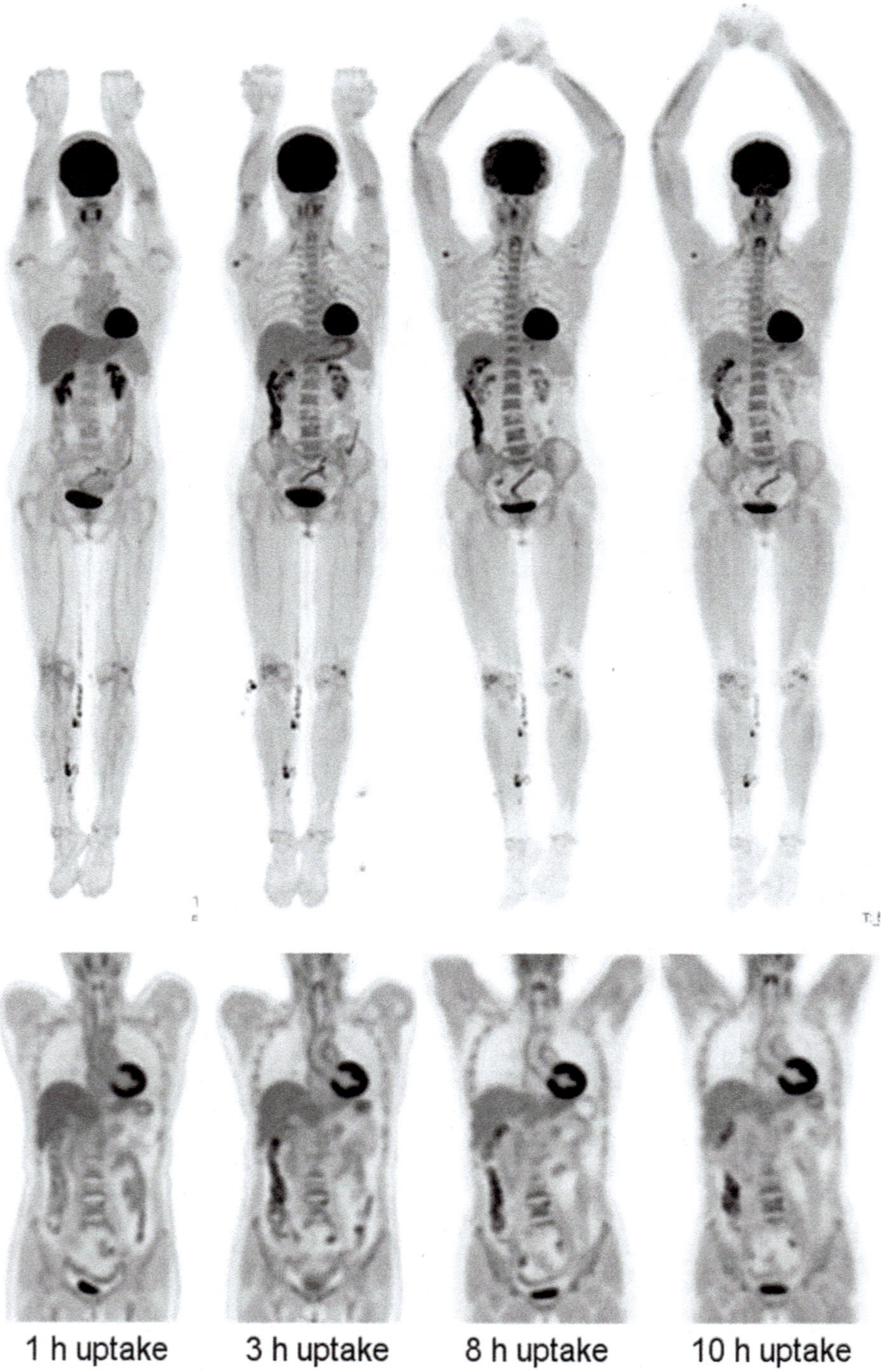

Fig. 9. Delayed imaging (256 MBq injected, 14 min scan duration). (*Left-to-right*) Images from scans performed at 1, 3, 8, and 10 h after injection. (*Top row*) maximum intensity projection (MIP) images. (*Bottom row*) Coronal views of thorax and abdomen. Head motion artifacts are visible in 8-h scan. This research was originally published in *JNM*. (This research was originally published in JNM. Badawi RD, Shi H, Hu P, Chen S, Xu T, Price PM, Ding Y, Spencer BA, Nardo L, Liu W, Bao J, Jones T, Li H, Cherry SR (2019) First Human Imaging Studies with the EXPLORER Total-Body PET Scanner. J Nucl Med 60, 299-303. © SNMMI.[30])

its role has substantially expanded over the years to other important domains. Soon after the first application of FDG in human beings, it was noted that both infectious and inflammatory processes were noted to have significant uptake of this compound at the affected sites (**Fig. 10**).[40–42] This observation has opened up a major domain for expanding the role of PET to the day-to-day

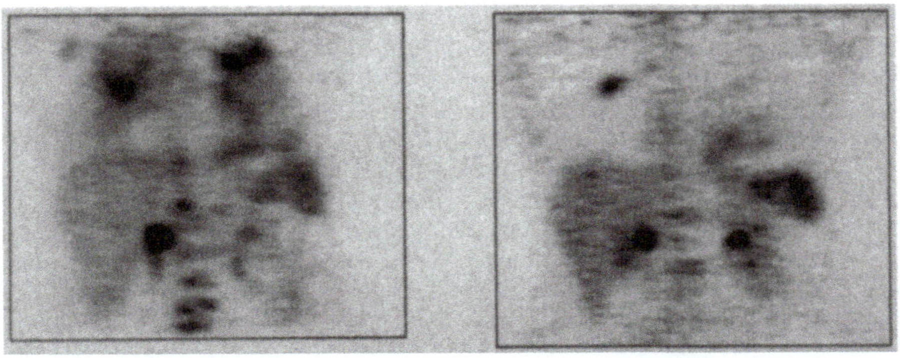

Fig. 10. This patient with proven sarcoidosis had intense uptake of FDG bilaterally in the upper lobes of both lungs on the baseline scan (left), which dissipated substantially following treatment. A repeat scan performed 11 months later, shows a small focus of uptake in the right upper lung and moderate disease activity in the spleen (Hongming Zhuang, Abass Alavi, 18-Fluorodeoxyglucose positron emission tomographic imaging in the detection and monitoring of infection and inflammation, Seminars in Nuclear Medicine, 32 (1), 2002, 47-59, https://doi.org/10.1053/snuc.2002.29278. [40])

practice of medicine because infection and inflammation are the two most common diseases of mankind. FDG-PET has been particularly useful in assessing patients with fever of unknown origin (FUO),[43,44] musculoskeletal infections,[40] and rheumatologic disorders (**Fig. 11**).[45] This has been of great importance in assessing response to various treatment modalities of patients with infection and inflammation. FDG-PET has revolutionized this discipline in medicine since determining the efficacy of modern drugs for treating such entities was unavailable until clinical use of PET became a reality.[46,47]

The impact of FDG-PET has been unmatched by any other technique introduced during the past 5 decades. The success of FDG-PET has led to the development of numerous positron-emitting radiotracers that have improved management of many serious disorders.

In addition, FDG-PET has warranted the installation of cyclotrons in many centers, which have also paved the way for the synthesis of other PET tracers for routine clinical applications as well as research. Moreover, institutions engaged in PET instrumentational research have expanded their domain of research and this has also accelerated the advancement and implementation of this technology to research.

Based on what is described in this communication, it is clear that the introduction of FDG to medicine has been revolutionary during the past 5 decades, and its impact rivals that of other technical advances that have been made in medicine during the past century (**Fig. 12**).[48] Therefore, it is timely to celebrate the impact of this unique tracer and its critical role in so many domains of medicine. It is also time to applaud Henry Wagner, a pioneer in Nuclear Medicine, who called FDG *the molecule of the century*.

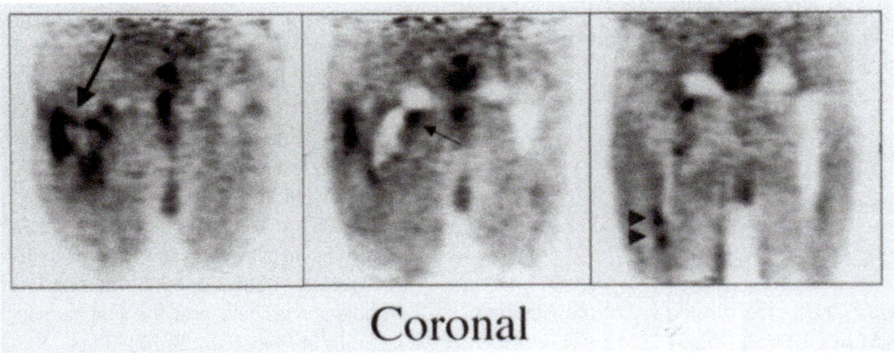

Fig. 11. Coronal images of 63-year-old man with painful right hip prosthesis. Loosening (*short arrow*), infection (*arrowheads*), and fistula (*long arrow*) are shown. This research was originally published in *JNM*. (This research was originally published in JNM. Zhuang H, Duarte PS, Pourdehnad M, Maes A, Van Acker F, Shnier D, Garino JP, Fitzgerald RH, Alavi A (2001) The promising role of 18F-FDG PET in detecting infected lower limb prosthesis implants. J Nucl Med 42, 44-48. © SNMMI.[45])

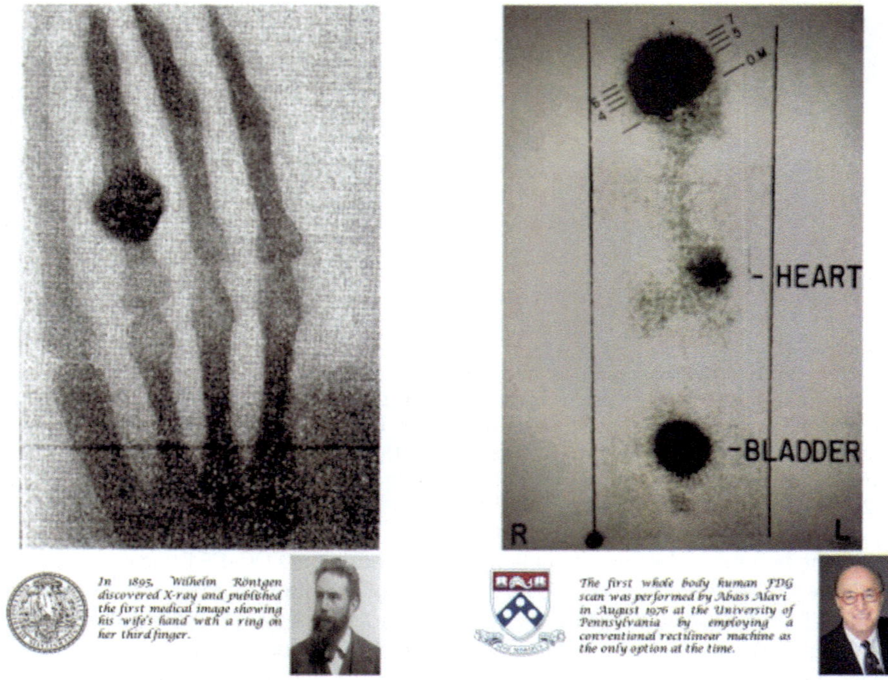

Fig. 12. Introduction of X-ray to medicine by Röntgen in 1895 (*left*) has had a substantial impact on the day-to-day practice of medicine. Similarly, imaging with FDG (*right*) has been another major step forward by enhancing the role of medical imaging and this has led to an unparalleled impact on both research and patient care. (Alavi, A., Hess, S., Werner, T.J. et al. An update on the unparalleled impact of FDG-PET imaging on the day-to-day practice of medicine with emphasis on management of infectious/inflammatory disorders. Eur J Nucl Med Mol Imaging 47, 18–27 (2020). https://doi.org/10.1007/s00259-019-04490-6.[48])

CLINICS CARE POINTS

- The evolution of FDG-PET imaging and its introduction to medicine has revolutionized many disciplines including neurology, psychiatry, oncology, infection/inflammation, and theranostics.
- The introduction of FDG-PET has led to the survival of this technology in medicine as well as the development of many other radiotracers and sophisticated instruments over the past 5 decades.

DISCLOSURE

Nothing to disclose.

REFERENCES

1. Rosenow UF. Notes on the legacy of the Röntgen rays. Med Phys 1995;22:1855–67.
2. Kevles BH. Naked to the Bone: Medical Imaging in the Twentieth Century - Softcover. New York: Basic Books; 1998.
3. Kuhl DE, Edwards RQ. Image separation radioisotope scanning. Radiology 1963;80:653–62.
4. Kuhl DE, Edwards RQ, Ricci AR, et al. The Mark IV system for radionuclide computed tomography of the brain. Radiology 1976;121:405–13.
5. Ter-Pogossian MM, Phelps ME, Hoffman EJ, et al. A positron-emission transaxial tomograph for nuclear imaging (PETT). Radiology 1975;114:89–98.
6. Brownell GL, Budinger TF, Lauterbur PC, et al. Positron tomography and nuclear magnetic resonance imaging. Science 1982;215:619–26.
7. Hounsfield GN. Computerized transverse axial scanning (tomography). 1. Description of system. Br J Radiol 1973;46:1016–22.
8. Greenberg JH. Autoradiography and cerebral function. In: Imaging and correlative physicochemical techniques. Springer; 1988. p. 107–78.
9. Alavi A, Reivich M. Guest editorial: the conception of FDG-PET imaging. Semin Nucl Med 2002;32:2–5.
10. Hess S, Høilund-Carlsen PF, Alavi A. Historic images in nuclear medicine: 1976: the first issue of clinical nuclear medicine and the first human FDG study. Clin Nucl Med 2014;39:701–3.
11. Rich DA. A brief history of positron emission tomography. J Nucl Med Technol 1997;25:4–11.
12. Jones T, Townsend D. History and future technical innovation in positron emission tomography. J Med Imaging 2017;4:011013.

13. Townsend DW, Beyer T. A combined PET/CT scanner: the path to true image fusion. Br J Radiol 2002;75:S24–30. Spec No.
14. Townsend DW. A combined PET/CT scanner: the choices. J Nucl Med 2001;42:533–4.
15. Kuhl DE, Metter EJ, Riege WH, et al. Effects of human aging on patterns of local cerebral glucose utilization determined by the [18F] fluorodeoxyglucose method. J Cereb Blood Flow Metab 1982;2:163–71.
16. Alavi A, Newberg AB, Souder E, et al. Quantitative analysis of PET and MRI data in normal aging and Alzheimer's disease: atrophy weighted total brain metabolism and absolute whole brain metabolism as reliable discriminators. J Nucl Med 1993;34:1681–7.
17. Alavi A, Reivich M, Ferris S, et al. Regional cerebral glucose metabolism in aging and senile dementia as determined by 18F-deoxyglucose and positron emission tomography. Exp Brain Res 1982;(Suppl 5):187–95.
18. Fazekas F, Alavi A, Chawluk JB, et al. Comparison of CT, MR, and PET in Alzheimer's dementia and normal aging. J Nucl Med 1989;30:1607–15.
19. Kim CK, Alavi JB, Alavi A, et al. New grading system of cerebral gliomas using positron emission tomography with F-18 fluorodeoxyglucose. J Neuro Oncol 1991;10:85–91.
20. Phelps ME, Huang SC, Hoffman EJ, et al. Tomographic measurement of local cerebral glucose metabolic rate in humans with (F-18)2-fluoro-2-deoxy-D-glucose: validation of method. Ann Neurol 1979;6:371–88.
21. Kuhl DE, Engel J Jr, Phelps ME, et al. Epileptic patterns of local cerebral metabolism and perfusion in humans determined by emission computed tomography of 18FDG and 13NH3. Ann Neurol 1980;8:348–60.
22. Sperling MR, Gur RC, Alavi A, et al. Subcortical metabolic alterations in partial epilepsy. Epilepsia 1990;31:145–55.
23. Alavi A, Dann R, Chawluk J, et al. Positron emission tomography imaging of regional cerebral glucose metabolism. Semin Nucl Med 1986;16:2–34.
24. Kumar A, Newberg A, Alavi A, et al. Regional cerebral glucose metabolism in late-life depression and Alzheimer disease: a preliminary positron emission tomography study. Proc Natl Acad Sci U S A 1993; 90:7019–23.
25. Buchsbaum MS, Ingvar DH, Kessler R, et al. Cerebral glucography with positron tomography. Use in normal subjects and in patients with schizophrenia. Arch Gen Psychiatry 1982;39:251–9.
26. Cavaliere C, Galli A, Meneghini C, et al. Molecular connectivity studies of cerebral glucose metabolism and blood flow: a scoping review. Neurosci Biobehav Rev 2026;185:106623.
27. Hustinx R, Bénard F, Alavi A. Whole-body FDG-PET imaging in the management of patients with cancer. Semin Nucl Med 2002;32:35–46.
28. Beyer T, Townsend DW, Brun T, et al. A combined PET/CT scanner for clinical oncology. J Nucl Med 2000;41:1369–79.
29. Cherry SR, Jones T, Karp JS, et al. Total-body PET: maximizing sensitivity to create new opportunities for clinical research and patient care. J Nucl Med 2018;59:3–12.
30. Badawi RD, Shi H, Hu P, et al. First human imaging studies with the EXPLORER total-body PET scanner. J Nucl Med 2019;60:299–303.
31. Vandenberghe S, Moskal P, Karp JS. State of the art in total body PET. EJNMMI Phys 2020;7:35.
32. Alavi A, Saboury B, Nardo L, et al. Potential and Most relevant applications of total body PET/CT imaging. Clin Nucl Med 2022;47:43–55.
33. Torigian DA, Zaidi H, Kwee TC, et al. PET/MR imaging: technical aspects and potential clinical applications. Radiology 2013;267:26–44.
34. Catana C. Development of dedicated brain PET imaging devices: recent advances and future perspectives. J Nucl Med 2019;60:1044–52.
35. Narayanan D, Berg WA. Dedicated breast gamma camera imaging and breast PET: current status and future directions. Pet Clin 2018;13:363–81.
36. Basu S, Zaidi H, Houseni M, et al. Novel quantitative techniques for assessing regional and global function and structure based on modern imaging modalities: implications for normal variation, aging and diseased states. Semin Nucl Med 2007;37: 223–39.
37. Zaidi H, Alavi A, Naqa IE. Novel quantitative PET techniques for clinical decision support in oncology. Semin Nucl Med 2018;48:548–64.
38. Cheson BD, Fisher RI, Barrington SF, et al, Alliance, Australasian Leukaemia and Lymphoma Group, Eastern Cooperative Oncology Group, European Mantle Cell Lymphoma Consortium, Italian Lymphoma Foundation, European Organisation for Research, Treatment of Cancer/Dutch Hemato-Oncology Group, Grupo Español de Médula Ósea, German High-Grade Lymphoma Study Group, German Hodgkin's Study Group, Japanese Lymphorra Study Group, Lymphoma Study Association, NCIC Clinical Trials Group, Nordic Lymphoma Study Group, Southwest Oncology Group, United Kingdom National Cancer Research Institute. Recommendations for initial evaluation, staging, and response assessment of Hodgkin and non-Hodgkin lymphoma: the Lugano classification. J Clin Oncol 2014;32:3059–68.
39. Pak K, Cheon GJ, Nam HY, et al. Prognostic value of metabolic tumor volume and total lesion glycolysis in head and neck cancer: a systematic review and meta-analysis. J Nucl Med 2014;55:884–90.
40. Zhuang H, Alavi A. 18-fluorodeoxyglucose positron emission tomographic imaging in the detection and monitoring of infection and inflammation. Semin Nucl Med 2002;32:47–59.

41. Jaleel J, Sagar S, Kumar R. Utility of PET/computed tomography in infection and inflammation imaging. Pet Clin 2022;17:533–42.
42. Abikhzer G, Treglia G, Pelletier-Galarneau M, et al. EANM/SNMMI guideline/procedure standard for [18F] FDG hybrid PET use in infection and inflammation in adults v2. 0. Eur J Nucl Med Mol Imag 2025; 52:510–38.
43. Hess S, Noriega-Álvarez E, Leccisotti L, et al. EANM consensus document on the use of [18F] FDG PET/CT in fever and inflammation of unknown origin. Eur J Nucl Med Mol Imag 2024;51:2597–613.
44. Treglia G, Albano D, Wittebole X, et al. Diagnostic value of [18F] FDG PET/CT for detection of infectious and inflammatory foci in critically ill patients: a systematic review and meta-analysis. Eur J Nucl Med Mol Imag 2026;1–12.
45. Zhuang H, Duarte PS, Pourdehnad M, et al. The promising role of 18F-FDG PET in detecting infected lower limb prosthesis implants. J Nucl Med 2001;42: 44–8.
46. Singh SB, Bhandari S, Bhandari S, et al. Role of PET/CT in diagnosing and monitoring disease activity in rheumatoid arthritis: a review. Ann Nucl Med 2024; 38:165–75.
47. Subesinghe M, Bhuva S, Arumalla N, et al. 2-deoxy-2 [18F] fluoro-D-glucose positron emission tomography–computed tomography in rheumatological diseases. Rheumatology 2022;61:1769–82.
48. Alavi A, Hess S, Werner TJ, et al. An update on the unparalleled impact of FDG-PET imaging on the day-to-day practice of medicine with emphasis on management of infectious/inflammatory disorders. Eur J Nucl Med Mol Imaging 2020;47:18–27.

Normal Patterns and Variants in PET Brain Imaging from Childhood to Aging

Sahar Darabi Monadi, MD[a], Thomas J. Werner, MSE[b], Abass Alavi, MD[c], Andrew B. Newberg, MD[d,e,*]

KEYWORDS

- Positron emission tomography (PET) • FDG (18F-fluorodeoxyglucose)
- Cerebral glucose metabolism (CMRGlc) • Normal variation • Brain function • Aging and cognition
- Neuropsychiatric disorders • Functional imaging

KEY POINTS

- Interpretation of fluorodeoxyglucose (FDG) PET brain scans requires careful accounting for normal variability related to mental state, sensory stimulation, emotional status, and age-related changes.
- Advancements in PET significantly improved functional brain imaging, particularly using positron emitting tracers like FDG that allow high resolution assessment of cerebral glucose metabolism.
- Despite technological progress, limited data on normal and longitudinal variability remain a challenge, constraining, the full clinical and research utility of PET in neuropsychiatric disorders.

INTRODUCTION

Precise clinical and research interpretation of brain PET requires a clear definition of normal variation, which is inherently complicated by diverse mental states. This article reviews the technical and neurophysiological factors influencing normal findings, including the radiopharmaceuticals used to measure cerebral blood flow (CBF), metabolism, and neurotransmitter systems. It further evaluates how baseline cognitive, sensory, and emotional states, along with age-related neurologic shifts across the lifespan, alter the parameters of a *normal* scan.

Brain tomography began in the 1960s with Kuhl and Edwards'[1] development of single photon emission computed tomography (SPECT), enabling the first transaxial reconstructions of cerebral radionuclide distribution. SPECT provided early insights into neuropsychiatric conditions,[2,3] evolving from early ^{123}I and ^{99}mTc substrates to modern CBF tracers like Technetium 99m hexamethyl propylene amine oxime (HMPAO) and Technetium 99m ethylene cysteinate dimer. Subsequent PET and SPECT radiopharmaceuticals now evaluate various functional parameters, including neurotransmitter systems[4,5] (**Table 1**). While not yet clinical standards, these tracers

[a] Department of Radiology, Thomas Jefferson University, Philadelphia, PA, USA; [b] Department of Radiology, Hospital of the University of Pennsylvania, Philadelphia, PA, USA; [c] Division of Nuclear Medicine, Department of Radiology, Hospital of the University of Pennsylvania, University of Pennsylvania Perelman School of Medicine, Philadelphia, PA, USA; [d] Department of Radiology, Sidney Kimmel Medical College, Thomas Jefferson University, Philadelphia, PA, USA; [e] Department of Integrative Medicine and Nutritional Sciences, Sidney Kimmel Medical College, Thomas Jefferson University, Philadelphia, PA, USA
* Corresponding author. Department of Integrative Medicine, 789 East Lancaster Avenue, Suite 110, Villanova, PA 19085.
E-mail address: Andrew.newberg@jefferson.edu

PET Clin 21 (2026) 471–482
https://doi.org/10.1016/j.cpet.2026.04.003

Abbreviations

CBF	cerebral blood flow
FDG	18F-fluorodeoxyglucose
HMPAO	hexamethyl propylene amine oxime
OEF	oxygen extraction fraction
PVC	partial volume correction
SPECT	single photon emission computed tomography

represent essential future diagnostic tools for neuropsychiatric disorders.

While SPECT proved valuable, positron-emitting radionuclides significantly expanded radiopharmaceutical development. Isotopes such as 11C, 18F, and 13N are able to bind to natural biological molecules, enabling an array of tracers for studying diverse physiologic processes.[3] Notably, 18F-fluorodeoxyglucose (FDG) was developed to measure regional cerebral glucose metabolism (CMRGlc).[6] The physics of 18F decay—positron emission followed by annihilation—produces 2 511-keV gamma rays. This principle allows PET a theoretic spatial resolution of 2 to 3 mm, vastly superior to SPECT's 8 to 10 mm, with modern technology continually approaching this limit.[7–9]

FDG is the primary neurologic PET tracer, measuring CMRGlc (**Fig. 1**).[10] Currently, it is the only clinically approved tracer for evaluating seizures, brain tumors, and dementia (it should be noted that there are now 3 amyloid PET tracers for the evaluation of Alzheimer's but these do not aid the detection of other neurodegenerative disorders such as frontotemporal dementia). FDG PET also has been pivotal in researching neuropsychiatric disorders.[11,12] While newer positron-emitting analogs now facilitate the study of various neurophysiological processes, literature remains limited regarding normal variants and longitudinal changes in healthy cohorts.

NORMAL VARIANTS IN FUNCTIONAL NEUROIMAGING STUDIES

Accurately identifying abnormalities requires defining the spectrum of normal variation. Establishing a *baseline* is challenging, as recent factors affecting a given patient significantly influence imaging outcomes. Consequently, activation studies use healthy controls performing sensorimotor, cognitive, or emotional tasks to delineate these states. For instance, the transition from eyes-closed to eyes-open states markedly increases visual cortex activation, which scales with scene complexity.[13,14] Environmental motion further engages the visual, medial prefrontal, and extrastriate cortices, alongside the temporoparietal junction and basal temporal regions.[15,16] Similarly, auditory stimuli modulate activity based on complexity: pure tones primarily activate the left transverse temporal gyrus, whereas speech and music engage broad bilateral associative auditory regions.[17,18]

Higher-order cognitive processes significantly affect cerebral activity patterns (**Fig. 2**).[19] Research indicates that attention, problem-solving, and meditative practices selectively recruit or suppress specific regions.[20,21] For example, tasks requiring focused attention typically increase prefrontal and

Table 1
A partial listing of radioligands used in neurologic PET imaging

Compound	Application
[15O] H2O	Blood flow
[18F] Fluorodeoxyglucose*	Glucose metabolism
15O2	Oxygen metabolism
[11C] L-methionine	Amino acid metabolism
[11C] raclopride, [11C] methylspiperone, [18F] fluorodopa*, [18F] spiperone	Dopamine receptor activity
[18F] Florbetapir (Amyvid)*, [18F] Flutemetamol F18 (Vizamyl)*, [18F] Florbetaben F18 (Neuraceq)*	Amyloid accumulation for Alzheimer's
Flortaucipir (18F-AV-1451/TAUVID)*	Tau protein accumulation
[11C] carfentanil, [11C] etorphine	Opiate receptor activity
[11C] flunitrazepam	Benzodiazepine receptor activity
[11C] scopolamine, [11C] quinuclidinyl benzilate	Muscarinic cholinergic receptors
6-[18F] fluoro-L-DOPA*, 4-[18F] flouro-m-tyrosine	Presynaptic dopaminergic system
[11C] ephedrine, [18F] fluorometaraminol	Adrenergic terminals

* These are tracers that are currently approved for clinical use by the FDA.

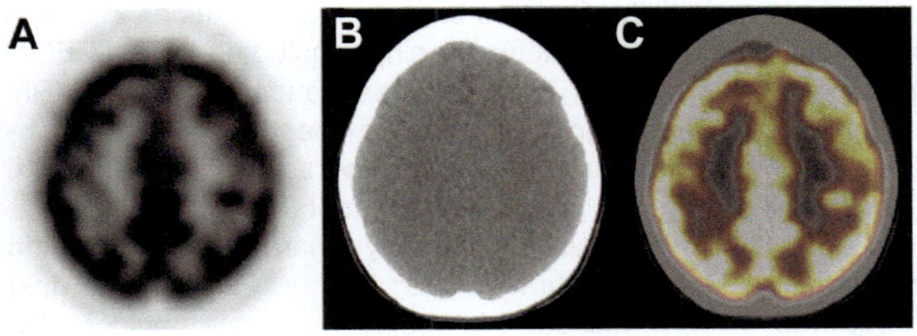

Fig. 1. (*A–C*) Axial PET (*A*), x-ray computed tomography (CT) (*B*), and fused PET/CT (*C*) images through frontal lobe of adult brain. (Paul C. Tumeh et al., Structural and Functional Imaging Correlates for Age-Related Changes in the Brain, Seminars in Nuclear Medicine, 37 (2), 2007, 69-87, https://doi.org/10.1053/j.semnuclmed.2006.10.002.[10])

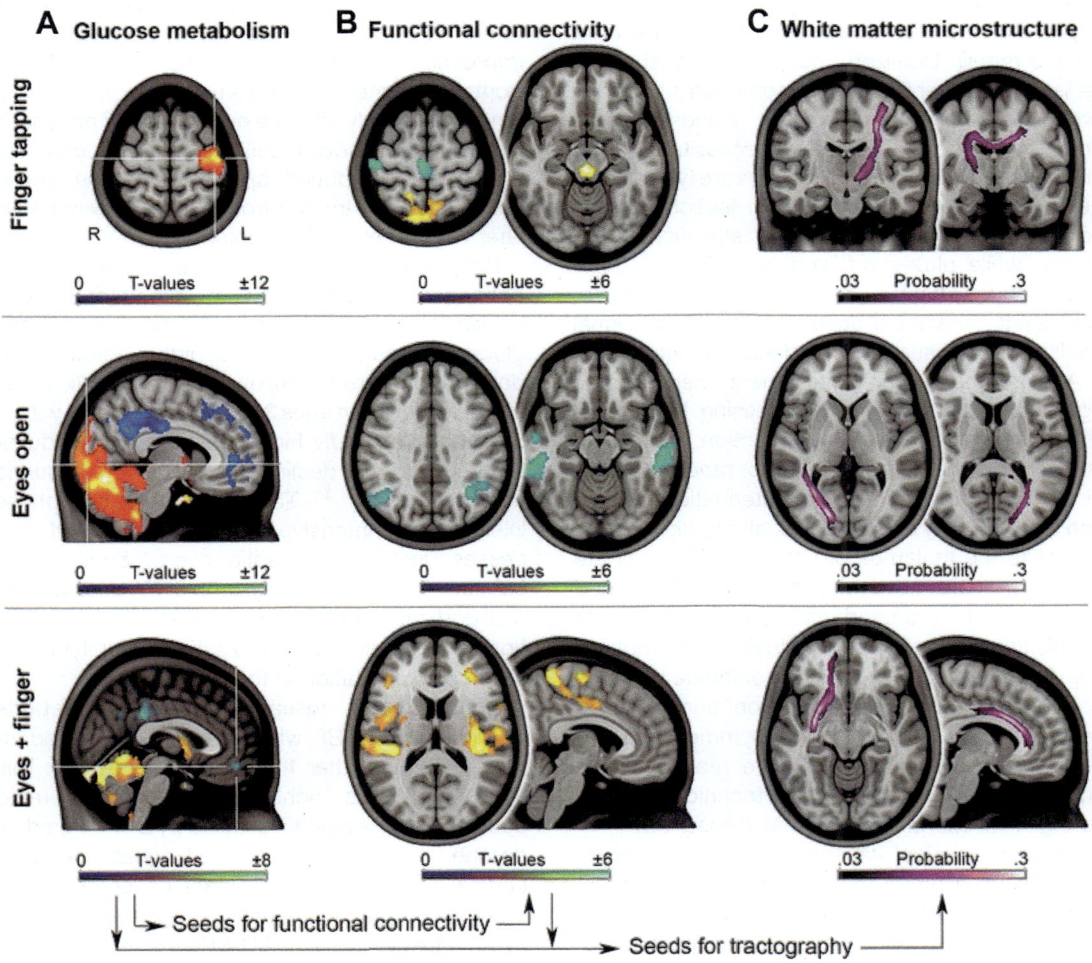

Fig. 2. (*A–C*) Task-specific changes in glucose metabolism, functional connectivity, and the corresponding white matter fiber tracts. (*A*) Significant changes in glucose metabolism during task performance served as seed regions for functional connectivity ($P<.05$ family wise error [FWE]-corrected, seeds marked by crosshair). Common changes of both conditions were assessed by conjunction analysis. (*B*) Compared to rest, widespread changes in functional connectivity were observed beyond the primary resting-state networks ($P<.05$ FWE-corrected). (*C*) White matter fiber tracts as modeled by probabilistic tractography exhibited task-related changes in radial and axial diffusivity during finger tapping and when eyes were opened, respectively. (Hahn, A., Gryglewski, G., Nics, L. et al. Task-relevant brain networks identified with simultaneous PET/MR imaging of metabolism and connectivity. Brain Struct Funct 223, 1369–1378 (2018). https://doi.org/10.1007/s00429-017-1558-0.[19])

anterior cingulate gyrus activity.[21,22] Emotional responses engage the limbic system, particularly the amygdala, across multiple neurotransmitter pathways.[18,23,24] These findings have critical clinical implications. A subject's mental state during radiotracer administration alters the subsequent imaging results. For instance, tension increases muscular FDG uptake, while anxiety or personal preoccupation can shift cerebral patterns compared to a calm state. Consequently, cognitive and emotional variables introduce *normal variants* reflecting specific peri-imaging mental activity.[25,26]

Technical variables significantly influence brain perfusion assessment and can introduce artifacts or *normal variants*. Critical factors include injection-to-scan latency, administered dose, image processing filters, and test-retest reliability.[12] While ideal tracers remain localized, most exhibit washout or redistribution over time—a phenomenon particularly pronounced in neurotransmitter ligands. Due to short half-lives, PET imaging necessitates strict timing; for example, 18F-FDG scans are typically acquired 30 to 60 minutes postinjection. Delays compromise image sensitivity, specificity, and clarity, while ultra-short-lived isotopes like 15O-H2O require near-immediate scan acquisition. Additionally, the tracer dose directly impacts signal quality and the visualization of deep brain structures.

Accurate cerebral assessment necessitates rigorous image filtering and processing. PET acquisition requires attenuation correction, dead-time adjustment, and compensation for random events or single-photon detections. Attenuation correction is particularly critical for visualizing deep structures like the thalamus or brainstem. To mitigate patient motion, head stabilization or shortened scan durations are used; alternatively, multiframe acquisition allows the exclusion of motion-corrupted data. While advanced software provides post-hoc motion and tilt correction, unrecognized head tilt can simulate structural asymmetry (eg, uneven thalami). Although software realignment is often effective, identifying these technical artifacts during initial interpretation remains essential.

Despite technical variables, CBF, metabolism, and neurotransmitter studies demonstrate robust test-retest reliability. In healthy controls, repeat imaging typically yields regional and absolute activity values with minimal variability, generally within 5% to 10%.[27,28]

NEUROIMAGING IN THE STUDY OF AGING FROM INFANCY TO ADULTHOOD

Neuroimaging is essential for investigating cerebral development and maturation from infancy through adulthood. While postmortem studies initially identified biochemical alterations in aging, functional neuroimaging—including PET, SPECT, functional magnetic resonance imaging (fMRI), and magnetic resonance spectroscopy—now enables the longitudinal *in vivo* assessment of human cerebral physiology and metabolism.

PET has significantly characterized pediatric brain maturation (**Fig. 3**).[29,30] During the first year, glucose metabolism follows a phylogenetic sequence: evolutionarily older regions mature functionally before more recent structures.[31,32] These metabolic shifts parallel behavioral milestones. For example, maturation of visuospatial and primitive reflex functions coincides with increased glucose metabolism in the parietal and temporal cortices, cerebellum, and primary visual areas, while basal ganglia activity corresponds to improved sensorimotor integration.[33] Conversely, frontal lobe metabolism remains low in early infancy, rising only with the emergence of advanced cognitive and social abilities. By age one, the metabolic distribution approximates the young adult pattern,[34] though frontal lobe activity peaks later than other cortical regions.[35]

Despite qualitative similarities, absolute metabolic rates in infants differ significantly from adult values. Recent PET data indicate that cerebral glucose consumption is low at birth, approximately doubling during early childhood.[30] Metabolic activity peaks between ages 3 and 9 with regional values remaining markedly higher than in young adults-before gradually declining to adult levels during adolescence.[30,31,36] This hypermetabolic phase likely reflects intensive neurodevelopmental processes, including synaptic overproduction and subsequent pruning. For example, the decline in visual cortical metabolism correlates with the cessation of heightened neural plasticity, signifying the functional maturation of the visual system.[34]

Normal aging research consistently reports declining global CBF, with more pronounced reductions in gray matter than white matter.[37,38] This decline appears nonlinear, featuring a rapid decrease before age 36 followed by a more gradual decline.[39] Waldemar and colleagues identified cortical atrophy as the primary driver of whole-brain CBF reductions, confirming age-related frontal hypoperfusion via HMPAO-SPECT.[37] Conversely, using 133Xe inhalation SPECT, global blood flow did not correlate directly with age. While atrophy increased with senescence, age alone was not a predictor of whole-brain CBF. Approximately 70% of global flow variance remained unexplained by age, sex, or atrophy.[40]

An age-related decline in bilateral frontal lobe perfusion is consistently observed in PET imaging.[41] PET imaging further demonstrates reduced

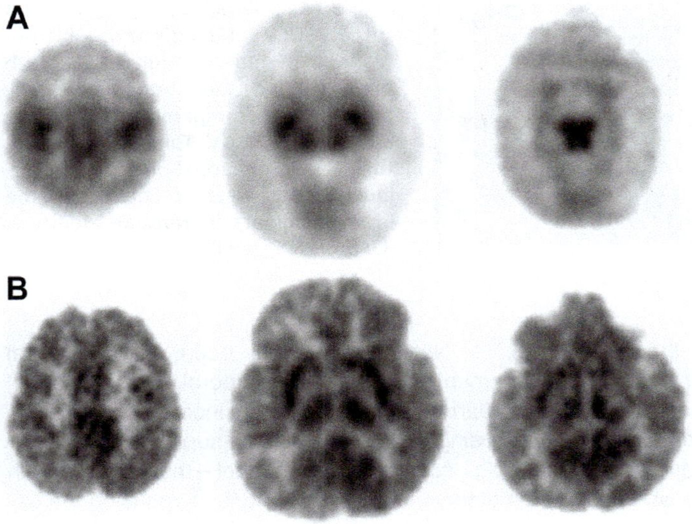

Fig. 3. (*A, B*) CMRGlc during infancy. (*A*) represents PET images of glucose metabolism using FDG in a term newborn infant at postnatal day 4 of age. (*B*) represents images of glucose uptake in a 12-month-old infant. Increased glucose uptake is noted in the primary sensory and motor cortex, thalamus, basal ganglia, and brainstem with decreased activity in the cerebral cortex in the newborn. (Sujatha Kannan, Harry T. Chugani, Applications of Positron Emission Tomography in the Newborn Nursery, Seminars in Perinatology, 34 (1), 2010, 39-45, https://doi.org/10.1053/j.semperi.2009.10.004.[29])

regional CBF in the cingulate and parahippocampal gyri, superior temporal and medial frontal regions, and posterior parietal cortex.[42] These decreases are most prominent in limbic and association cortices, potentially underlying age-related cognitive shifts.[43] Significant CBF reductions in the left superior temporal region suggest a specific hemispheric vulnerability to aging.[41,43]

Using SPECT with statistical parametric mapping, researchers identified age-associated reductions in tracer uptake within the anterior cingulate, basal ganglia, left prefrontal/lateral frontal cortex, and the left superior temporal and insular region.[44] Findings also revealed increasing right-to-left asymmetry with age, particularly in the frontal and temporal neocortex. Sex-related differences were significant with women exhibiting higher right parietal uptake, while men showed greater uptake in the cerebellum and the left anterior temporal and orbitofrontal regions.

FDG-PET studies consistently show declining global cerebral glucose metabolism (CMRGlc) with age (much like the findings with CBF), particularly in the temporal, parietal, and somatosensory cortices, with maximal reduction in the frontal lobes (**Fig. 4**).[10,45–52] A summary of age-related regional metabolic changes is presented in **Box 1**. Kuhl and colleagues[53] reported a progressive decline, noting a 26% reduction by age 78 compared to age 18. Alavi and colleagues[54] confirmed these regional decreases and found that minor medical conditions did not significantly alter global or regional CMRGlc. However, areas such as the pons and cerebellum may have increased metabolism with age (**Fig. 5**).[55]

Yoshii and colleagues[49] examined CMRGlc relative to age, gender, brain volume, and vascular risk. Initial findings showed lower mean CMRGlc in older cohorts—notably in frontal, parietal, and temporal regions—and higher rates in women. However, when adjusting for age-related brain volume loss, age and gender effects became nonsignificant. While atrophy is a key factor in statistical normalization, it accounted for only 21% of CMRGlc variability; cerebrovascular risk factors had no measurable impact.

A high-resolution FDG-PET study of 120 healthy participants (ages 19–79) identified reduced cortical metabolism as the most consistent hallmark of normal aging, with the frontal lobe showing the most significant decline.[56] Subtirelu and colleagues recently corroborated this, specifically localizing significant metabolic reduction to the lateral orbital gyrus.[55] While some evidence suggests particular temporal lobe vulnerability,[57] other cortical regions—parietal, occipital, and temporal—exhibit high intergroup and intragroup variability. Collectively, these age-related shifts manifest as elevated cerebellum-to-cortex metabolic ratios and an increased anterior–posterior metabolic gradient.

High-resolution FDG-PET confirms that frontal, parietal, and occipital metabolism remains symmetric across the lifespan, whereas the left temporal lobe consistently exhibits lower activity than the right.[56] The basal ganglia, thalami, hippocampi, cerebellum, and posterior cingulate remain stable and symmetric, and the visual cortices are notably, but consistently hypermetabolic.[45,56,58] Brainstem activity increases with age, potentially driven by dopaminergic alterations.[55]

Regarding sex-related differences, recent data move beyond early reports of parity[59] to identify gender-specific *fingerprints*. Males typically

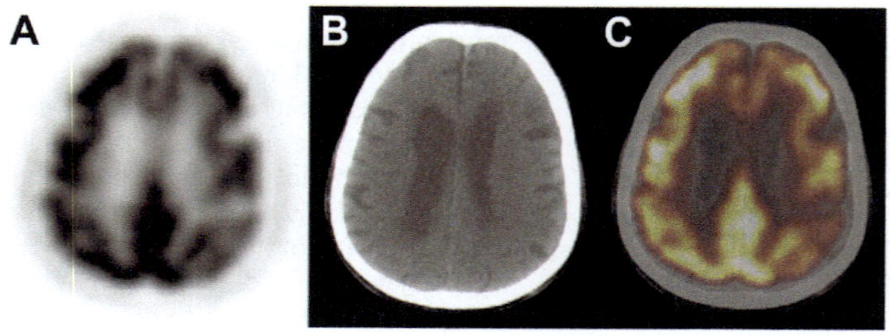

Fig. 4. (*A–C*) Axial PET (*A*), CT (*B*), and fused PET/CT (*C*) images through frontal lobe of elderly adult brain. Both brain volume and metabolic activity are decreased compared with younger adult brain. (Paul C. Tumeh et al., Structural and Functional Imaging Correlates for Age-Related Changes in the Brain, Seminars in Nuclear Medicine, 37 (2), 2007, 69-87, https://doi.org/10.1053/j.semnuclmed.2006.10.002.[10])

exhibit higher baseline metabolism in the right insula, middle temporal, and medial frontal regions, while females show higher hypothalamic activity.[60] Aging effects also diverge: men experience accelerated decline in the left thalamus and caudate nucleus during their 60s and 70s, whereas women show primary reductions in the occipital lobe and a slower overall metabolic decline.[60,61]

While early hypotheses suggested that age-related FDG uptake declines resulted from altered neuronal transport or phosphorylation kinetics,[53] subsequent kinetic modeling proved these rate constants remain stable.[62,63] Consequently, reduced FDG uptake likely represents a genuine decrease in cerebral metabolic activity, a finding recently corroborated by high-resolution PET/CT studies accounting for structural atrophy and global metabolic shifts.[52,55]

Data on oxygen metabolism ($CMRO_2$) remain divergent. While global rates may appear stable[64] 15O PET studies identify age-associated gray matter declines, particularly in those over age 50.[65,66] Notable reductions occur in the bilateral putamen and left supratemporal, inferior frontal, and parietal cortices. Despite inconsistent findings regarding CBF,[66–68] research supports a *hemodynamic compensation* model—the aging brain maintains metabolic stability by increasing the oxygen extraction fraction (OEF) to offset reduced perfusion.[69–71] Furthermore, high cardiorespiratory fitness may preserve CBF, mitigating the need for compensatory OEF elevation.[72]

Interpreting geriatric PET data are complicated by age-related atrophy, which can artificially lower measured metabolic activity due to signal averaging with CSF spaces. Foundational MRI studies[73–75] established that ventricular and total brain volumes correlate strongly with age. Notably, healthy men exhibit greater age-related atrophy—particularly in the left hemisphere—compared to the more symmetric changes seen in women.[76] While these anatomic shifts contribute to observed metabolic declines, modern research using partial volume correction (PVC) confirms that regional hypometabolism in the frontal and cingulate cortices remains a biological reality, not merely a structural artifact.[55,77] However, contemporary longitudinal analyses suggest that PVC can sometimes introduce noise, prompting some researchers to favor noncorrected images for stable metabolic tracking.[78] Consequently, current PET/SPECT reviews advocate for tailored correction strategies to balance measurement bias and precision.[79] Despite the consistent link between frontal atrophy and aging, it remains unclear if structural loss fully accounts for observed frontal hypometabolism.

Box 1
Regions observed to have significant hypometabolism with aging

- Anterior corpus callosum
- Cingulate gyrus
- Frontal lobe
- Frontal eye fields
- Orbital Frontal gyrus
- Middle frontal gyrus
- Middle temporal gyrus
- Parietal lobe
- Primary sensory cortex
- Sensorimotor
- Superior parietal gyrus
- Temporal lobe

Regions of interest significant at $P = .001$.

NEUROTRANSMITTER FUNCTION IN AGING

PET, and SPECT, facilitate the *in vivo* evaluation of aging neurotransmitter systems (see **Table 1**). The nigrostriatal dopaminergic pathway is a primary focus due to its role in extrapyramidal function and Parkinson's disease.

Nigrostriatal research shows postmortem age-related D2 receptor reductions.[80–82] Imaging of D1

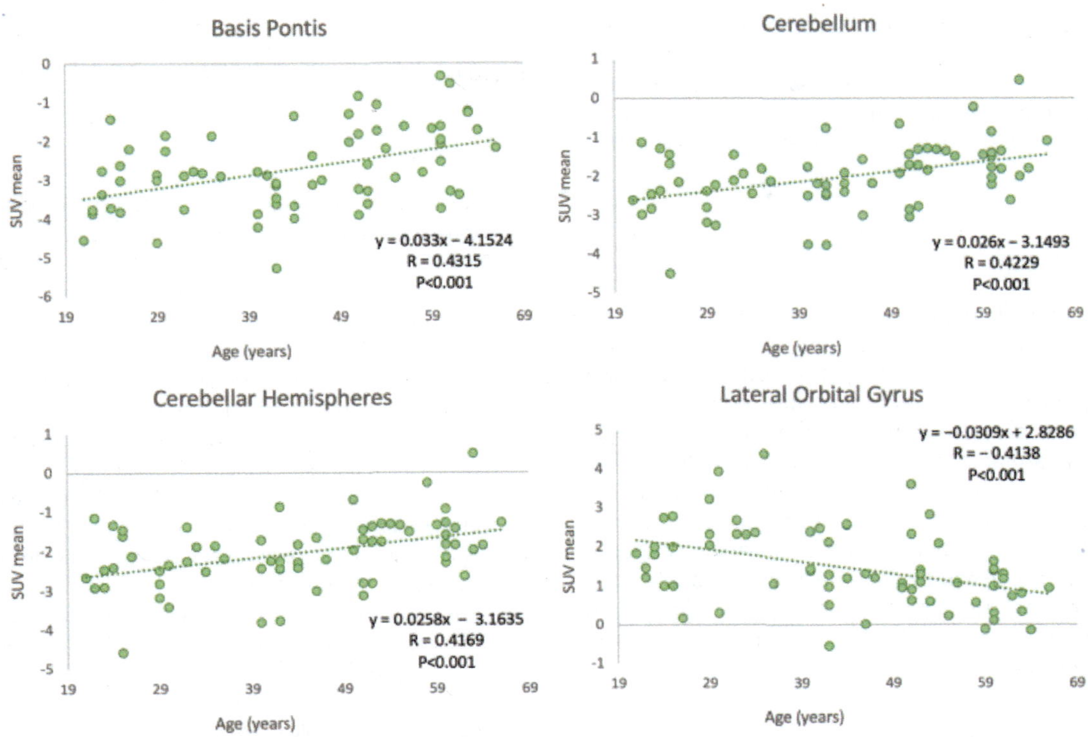

Fig. 5. Correlation between age and PET-FDG uptake in various cerebral regions. (Subtirelu, R.C. et al., Aging and Cerebral Glucose Metabolism: 18F-FDG-PET/CT Reveals Distinct Global and Regional Metabolic Changes in Healthy Patients. Life 2023, 13, 2044. https://doi.org/10.3390/life13102044.[55])

receptors initially yielded mixed results,[82,83] but meta-analyses confirm significant lifespan declines for D1 and D2 availability, despite preserved presynaptic synthesis.[84] D1 loss is biphasic, pivoting toward decline around age 40.[85] Longitudinal evidence indicates striatal and cortical receptor binding decreases by ~7% per decade[86] Striatal [18F]FD uptake, a D2-related dopamine analog, declines by roughly 0.35% annually,[87–89] mirroring estimated nigral neuronal loss.[85,90,91] While most studies document age-related D2 decreases,[92,93] earlier failures to detect this[94,95] likely stemmed from methodological issues regarding regions of interest.[96] [11C]raclopride confirms D2 density declines by 0.6% per year after age 30,[97–99] extending to extrastriatal regions.[100] Finally, dopamine transporter availability declines with age,[101] with β-CIT SPECT showing an 8% loss per decade[102,103] and TRODAT-1 revealing a nonlinear reduction that is steepest before age 40.[104]

The serotonergic system exhibits significant age-related decline, with reuptake sites decreasing by ~10% per decade in the thalamus and midbrain.[105] While women may experience slower transporter reductions,[106] serotonin 1A receptor activity declines at roughly 10% per decade across most cortical regions.[107] This 1 A decline may be gender-specific, appearing more pronounced in men.[108] Similarly, serotonin 2A receptors show substantial loss-up to 42% between ages 23 and 60.[109] This decline follows a nonlinear, mid-life-dominant trajectory[110] that persists after adjusting for cerebral atrophy.[111]

Among less-studied systems, the vesicular acetylcholine transporter shows a modest 3.7% reduction per decade.[112] In contrast, muscarinic cholinergic receptor ligands reveal a 45% to 50% decrease across the lifespan.[113–115] Finally, monoamine oxidase activity is noted to increase with advancing age.[116]

Multimodal FDG and neurotransmitter PET investigations reveal that D2 receptor loss correlates directly with decreased glucose metabolism in the frontal cortex and anterior cingulate, identifying dopaminergic decline as a primary driver of reduced brain function.[117] Genetic variation influences this trajectory, as the DRD4-7R allele appears to protect against age-related metabolic decline in frontal and temporal regions.[118] The DyNAMiC project, which integrates FDG PET, D1/D2 receptor PET, and fMRI, confirms that steady receptor loss reduces frontal glucose metabolism and degrades both functional network stability and striatal-hippocampal connectivity.[86]

The expanding array of PET and SPECT radioligands (see **Box 1**, **Table 1**) offers significant potential to clarify neurotransmitter alterations in normal aging and neuropsychiatric disorders. While key pathways have been identified, many systems remain insufficiently characterized within the context of age-related neurobiological shifts.

SUMMARY

Functional imaging, particularly PET, enables the *in vivo* assessment of cerebral biochemical processes and the impact of various interventions on normal aging. Accurate interpretation necessitates a rigorous understanding of both technical artifacts and baseline age-related shifts. Because aging alters CBF, oxygen and glucose metabolism, and neurotransmitter systems, establishing comprehensive reference ranges is essential. Recognizing the normal spectrum of functional neuroimaging findings remains critical for both clinical diagnosis and valid research interpretation.

CLINICS CARE POINTS

- FDG PET brain imaging is most clinically useful when interpreted alongside the patient's neurological examination, cognitive testing, MRI findings, and clinical history rather than as a standalone diagnostic tool.
- Interpretation requires awareness of normal metabolic variability related to age, medications, sensory stimulation, emotional state, glucose levels, and recent cognitive activity, all of which can affect regional FDG uptake patterns.
- Characteristic metabolic patterns may help differentiate neurodegenerative disorders such as Alzheimer's disease, Frontotemporal dementia, and Lewy body dementia, but overlap between disorders and atypical presentations remain important diagnostic pitfalls.
- Seizure disorders require careful timing considerations because interictal and ictal FDG PET scans may show very different metabolic findings, potentially affecting localization and interpretation.
- Technical and physiologic confounders—including patient motion, hyperglycemia, sedating medications, psychiatric conditions, and partial-volume effects from brain atrophy—can significantly alter scan interpretation and should always be considered before drawing clinical conclusions.

DISCLOSURE

There is nothing to disclose for any of the authors.

REFERENCES

1. Kuhl DE, Edwards RQ. Image separation radioisotope scanning. Radiology 1963;80(4):653–62.
2. Kuhl DE, Edwards RQ, Ricci AR, et al. The mark IV system for radionuclide computed tomography of the brain. Radiology 1976;121(2):405–13.
3. Alavi A, Hirsch LJ. Studies of central nervous system disorders with single photon emission computed tomography and positron emission tomography: evolution over the past 2 decades. In: Seminars in nuclear medicine. Elsevier; 1991.
4. Crişan G, Moldovean-Cioroianu NS, Timaru DG, et al. Radiopharmaceuticals for PET and SPECT imaging: a literature review over the last decade. Int J Mol Sci 2022;23(9):5023.
5. Kung HF. Overview of radiopharmaceuticals for diagnosis of central nervous disorders. Crit Rev Clin Lab Sci 1991;28(4):269–86.
6. Sandler MP. Diagnostic nuclear medicine. Lippincott Williams & Wilkins; 2003.
7. Davis KM, Ryan JL, Aaron VD, et al. PET and SPECT imaging of the brain: history, technical considerations, applications, and radiotracers. In: Seminars in ultrasound, CT and MRI. Elsevier; 2020.
8. Meikle SR, Sossi V, Roncali E, et al. Quantitative PET in the 2020s: a roadmap. Phys Med Biol 2021;66(6):06RM01.
9. Alavi A, Surti KS, Newberg A. Preliminary report of performance of high resolution Gadalinium Orthosilicate (GSO)- based dedicated brain PET scanner. J Nucl Med 2002;43:296. Abstract.
10. Tumeh PC, Alavi A, Houseni M, et al. Structural and functional imaging correlates for age-related changes in the brain. Semin Nucl Med 2007; 37(2):69–87.
11. Newberg A, Alavi A, Reivich M. Determination of regional cerebral function with FDG-PET imaging in neuropsychiatric disorders. In: Seminars in nuclear medicine. Elsevier; 2002.
12. Guedj E, Varrone A, Boellaard R, et al. EANM procedure guidelines for brain PET imaging using [18F] FDG, version 3. Eur J Nucl Med Mol Imag 2022;49(2):632–51.
13. Catafau A, Parellada E, Lomeña F, et al. Baseline, visual deprivation and visual stimulation 99TCm-HMPAO-related changes in visual cortex can be detected with a single-head SPET system. Nucl Med Commun 1996;17(6):480–4.
14. Riedl V, Bienkowska K, Strobel C, et al. Local activity determines functional connectivity in the resting human brain: a simultaneous FDG-PET/fMRI study. J Neurosci 2014;34(18):6260–6.

15. Beer J, Blakemore C, Previc FH, et al. Areas of the human brain activated by ambient visual motion, indicating three kinds of self-movement. Exp Brain Res 2002;143(1):78–88.
16. Castelli F, Happé F, Frith U, et al. Movement and mind: a functional imaging study of perception and interpretation of complex intentional movement patterns. In: Social neuroscience. Psychology Press; 2013. p. 155–69.
17. Mirz F, Ovesen T, Ishizu K, et al. Stimulus-dependent central processing of auditory stimuli: a PET study. Scand Audiol 1999;28(3):161–9.
18. Putkinen V, Hahn A, Tuisku J, et al. Cerebral glucose utilisation during musical emotions: a multimodal functional pet/MRI study. bioRxiv 2025. 2025.08. 28.672829.
19. Hahn A, Gryglewski G, Nics L, et al. Task-relevant brain networks identified with simultaneous PET/MR imaging of metabolism and connectivity. Brain Struct Funct 2018;223(3):1369–78.
20. Rischka L, Gryglewski G, Pfaff S, et al. Reduced task durations in functional PET imaging with [18F] FDG approaching that of functional MRI. Neuroimage 2018;181:323–30.
21. Godbersen GM, Klug S, Wadsak W, et al. Task-evoked metabolic demands of the posteromedial default mode network are shaped by dorsal attention and frontoparietal control networks. eLife 2023;12:e84683.
22. Hahn A, Breakspear M, Rischka L, et al. Reconfiguration of functional brain networks and metabolic cost converge during task performance. eLife 2020;9:e52443.
23. Karjalainen T, Tuominen L, Manninen S, et al. Behavioural activation system sensitivity is associated with cerebral μ-opioid receptor availability. Soc Cognit Affect Neurosci 2016;11(8):1310–6.
24. Kantonen T, Karjalainen T, Isojärvi J, et al. Interindividual variability and lateralization of μ-opioid receptors in the human brain. Neuroimage 2020;217:116922.
25. Verger A, Guedj E. The renaissance of functional 18F-FDG PET brain activation imaging. Eur J Nucl Med Mol Imag 2018;45(13):2338–41.
26. Vogel WV, Valdés Olmos RA, Tijs TJW, et al. Intervention to lower anxiety of 18F-FDG PET/CT patients by use of audiovisual imagery during the uptake phase before imaging. J Nucl Med Technol 2012;40(2):92–8.
27. Kurland BF, Peterson LM, Shields AT, et al. Test–retest reproducibility of 18F-FDG PET/CT uptake in cancer patients within a qualified and calibrated local network. J Nucl Med 2019;60(5):608–14.
28. Vriens D, Visser EP, de Geus-Oei LF, et al. Methodological considerations in quantification of oncological FDG PET studies. Eur J Nucl Med Mol Imag 2010;37(7):1408–25.
29. Kannan S, Chugani HT. Applications of positron emission tomography in the newborn nursery. Semin Perinatol 2010;34(1):39–45.
30. Wang Y, Mo J, Sun Y, et al. Establishment of a normal control model of children's brain 18-fluorodeoxyglucose positron emission tomography and analysis of the changing pattern in patients aged 0–14 years. Quant Imag Med Surg 2024;14(7):4703.
31. Chugani HT, Phelps ME, Mazziotta JC. Positron emission tomography study of human brain functional development. Ann Neurol 1987;22(4):487–97.
32. Chugani HT, Phelps ME. Maturational changes in cerebral function in infants determined by 18FDG positron emission tomography. Science 1986;231(4740):840–3.
33. Barber TW, Veysey D, Billah B, et al. Normal brain metabolism on FDG PET/MRI during childhood and adolescence. Nucl Med Commun 2018;39(11):1022–32.
34. Chugani HT. Functional brain imaging in pediatrics. Pediatr Clin 1992;39(4):777–99.
35. Takahashi T, Shirane R, Sato S, et al. Developmental changes of cerebral blood flow and oxygen metabolism in children. Am J Neuroradiol 1999;20(5):917–22.
36. Goyal MS, Hawrylycz M, Miller JA, et al. Aerobic glycolysis in the human brain is associated with development and neotenous gene expression. Cell Metab 2014;19(1):49–57.
37. Takahashi K, Yamaguchi S, Kobayashi S, et al. Effects of aging on regional cerebral blood flow assessed by using technetium Tc 99m hexamethylpropyleneamine oxime single-photon emission tomography with 3D stereotactic surface projection analysis. Am J Neuroradiol 2005;26(8).
38. Mokhber N, Shariatzadeh A, Avan A, et al. Cerebral blood flow changes during aging process and in cognitive disorders: a review. NeuroRadiol J 2021;34(4):300–7.
39. Mozley PD, Sadek AM, Alavi A, et al. Effects of aging on the cerebral distribution of technetium-99m hexamethylpropylene amine oxime in healthy humans. Eur J Nucl Med 1997;24(7):754–61.
40. Waldemar G, Hasselbalch SG, Andersen AR, et al. 99mTc-d, l-HMPAO and SPECT of the brain in normal aging. J Cereb Blood Flow Metab 1991;11(3):508–21.
41. Inoue K, Nakagawa M, Goto R, et al. Regional differences between 99mTc-ECD and 99mTc-HMPAO SPET in perfusion changes with age and gender in healthy adults. Eur J Nucl Med Mol Imag 2003;30(11):1489–97.
42. Aanerud J, Borghammer P, Rodell A, et al. Sex differences of human cortical blood flow and energy metabolism. J Cereb Blood Flow Metab 2017;37(7):2433–40.

43. Petit-Taboue M, Landeau B, Desson JF, et al. Effects of healthy aging on the regional cerebral metabolic rate of glucose assessed with statistical parametric mapping. Neuroimage 1998;7(3):176–84.
44. Van Laere K, Versijpt J, Audenaert K, et al. 99mTc-ECD brain perfusion SPET: variability, asymmetry and effects of age and gender in healthy adults. Eur J Nucl Med 2001;28(7):873–87.
45. Chawluk J, Alavi A, Hurtig H. Altered patterns of regional cerebral glucose metabolism in aging and dementia. J Cereb Blood Flow Metab 1985;5-(Suppl 1):S121–2.
46. de Leon MJ, George AE, Tomanelli J, et al. Positron emission tomography studies of normal aging: a replication of PET III and 18-FDG using PET VI and 11-CDG. Neurobiol Aging 1987;8(4):319–23.
47. Chawluk JB, Alavi A, Dann R, et al. Positron emission tomography in aging and dementia: effect of cerebral atrophy. J Nucl Med 1987;28(4):431–7.
48. Weiss D, Souder E, Alavi A. Effects of normal aging on whole brain and regional glucose metabolism as assessed by F-18 positron emission tomography. J Nucl Med 1990;31:771.
49. Yoshii F, Barker WW, Chang JY, et al. Sensitivity of cerebral glucose metabolism to age, gender, brain volume, brain atrophy, and cerebrovascular risk factors. J Cereb Blood Flow Metab 1988;8(5):654–61.
50. Goyal MS, Vlassenko AG, Blazey TM, et al. Loss of brain aerobic glycolysis in normal human aging. Cell Metab 2017;26(2):353–60.e3.
51. De Leon M, Convit A, Wolf OT, et al. Prediction of cognitive decline in normal elderly subjects with 2-[18F] fluoro-2-deoxy-D-glucose/positron-emission tomography (FDG/PET). Proc Natl Acad Sci 2001; 98(19):10966–71.
52. Deery HA, Di Paolo R, Moran C, et al. Lower brain glucose metabolism in normal ageing is predominantly frontal and temporal: a systematic review and pooled effect size and activation likelihood estimates meta-analyses. Hum Brain Mapp 2023; 44(3):1251–77.
53. Kuhl DE, Metter EJ, Riege WH, et al. Effects of human aging on patterns of local cerebral glucose utilization determined by the [18F] fluorodeoxyglucose method. J Cereb Blood Flow Metab 1982;2(2):163–71.
54. Alavi A, Jolles PR, Jamison DO, et al. Anatomic and functional changes of the brain in normal aging and dementia as demonstrated by MRI, CT, and PET. Nucl Med Ann 1989;49–79.
55. Subtirelu RC, Teichner EM, Su Y, et al. Aging and cerebral glucose metabolism: 18F-FDG-PET/CT reveals distinct global and regional metabolic changes in healthy patients. Life 2023;13(10):2044.
56. Loessner A, Alavi A, Lewandrowski KU, et al. Regional cerebral function determined by FDG-PET in healthy volunteers: normal patterns and changes with age. J Nucl Med 1995;36(7):1141–9.
57. Eberling J, Nordahl TE, Kusubov N, et al. Reduced temporal lobe glucose metabolism in aging. J Neuroimaging 1995;5(3):178–82.
58. Alavi A, Chawluk JB, Hurtig H, et al. Determination of patterns of regional cerebral glucose metabolism in normal aging and dementia. J Nucl Med 1985;26. CONF-850611-).
59. Miura S, Schapiro MB, Grady CL, et al. Effect of gender on glucose utilization rates in healthy humans: a positron emission tomography study. J Neurosci Res 1990;27(4):500–4.
60. Kawachi T, Ishii K, Sakamoto S, et al. Gender differences in cerebral glucose metabolism: a PET study. J Neurol Sci 2002;199(1–2):79–83.
61. Feng B, Cao J, Yu Y, et al. Gender-related differences in regional cerebral glucose metabolism in normal aging brain. Front Aging Neurosci 2022; 14:809767.
62. Kuhl DE, Metter EJ, Riege WH, et al. The effect of normal aging on patterns of local cerebral glucose utilization. Ann Neurol 1984;15(S1):133–7.
63. Hawkins RA, Mazziotta JC, Phelps ME, et al. Cerebral glucose metabolism as a function of age in man: influence of the rate constants in the fluorodeoxyglucose method. J Cereb Blood Flow Metab 1983;3(2):250–3.
64. Dastur DK. Cerebral blood flow and metabolism in normal human aging, pathological aging, and senile dementia. J Cereb Blood Flow Metab 1985; 5(1):1–9.
65. Yamaguchi T, Kanno I, Uemura K, et al. Reduction in regional cerebral metabolic rate of oxygen during human aging. Stroke 1986;17(6):1220–8.
66. Takada H, Nagata K, Hirata Y, et al. Age-related decline of cerebral oxygen metabolism in normal population detected with positron emission tomography. Neurol Res 1992;14(2):128–31.
67. Leenders K, Perani D, Lammertsma AA, et al. Cerebral blood flow, blood volume and oxygen utilization: normal values and effect of age. Brain 1990; 113(1):27–47.
68. Martin AJ, Friston KJ, Colebatch JG, et al. Decreases in regional cerebral blood flow with normal aging. J Cereb Blood Flow Metab 1991;11(4):684–9.
69. Frackowiak R, Gibbs J. Cerebral metabolism and blood flow in normal and pathologic aging. New York, Raven: Functional Radionuclide Imaging of the Brain; 1983. p. 305–9.
70. Jiang D, Lu H. Cerebral oxygen extraction fraction MRI: techniques and applications. Magn Reson Med 2022;88(2):575–600.
71. Wu J, Oishi K, Soldan A, et al. Longitudinal changes in cerebral metabolic rate of oxygen in older adults without and with cognitive impairment. Alzheimer's Dement 2024;20:e085554.
72. Sanami S, Rezaei A, Tremblay SA, et al. Greater cardiorespiratory fitness is associated with higher

cerebral blood flow and lower oxygen extraction fraction in healthy older adults. J Cereb Blood Flow Metab 2026;0271678X251413924.
73. Wahlund L, Agartz I, Almqvist O, et al. The brain in healthy aged individuals: MR imaging. Radiology 1990;174(3):675–9.
74. Jernigan TL, Archibald SL, Berhow MT, et al. Cerebral structure on MRI, part I: localization of age-related changes. Biol Psychiatry 1991;29(1):55–67.
75. Tanna NK, Kohn MI, Horwich DN, et al. Analysis of brain and cerebrospinal fluid volumes with MR imaging: impact on PET data correction for atrophy. Part II. Aging and Alzheimer dementia. Radiology 1991;178(1):123–30.
76. Gur RC, Mozley PD, Resnick SM, et al. Gender differences in age effect on brain atrophy measured by magnetic resonance imaging. Proc Natl Acad Sci 1991;88(7):2845–9.
77. Greve DN, Salat DH, Bowen SL, et al. Different partial volume correction methods lead to different conclusions: an 18F-FDG-PET study of aging. Neuroimage 2016;132:334–43.
78. Sanabria Bohórquez SM, Baker S, Manser PT, et al. Evaluation of partial volume correction and analysis of longitudinal [18F] GTP1 tau PET imaging in Alzheimer's disease using linear mixed-effects models. Frontiers in Neuroimaging 2024; 3:1355402.
79. Azimi MS, Rahmim A, Arabi H, et al. Critical review of partial volume correction methods in PET and SPECT imaging: benefits, pitfalls, challenges, and future outlook. Eur J Nucl Med Mol Imag 2025;1–32.
80. Rinne JO, Lönnberg P, Marjamäki P. Age-dependent decline in human brain dopamine D1 and D2 receptors. Brain Res 1990;508(2):349–52.
81. Rinne J. Muscarinic and dopaminergic receptors in the aging human brain. Brain Res 1987;404(1–2): 162–8.
82. Morgan DG, Marcusson JO, Nyberg P, et al. Divergent changes in D-1 and D-2 dopamine binding sites in human brain during aging. Neurobiol Aging 1987;8(3):195–201.
83. Wang Y, Chan GL, Holden JE, et al. Age-dependent decline of dopamine D1 receptors in human brain: a PET study. Synapse 1998;30(1):56–61.
84. Karrer TM, Josef AK, Mata R, et al. Reduced dopamine receptors and transporters but not synthesis capacity in normal aging adults: a meta-analysis. Neurobiol Aging 2017;57:36–46.
85. Johansson J, Nordin K, Pedersen R, et al. Biphasic patterns of age-related differences in dopamine D1 receptors across the adult lifespan. Cell Rep 2023; 42(9).
86. Nordin K, Gorbach T, Pedersen R, et al. DyNAMiC: a prospective longitudinal study of dopamine and brain connectomes: a new window into cognitive aging. J Neurosci Res 2022;100(6):1296–320.
87. Cordes M, Snow BJ, Cooper S, et al. Age-dependent decline of nigrostriatal dopaminergic function: a positron emission tomographic study of grandparents and their grandchildren. Ann Neurol 1994; 36(4):667–70.
88. Bhatt MH, Snow BJ, Martin WR, et al. Positron emission tomography suggests that the rate of progression of idiopathic parkinsonism is slow. Ann Neurol 1991;29(6):673–7.
89. Martin W, Palmer MR, Patlak CS, et al. Nigrostriatal function in humans studied with positron emission tomography. Ann Neurol 1989;26(4):535–42.
90. McGeer PL, McGeer EG, Suzuki JS. Aging and extrapyramidal function. Arch Neurol 1977;34(1): 33–5.
91. Gibb W, Lees A. Anatomy, pigmentation, ventral and dorsal subpopulations of the substantia nigra, and differential cell death in Parkinson's disease. J Neurol Neurosurg Psychiatr 1991;54(5):388–96.
92. Inoue M, Suhara T, Sudo Y, et al. Age-related reduction of extrastriatal dopamine D2 receptor measured by PET. Life Sci 2001;69(9):1079–84.
93. Kaasinen V, Kemppainen N, Någren K, et al. Age related loss of extrastriatal dopamine D2-like receptors in women. J Neurochem 2002;81(5):1005–10.
94. Sawle G, Colebatch JG, Shah A, et al. Striatal function in normal aging: implications for Parkinson's disease. Ann Neurol 1990;28(6):799–804.
95. Eidelberg D, Takikawa S, Dhawan V, et al. Striatal 18F-dopa uptake: absence of an aging effect. J Cereb Blood Flow Metab 1993;13(5):881–8.
96. Vingerhoets FJ, Snow BJ, Schulzer M, et al. Reproducibility of fluorine-18-6-fluorodopa positron emission tomography in normal human subjects. J Nucl Med 1994;35(1):18–24.
97. Rinne JO, Hietala J, Ruotsalainen U, et al. Decrease in human striatal dopamine D2 receptor density with age: a PET study with [11C] raclopride. J Cereb Blood Flow Metab 1993;13(2):310–4.
98. Volkow ND, Wang GJ, Fowler JS, et al. Measuring age-related changes in dopamine D2 receptors with 11C-raclopride and 18F-N-methylspiroperidol. Psychiatr Res Neuroimaging 1996;67(1):11–6.
99. Antonini A, Leenders KL. Dopamine D2 receptors in normal human brain: effect of age measured by Positron Emission Tomography (PET) and [11C] raclopride a. Ann N Y Acad Sci 1993;695(1):81–5.
100. Kaasinen V, Vilkman H, Hietala J, et al. Age-related dopamine D2/D3 receptor loss in extrastriatal regions of the human brain. Neurobiol Aging 2000; 21(5):683–8.
101. Tedroff J, Aquilonius SM, Hartvig P, et al. Monoamine re-uptake sites in the human brain evaluated in vivo by means of 11C-nomifensine and positron emission tomography: the effects of age and Parkinson's disease. Acta Neurol Scand 1988;77(3): 192–201.

102. van Dyck CH, Seibyl JP, Malison RT, et al. Age-related decline in striatal dopamine transporter binding with iodine-123-b-CIT SPECT. J Nucl Med 1995;36(7):1175–81.
103. Marcusson JO, Alafuzoff I, Bäckström IT, et al. 5-Hydroxytryptamine-sensitive [3H] imipramine binding of protein nature in the human brain.: II. Effect of normal aging and dementia disorders. Brain Res 1987;425(1):137–45.
104. Mozley PD, Acton PD, Barraclough ED, et al. Effects of age on dopamine transporters in healthy humans. J Nucl Med 1999;40(11):1812–7.
105. Yamamoto M, Suhara T, Okubo Y, et al. Age-related decline of serotonin transporters in living human brain of healthy males. Life Sci 2002;71(7):751–7.
106. Kuikka JT, Tammela L, Bergström KA, et al. Effects of ageing on serotonin transporters in healthy females. Eur J Nucl Med 2001;28(7):911–3.
107. Tauscher J, Verhoeff NP, Christensen BK, et al. Serotonin 5-HT1A receptor binding potential declines with age as measured by [11C] WAY-100635 and PET. Neuropsychopharmacology 2001;24(5):522–30.
108. Meltzer CC, Drevets WC, Price JC, et al. Gender-specific aging effects on the serotonin 1A receptor. Brain Res 2001;895(1–2):9–17.
109. Baeken C, D'haenen H, Flamen P, et al. 123I-5-I-R91150, a new single-photon emission tomography ligand for 5-HT2A receptors: influence of age and gender in healthy subjects. Eur J Nucl Med 1998;25(12):1617–22.
110. Sheline Y, Mintun M, Moerlein S. Greater loss of 5-HT2A receptors in midlife than in late life. Year Bk Psychiatr Appl Ment Health 2003;2003(1):310–1.
111. Meltzer CC, Smith G, Price JC, et al. Reduced binding of [18F] altanserin to serotonin type 2A receptors in aging: persistence of effect after partial volume correction. Brain Res 1998;813(1):167–71.
112. Kuhl DE, Minoshima S, Fessler JA, et al. In vivo mapping of cholinergic terminals in normal aging, Alzheimer's disease, and Parkinson's disease. Ann Neurol 1996;40(3):399–410.
113. Suhara T, Inoue O, Kobayashi K, et al. Age-related changes in human muscarinic acetylcholine receptors measured by positron emission tomography. Neurosci Lett 1993;149(2):225–8.
114. Lee KS, Frey KA, Koeppe RA, et al. In vivo quantification of cerebral muscarinic receptors in normal human aging using positron emission tomography and [11C] tropanyl benzilate. J Cereb Blood Flow Metab 1996;16(2):303–10.
115. Dewey S, Volkow ND, Logan J, et al. Age-related decreases in muscarinic cholinergic receptor binding in the human brain measured with positron emission tomography (PET). J Neurosci Res 1990;27(4):569–75.
116. Fowler J, Volkow ND, Wang GJ, et al. Age-related increases in brain monoamine oxidase B in living healthy human subjects. Neurobiol Aging 1997;18(4):431–5.
117. Volkow ND, Logan J, Fowler JS, et al. Association between age-related decline in brain dopamine activity and impairment in frontal and cingulate metabolism. Am J Psychiatr 2000;157(1):75–80.
118. Volkow ND, Tomasi D, Wang GJ, et al. Association between dopamine D4 receptor polymorphism and age related changes in brain glucose metabolism. PLoS One 2013;8(5):e63492.

FDG-PET in Cognitive Impairment and Dementia

Julie Hong, MD[a], Daniel H.S. Silverman, MD, PhD[a,b,*]

KEYWORDS

• Fluorodeoxyglucose • Positron emission tomography • Alzheimer's • Dementia • Amyloid • Tau • Mild decline in cognition

KEY POINTS

- 2-[F-18]fluoro-2-deoxy-d-glucose-PET (FDG-PET) is the imaging modality with the greatest overall accuracy in the differential diagnosis of neurodegenerative disease in appropriately selected patients.
- Used in conjunction with other imaging modalities and/or fluid biomarkers, FDG-PET can provide guidance in selecting the most effective, safe use of available therapeutic strategies.
- An integrated algorithm based on best available evidence of the complementary roles for FDG-, amyloid- and tau- PET, as well as fluid biomarkers, is presented.

INTRODUCTION

Dementia is a growing global health challenge, affecting an estimated 57.4 million individuals worldwide and contributing substantially to disability, caregiver burden, and health care expenditures.[1] The majority of dementia cases are attributed to Alzheimer's disease (AD), which is characterized histopathologically by the extracellular accumulation of amyloid-beta (Aβ) plaques and intracellular neurofibrillary tangles composed of hyperphosphorylated tau protein.[2,3] Additional pathogenic mechanisms including mitochondrial dysfunction, oxidative stress, neuroinflammation, and synaptic loss contribute to progressive neuronal injury, cognitive decline, and eventual loss of functional independence for patients with AD.[4] The 2024 Lancet Commission on Dementia identified 14 modifiable risk factors that collectively account for approximately 45% of dementia risk, underscoring the scale of the public health challenge.[5]

The clinical diagnosis of AD remains challenging, especially in its earlier stages. Multiple neurodegenerative diseases can produce overlapping cognitive and behavioral symptoms, and co-occurrence of AD with dementia with Lewy bodies (DLB) or frontotemporal lobar dementia (FTLD) neurodegenerative processes, as well as with cerebrovascular compromise, is common.[6,7] The diagnostic challenge has been further complicated by the recognition of limbic-predominant age-related TDP-43 encephalopathy neuropathologic change (LATE-NC), a proteinopathy most prevalent in older adults that produces an amnestic dementia syndrome closely mimicking AD clinically but typically progressing more slowly and driven by TDP-43 rather than amyloid or tau pathology.[8,9] Neuropathological studies have consistently demonstrated limited consistency between clinical and autopsy-confirmed diagnoses, which further emphasizes the need for objective biomarkers that can improve diagnostic accuracy in living patients.[10]

The National Institute on Aging and Alzheimer's Association (NIA-AA) has progressively redefined diagnostic criteria to incorporate biomarker evidence across the AD continuum, from preclinical through dementia stages.[11,12] A recent longitudinal study has refined the preclinical timeline of

[a] Department of Nuclear Medicine and Theranostics, David Geffen School of Medicine at UCLA, University of California, Los Angeles, USA; [b] Department of Molecular and Medical Pharmacology, David Geffen School of Medicine at UCLA, University of California, Los Angeles, USA
* Corresponding author.
E-mail address: dsilver@ucla.edu

PET Clin 21 (2026) 483–497
https://doi.org/10.1016/j.cpet.2026.07.001

Abbreviations

Aβ	amyloid-beta
AD	Alzheimer's disease
ADNI	Alzheimer's Disease Neuroimaging Initiative
APOE	apolipoprotein E
ARIA	amyloid-related imaging abnormalities
AUC	area under the curve
DL	deep learning
DLB	dementia with Lewy bodies
EANM	European Association of Nuclear Medicine
FTLD	frontotemporal lobar degeneration
IDEAS	Imaging Dementia—Evidence for Amyloid Scanning
LATE-NC	limbic-predominant age-related TDP-43 encephalopathy neuropathologic change
MCI	mild cognitive impairment
MTL	medial temporal lobe
NIA-AA	National Institute on Aging and Alzheimer's Association
p-tau217	phosphorylated tau-217
SNMMI	Society of Nuclear Medicine and Molecular Imaging
SWI	susceptibility-weighted imaging

AD: Cerebrospinal fluid (CSF) amyloid-β42 levels begin to diverge approximately 18 years before clinical diagnosis, phosphorylated tau at approximately 11 years, and measurable cognitive decline at approximately 6 years.[13] Most recently, the 2024 NIA-AA revised criteria have redefined AD as a biological entity diagnosed through specific biomarker profiles, with plasma phosphorylated tau-217 (p-tau217) receiving designation as a Core 1 biomarker alongside more established PET and CSF measures.[14] However, this position is not without debate. For example, the International Working Group has reaffirmed a clinical-biological construct in which AD diagnosis requires both a characteristic clinical phenotype and supporting biomarker evidence, arguing that biomarker-positive cognitively unimpaired individuals are better characterized as *at-risk* rather than having the disease.[15,16] This ongoing discussion carries direct implications for how neuroimaging and biomarkers are deployed in clinical practice.

Concurrently, the approval of monoclonal antibodies targeting Aβ, including lecanemab and donanemab, has transformed the clinical purpose of neuroimaging from a purely diagnostic endeavor into an integrated diagnostic and therapeutic means of approaching AD. Imaging now serves not only to identify and differentiate disease but also to select patients for treatment, monitor response, and guide decisions about therapy modification.

This article reviews the current utility of structural, functional, and molecular neuroimaging techniques in the evaluation of AD and related disorders. Each modality is discussed with respect to its diagnostic utility and role in treatment planning. The impact of blood-based biomarkers on imaging utilization is addressed, quantification tools that enhance clinical interpretation are reviewed, and an updated algorithm for integrating these imaging modalities in contemporary clinical practice is presented.

2-[F-18]FLUORO-2-DEOXY-D-GLUCOSE-PET

Role in the Biomarker Framework and Diagnostic Accuracy

2-[F-18]fluoro-2-deoxy-d-glucose-PET (FDG-PET) measures regional cerebral glucose metabolism, providing a topographic map of synaptic activity and neuronal function.[12] Under the controversial 2024 revised NIA-AA criteria, the diagnosis of AD relies on biological markers of amyloid and phosphorylated tau pathology.[14]

This revision does not diminish the clinical utility of FDG-PET, however, for which prognostic- and autopsy-based evidence confirms an established role in differential diagnosis among neurodegenerative disorders and for predicting the imminence of cognitive and functional decline. The diagnostic accuracy of FDG-PET for detecting progressive dementia has been demonstrated across multiple validation paradigms. In the largest study with autopsy-confirmed diagnoses, FDG-PET achieved a sensitivity of 94% and specificity of 73% for predicting progressive dementia.[17] Follow-up analyses using contemporary PET scanners showed that specificity improved to 87% for predicting which patients would progress to dementia.[18] A more recent autopsy-validated study of 101 patients with younger-onset dementia found that when FDG-PET and amyloid PET findings were concordant, diagnostic accuracy approached 100%.[19] A comprehensive examination of the FDG-PET literature confirmed its high sensitivity across clinical settings,[20] and a recent systematic review and meta-analysis reported a pooled area under the curve (AUC) of 0.864 for FDG-PET in differentiating AD from cognitively normal controls.[21]

Characteristic Metabolic Patterns and Differential Diagnosis

The regional distribution of hypometabolism on FDG-PET reflects the topography of neuronal dysfunction specific to each neurodegenerative disease, which enables pattern-based differential diagnosis. In AD, hypometabolism is typically first observed in the posterior cingulate cortex during the prodromal phase, subsequently extending to the parietotemporal association cortices as the disease progresses.[17,22] FDG-PET is useful for tracking disease progression, as metabolic deficits worsen with advancing pathology and predict declining cognitive abilities.[23,24] In early-onset AD compared to late-onset AD, FDG-PET demonstrates more pronounced glucose hypometabolism in parts of the parietal and precuneus/ posterior cingulate cortex, including Brodmann areas 7, 31, and 40.[25]

FDG-PET can also differentiate AD from other common dementias. Patients with vascular dementia typically show scattered, asymmetric metabolic deficits corresponding to affected vascular territories, in contrast to the characteristic parietotemporal pattern of AD.[20]

DLB (**Fig. 1**) is characterized by hypometabolism in the occipital cortex with relative preservation of the posterior cingulate sometimes described as the *cingulate island sign*.[26] Using postmortem validation, FDG-PET distinguished DLB from AD with an accuracy exceeding that of clinical diagnostic criteria.[27] More recently, a metabolic ratio comparing medial temporal and substantia nigra uptake achieved 94% sensitivity and 83% specificity for distinguishing prodromal DLB from prodromal AD, demonstrating the utility of FDG-PET well before the dementia stage.[28]

FTLD comprises an umbrella of diagnoses, with different pathologies, genetics and corresponding patterns of metabolism, but as its name implies have in common predominant effects on frontal and/or temporal lobes. Anterior temporal hypometabolism rather than the more posterior temporal hypometabolism seen in AD is characteristic (**Fig. 2**), and hypometabolism in the frontal cortex, caudate nuclei, and insula is also common. These metabolic patterns predict pathologic diagnosis better than clinical assessment can.[29,30]

A recent advance in differential diagnosis of dementia is the recognition of LATE-NC as a specific entity with a characteristic FDG-PET signature. LATE-NC is a highly prevalent proteinopathy in older adults that produces an amnestic dementia syndrome that can present itself in a manner that is clinically indistinguishable from AD.[8] Grothe and colleagues[9] examined antemortem FDG-PET scans from patients with autopsy-confirmed LATE-NC and identified a metabolic pattern markedly different from AD: pronounced hypometabolism in the medial temporal lobe (MTL), amygdala, and fronto-opercular/insular cortex, with relative sparing of the inferior temporal and lateral parietal regions typically affected in AD. Patients with this pattern are significantly older, have lower apolipoprotein E (APOE) ε4 frequency, lower AD-CSF biomarker burden, and a slower rate of cognitive decline compared to those with a typical AD metabolic signature. Because LATE-NC does not inherently involve Aβ or tau pathology, patients harboring this condition may not benefit from antiamyloid immunotherapies, making its identification through FDG-PET valuable for appropriate therapeutic decision-making and clinical trial enrichment.

Prognostic Value and Stratification of Mild Cognitive Impairment

FDG-PET has a well-established prognostic value for predicting which individuals with mild cognitive impairment (MCI) will progress to dementia. Decline in FDG uptake tends to precede and parallel declining cognitive abilities, and FDG-PET can predict rate of subsequent cognitive and functional decline in individuals who go on to develop AD.[24,31] A recent systematic review confirmed that FDG-PET and amyloid-PET are accurate molecular imaging biomarkers for predicting MCI-to-dementia conversion, with FDG-PET providing the highest positive predictive value for imminent clinical progression.[32] When combined with genetic risk markers such as APOE ε4 carrier status, the predictive accuracy of FDG-PET for conversion of amnestic MCI to AD dementia is further improved, with reported sensitivities approaching 100% in enriched cohorts.[32] FDG-PET is also particularly useful for evaluating highly intelligent individuals who may perform well on standard cognitive assessments despite harboring significant hypometabolism indicative of impending dementia.[17,33]

A major advance in the understanding of MCI heterogeneity has come from metabolic phenotyping with FDG-PET,[34,35] which used automated voxel-based algorithms to stratify a large cohort of amnestic MCI subjects into 3 biologically and clinically distinct subtypes based on their spatial hypometabolic profiles. The first subtype, characterized by hippocampal-sparing cortical hypometabolism, occurred in younger patients with the highest AD-CSF pathology burden and showed rapid progression to dementia. The second subtype, featuring combined hippocampal and cortical hypometabolism, was associated with higher prevalence for APOE ε4 carriers and followed a trajectory consistent with typical AD, with steady progression from MCI to dementia. The third subtype, displaying isolated MTL hypometabolism, was notable for a discordance between structure and pathology: despite exhibiting

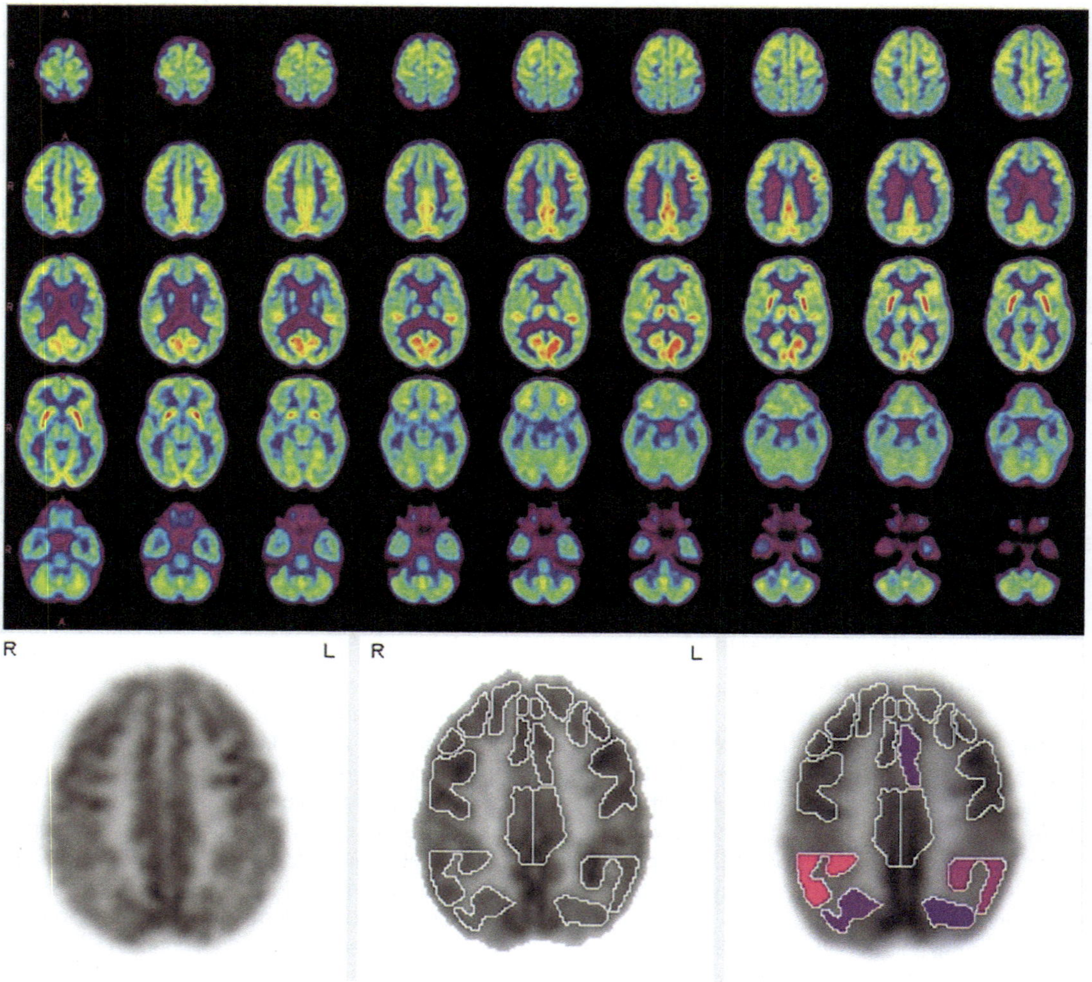

Fig. 1. Brain FDG-PET scan demonstrating metabolic features of DLB in a 75-year-old male. Diagnosis was further corroborated by DaT SPECT scan demonstrating the presynaptic dopaminergic deficit characteristic of DLB and other Parkinsonian conditions. *Top panel* illustrates transaxial planes represented at a slice angle along the anterior commissure-posterior commissure axis from superior to inferior levels in rainbow color scale. *Bottom panel* illustrates transaxial plane of brain of patient in a linear inverse gray scale (*left*), of template brain overlaid with standardized regions of interest (*middle*), and of the patient's brain PET data transformed to template space with standardized regions having abnormally low metabolism depicted in a color scale (*right*). In addition to parietotemporal hypometabolism, lateral occipital cortex is also seen to be hypometabolic while posterior cingulate metabolism is seen to be robustly preserved—oppositely to the pattern of metabolism typically seen in patients having parietotemporal hypometabolism due to AD.

severe structural hippocampal atrophy on MR imaging, these patients, who were generally older, possessed the lowest burden of AD-CSF pathology and demonstrated a largely stable clinical course with the lowest rate of progression to dementia among the 3 groups. This finding carries important implications for clinical trial design: isolated MTL hypometabolism on FDG-PET likely reflects non-AD pathology (potentially including LATE-NC), and patients displaying this pattern should be carefully evaluated before enrollment in antiamyloid therapeutic trials to avoid dilution of treatment effect sizes.

Deep Learning and Artificial Intelligence–Enhanced Interpretation

The application of deep learning (DL) architectures to FDG-PET interpretation has emerged as an active area of development since previous reviews of this topic. A 2025 systematic review and meta-analysis synthesizing data from 36 studies reported that DL-assisted FDG-PET achieves pooled AUC values of 0.98 for differentiating AD from cognitively normal controls, 0.95 for distinguishing AD from MCI, and 0.94 for classifying MCI from normal cognition.[36] These metrics

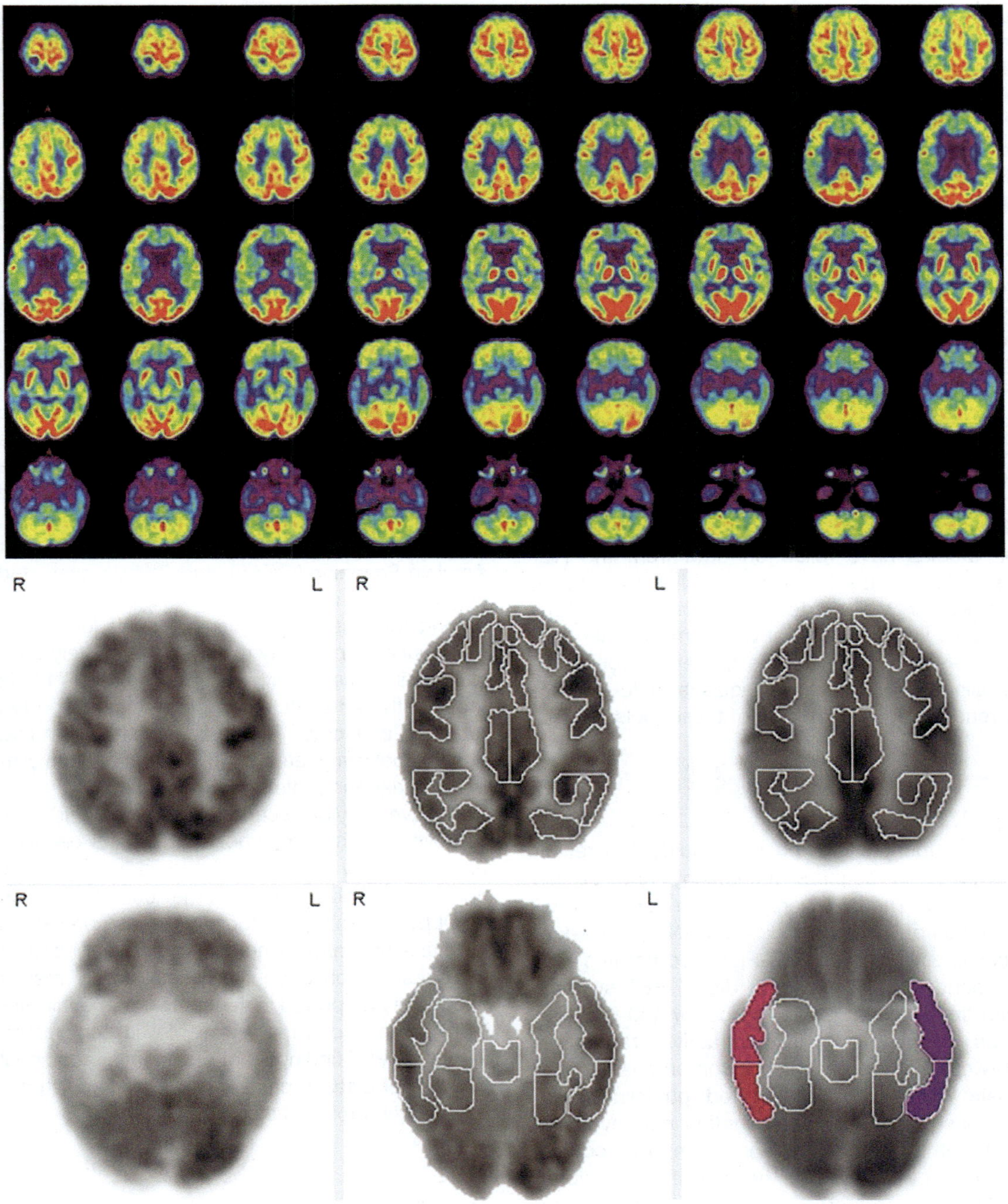

Fig. 2. Brain FDG-PET scan demonstrating anterior temporal-predominant hypometabolism, a characteristic feature of TDP-43 proteinopathy, as can occur in temporal-predominant FTLD or LATE. In this 70 year old female patient, a clinical diagnosis of frontotemporal dementia was further corroborated by particularly marked progression of temporal hypometabolism over a 2-year period, along with evolution of behavioral-predominant symptoms. *Top panel* illustrates transaxial planes in rainbow color scale from superior to inferior levels. *Middle panel* illustrates transaxial plane of brain in inverse linear gray scale, which, in contrast with the brain of the patient with DLB illustrated in Fig. 1, has well-preserved metabolism in parietotemporal and occipital cortex. *Bottom panel* illustrates a transaxial plane depicting the marked hypometabolism of bilateral anterior temporal lobes.

exceed the performance of conventional visual interpretation and traditional region-of-interest analyses. In a separate study, a three-dimensional convolutional neural network trained on FDG-PET data matched the classification accuracy of expert nuclear medicine physicians for multiclass differentiation among AD, DLB, MCI, and cognitively normal individuals.[37]

The advantage of DL models lies in their capacity to extract subvisual metabolic features directly from raw voxel intensities, detecting patterns of synaptic dysfunction that span distributed neural networks and may elude the human eye at early disease stages. Importantly, DL outputs derived from FDG-PET provide independent prognostic value even within subgroups already confirmed to be amyloid-positive, suggesting that the metabolic pattern captures information about functional trajectory beyond what amyloid status conveys. However, it should be noted that most published DL studies have relied on data from the Alzheimer's Disease Neuroimaging Initiative (ADNI) and similar well-curated research cohorts. Prospective validation in real-world, multicenter clinical settings with diverse patient populations remain an important prerequisite before widespread clinical deployment of these tools.

Updated Acquisition and Interpretation Standards

Recent updates to procedural guidelines reflect advances in scanner technology and clinical workflows. The third version of the European Association of Nuclear Medicine (EANM) procedure guidelines for brain FDG-PET incorporates recommendations for modern digital PET systems with time-of-flight resolution below 400 picoseconds, enabling administered activity reductions of twofold or greater without compromising diagnostic quality.[38] The updated guidelines also emphasize point spread function deconvolution during image reconstruction to improve cortical resolution and endorse the use of age-adapted statistical parametric mapping templates for more accurate identification of pathologic versus age-related metabolic changes. Complementing these technical standards, a European intersocietal Delphi consensus defined structured, patient-centered workflows for biomarker testing across 11 clinical syndromes, prioritizing FDG-PET early in the diagnostic workup for patients with nonamnestic cognitive deficits, dysexecutive syndromes, atypical parkinsonism, or early-onset rapidly progressive cognitive decline.[39] Updated practice guidelines jointly published by the Society of Nuclear Medicine and Molecular Imaging (SNMMI) and EANM further reaffirmed the role of FDG-PET for differential diagnosis, with additional recommendations for digital PET and PET/MR acquisition.[40]

AMYLOID PET IN THE THERAPEUTIC ERA

Diagnostic Fundamentals

Aβ deposition is typically considered to be an early event in the AD pathologic cascade. The development of PET tracers targeting fibrillar Aβ, including Pittsburgh Compound B labeled with carbon-11 and several fluorine-18 tracers (florbetapir, florbetaben, and flutemetamol in the United States), enabled in vivo detection of amyloid plaque burden.

A negative amyloid scan indicates sparse to no Aβ plaques and suggests that cognitive deficits are unlikely attributable to AD. Early studies of clinically diagnosed AD patients reported amyloid positivity rates of approximately 96%.[41] However, data from the Imaging Dementia—Evidence for Amyloid Scanning (IDEAS) study, which evaluated amyloid PET in diagnostically uncertain cases among Medicare beneficiaries, found lower and more variable positivity rates: approximately 50% to 56% in patients with MCI and 59% to 71% in those with dementia, depending on self-reported race and ethnicity.[42] These findings highlight that amyloid positivity rates are influenced by both clinical context and patient demographics.

Positive amyloid scans do not, on their own, establish a clinical diagnosis of AD, as elevated plaque density has been observed in cognitively normal older adults and in other conditions such as DLB.[43,44] Amyloid deposition is also present in normal aging and in non-AD neurodegenerative diseases.[45] Consequently, amyloid PET results should be interpreted in the context of the full clinical picture and, where available, in conjunction with FDG-PET findings that can identify additional patterns of disease pathology and distinguish between overlapping etiologies.

Clinical Utility and Cost Considerations

The clinical utility of amyloid PET has been evaluated in several large prospective studies. In the IDEAS study, amyloid PET results led to changes in clinical management in approximately 60% of cases involving patients with MCI or dementia of uncertain etiology.[46,47] The New IDEAS study extended these findings to a more racially and ethnically diverse cohort of 5757 participants, confirming that amyloid PET changed management in 59% of cases across demographic groups; following the approval of lecanemab, 233 participants were started on or recommended for antiamyloid therapy after a positive scan.[48]

The cost barrier historically associated with amyloid PET has been partially addressed by regulatory changes. In October 2023, the Centers for Medicare and Medicaid Services retired the prior one-scan-per-lifetime restriction on amyloid PET coverage, allowing local Medicare Administrative Contractors to determine coverage policies and enabling repeat scans for treatment monitoring.[49] Updated appropriate use criteria now rate amyloid PET for antiamyloid therapy eligibility assessment as *appropriate* with the highest consensus score of 8 out of 9.[50]

The emergence of blood-based biomarkers, particularly plasma p-tau217, has introduced a cost-effective prescreening layer that may reduce the overall need for amyloid PET. A 2-step workflow in which plasma p-tau217 is used as an initial screen, with confirmatory amyloid PET reserved for the approximately 20% of cases with intermediate blood test results, maintained greater than 95% diagnostic accuracy while reducing amyloid PET utilization by approximately 80%.[51]

Plasma p-tau217 has achieved diagnostic accuracy approaching that of established amyloid PET and CSF measures. In a multicenter diagnostic accuracy study, a commercially available blood test incorporating p-tau217 achieved 88% to 92% accuracy for identifying amyloid PET positivity in both primary and secondary care settings.[52] An independent study confirmed that plasma p-tau217 was similar in accuracy to U.S. Food and Drug Administration (FDA)-approved CSF assays, with an AUC of 0.95 to 0.97 for amyloid PET status.[53] Regulatory clearance has followed: the Lumipulse G p-tau217/Aβ42 blood test received FDA clearance in May 2025, and the Elecsys pTau181 assay was cleared in October 2025. It should be noted, however, that blood-based biomarkers do not provide the differential diagnostic, regional staging, or copathology information available through FDG-PET. A positive blood test can identify likely amyloid pathology, however it cannot distinguish AD from DLB, Frontotemporal Lobar Degeneration (FTLD), LATE-NC, or vascular dementia—a distinction that remains the domain of metabolic and structural imaging.

Limitations of Amyloid Imaging

Several limitations of amyloid PET should be recognized when interpreting its results in clinical practice. Aβ deposition can be an early event in the AD pathologic cascade, but accumulation eventually plateaus or declines. Evidence suggests a possible decoupling between amyloid deposition and the downstream processes that mediate neurodegeneration, which limits the utility of amyloid imaging as a marker of disease progression or dementia severity.[54,55] There is generally poor correlation between disease stage and Aβ levels in patients with established dementia, and amyloid PET provides limited prognostic information for asymptomatic individuals or those with AD risk factors alone.

The relationship between amyloid and clinical outcomes has been further debated in the context of antiamyloid therapy. Some investigators have noted that despite substantial reductions in amyloid PET signal following treatment with monoclonal antibodies, the associated clinical benefits are modest and accompanied by increased rates of amyloid-related imaging abnormalities, microhemorrhages, and accelerated brain volume loss.[56] This perspective suggests that amyloid plaque clearance, as measured by PET, may not directly correspond to neuroprotection, and functional imaging with FDG-PET may ultimately prove to be a more informative measure of therapeutic benefit. In group-based analyses, however, lecanemab and donanemab have demonstrated statistically significant slowing of clinical decline in well-powered Phase 3 trials,[57,58] and updated appropriate use criteria include the use of amyloid PET for treatment eligibility assessment.[50]

Additionally, research has shown that Aβ oligomers, rather than the fibrillar Aβ plaques detected by amyloid PET, may be the primary neurotoxic species initiating the neurodegenerative process.[59,60] In this context, it is important to note that oligomeric Aβ cannot be directly visualized with current amyloid PET tracers.

TAU PET

Tau Pathology, Synaptic Loss, and Prognostic Value

Tau PET is a molecular neuroimaging modality that targets aggregated tau protein, which is a hallmark of AD neuropathology. Interest in tau imaging has grown in part because tau pathology is more closely linked to synaptic loss and cognitive decline than amyloid deposition.[61] A multitracer PET study using [^{18}F]MK-6240 for tau, [^{11}C]UCB-J for synaptic density, and [^{18}F]AZD4694 for amyloid confirmed that tau burden was more closely associated with both cross-sectional and longitudinal synaptic loss than amyloid burden.[62]

The prognostic value of tau PET has been established across large multicenter cohorts. In a study of 1431 participants from 8 independent cohorts, tau PET outperformed both amyloid PET and structural MR imaging for predicting subsequent cognitive decline in individuals with MCI and preclinical AD.[63] Among cognitively unimpaired individuals, those who were positive for both amyloid and tau on PET were at substantially elevated risk of future cognitive decline compared to those positive for amyloid alone, establishing tau PET as a marker for identifying individuals at higher near-term risk of progression.[64] A recent mega-analysis of 12,048 participants across 42 cohorts characterized the prevalence of tau PET positivity, reporting rates of 1.1% to 4.4% in cognitively unimpaired Aβ-negative individuals compared to 17.4% to 22.2% in cognitively unimpaired Aβ-positive individuals.[65]

In Vivo Braak Staging

Neuropathological studies have long established that tau neurofibrillary tangles in AD accumulate in a hierarchical spatial pattern described by Braak and Braak (1991), beginning in the transentorhinal cortex (Braak stages I–II), spreading to limbic structures including the hippocampus and amygdala (stages III–IV), and eventually involving neocortical association areas (stages V–VI). Tau PET now allows approximation of this staging in living patients. Using [^{18}F]MK-6240, Therriault and colleagues[66] demonstrated that tau accumulation proceeds hierarchically in vivo, and that progression beyond Braak stage III occurs primarily in the presence of abnormal amyloid, which supports a model in which amyloid pathology gates the neocortical spread of tau.

The feasibility of in vivo Braak staging has been evaluated across multiple tau PET tracers. In a head-to-head comparison of 100 participants who underwent PET with both flortaucipir and [^{18}F]MK-6240, there was substantial agreement between tracers for Braak staging, though flortaucipir tended to overestimate early Braak stages due to choroid plexus spillover.[67] Tau PET staging has already influenced clinical trial design. In the TRAILBLAZER-ALZ 2 trial, stratification by tau PET burden was used to define enrollment subgroups, and patients with low-to-medium tau showed a greater treatment response to donanemab than those with high tau.[58] This precedent suggests that tau PET staging may inform individualized treatment decisions as additional therapies become available.

Tracer Landscape and Clinical Use Criteria

Flortaucipir ([18F]AV-1451), marketed as Tauvid, is currently the only FDA-cleared tau PET tracer (approved 2020) and received European Medicines Agency marketing authorization in August 2024. Although generally validated, flortaucipir exhibits recognized off-target binding in the choroid plexus and basal ganglia. Second-generation tracers, including [18F]MK-6240 (florquinitau), demonstrate reduced off-target signal and are approaching regulatory approval, expected in 2026.[68] In 2025, the first formal appropriate use criteria for tau PET were published by a joint committee of the Alzheimer's Association and the SNMMI, rating 5 of 17 clinical scenarios as appropriate, generally involving patients with confirmed amyloid pathology in whom tau staging could inform prognosis or treatment selection.[50] Tau PET was not recommended as a first-line diagnostic tool for typical cognitive impairment.

STRUCTURAL MR IMAGING

Atrophy Patterns, Differential Diagnosis, and Limitations

Structural MR imaging provides information about the amount, distribution, and rate of cerebral atrophy, which can serve as an indirect marker of neurodegeneration. Different neurodegenerative diseases tend to produce characteristic patterns of regional neuronal loss. Antemortem MR imaging scans of pathologically confirmed dementia cases have demonstrated that patients with AD primarily exhibit atrophy in temporoparietal association areas and the MTL, while DLB patients show atrophy in the bilateral amygdala, dorsal midbrain, and inferior temporal lobes, and FTLD is associated with predominant frontal and temporal lobe volume loss.[69] MTL atrophy is correlated with cognitive decline and has been widely used as a supportive diagnostic marker in clinical practice.

Recent applications of DL to structural MR imaging data have partially addressed the historical limitation of overlapping atrophy patterns across diseases. A multimodal DL framework trained on 8 independent datasets matched or exceeded the classification accuracy of practicing neurologists for differentiating AD, DLB, and other dementias from MR imaging and clinical data.[70] In a separate study using data from the ADNI, a DL MR imaging approach achieved an area under the receiver operating characteristic curve of 0.788 for classifying prodromal AD, outperforming CSF amyloid and tau biomarkers as individual predictors.[71] These findings suggest that DL may extract diagnostically relevant information from structural MR imaging that is not readily captured by conventional volumetric analysis.

Despite its wide availability and the absence of ionizing radiation, MR imaging has several recognized limitations in the evaluation of neurodegenerative diseases. MR imaging cannot directly detect the histopathological hallmarks of AD, has limited molecular specificity, and the atrophy patterns associated with different dementias overlap considerably.[41] Volume changes may also occur due to factors unassociated with disease progression, such as hydration status, corticosteroid use, or comorbid conditions, which can complicate longitudinal interpretation. Even when structural abnormalities are not detectable on MR imaging, changes in brain function because of neurodegenerative disease may be identified using PET, underscoring the complementary nature of structural and functional imaging.

MR Imaging in the Era of Antiamyloid Therapy

The approval of antiamyloid immunotherapies has affected the interpretation and application of structural MR imaging in 2 ways: it has introduced a new confounder for longitudinal volumetric assessments, and it has created an entirely new clinical role for MR imaging in treatment safety monitoring.

In the CLARITY AD trial, lecanemab-treated patients showed accelerated brain volume loss compared to the placebo group over 18 months, despite demonstrating clinical benefit overall on cognitive endpoints.[57] The mechanism of this treatment-related *pseudoatrophy* remains under investigation, but its presence adds complexity to the use of serial volumetric MR imaging for tracking disease progression in patients receiving antiamyloid therapy. Clinicians interpreting follow-up MR imaging scans in treated patients must account for the possibility that interval volume loss may reflect a treatment effect rather than disease advancement.

More consequentially, MR imaging has become the sole imaging modality for detecting amyloid-related imaging abnormalities (ARIA), which represents a spectrum of treatment-associated findings that includes vasogenic edema and sulcal effusions (ARIA-E), visible on FLAIR sequences, and microhemorrhages and superficial siderosis (ARIA-H), detected on T2*-weighted gradient echo or susceptibility-weighted imaging (SWI) sequences.[72] In the CLARITY AD trial, ARIA-E occurred in 12.6% of lecanemab-treated patients.[57] The incidence of ARIA is higher among APOE ε4 homozygotes, which is one reason APOE genotyping is recommended before initiating therapy.

Clinical practice guidelines for antiamyloid therapy mandate baseline MR imaging before treatment initiation and serial MR imaging monitoring during the first year, with a recommended minimum of 3 to 4 scans.[73] Three sequences are considered essential for ARIA surveillance: T2*-weighted gradient echo or SWI, FLAIR, and diffusion-weighted imaging.[72] Updated monitoring recommendations published in 2025 provide standardized MR imaging protocols and clinical workflows for ARIA detection across practice settings.[74] Following reports of serious ARIA-E events, including fatalities, in patients receiving lecanemab, the FDA issued an updated safety statement in August 2025 recommending an additional MR imaging before the third infusion. The integration of ARIA monitoring into routine clinical practice has substantial implications for radiology workflow and scanner capacity since each patient receiving antiamyloid therapy requires multiple dedicated brain MR imaging examinations during their treatment course.

CLINICAL INTEGRATION AND REVISED DIAGNOSTIC ALGORITHM

The preceding sections have reviewed the diagnostic capabilities and evolving clinical roles of individual neuroimaging modalities. The practical question for the clinician is how these tools should be sequenced and integrated in the evaluation of a patient presenting with cognitive concerns. An updated algorithm for this purpose is presented here (**Fig. 3**), reflecting changes in the diagnostic and therapeutic landscape since the previous version of this framework.[75] The revised algorithm incorporates blood-based biomarker screening, positions FDG-PET as the initial molecular imaging study in most patients for differential diagnosis, and adds decision nodes for antiamyloid therapy eligibility and treatment monitoring.

Clinical Evaluation and Structural Imaging

The initial step remains a thorough history and physical examination. If the clinician or a reliable informant identifies cognitive deficits, personality changes, or behavioral disturbances, the evaluation should proceed to determine whether suspicious historical features or focal neurologic findings are present. If so, structural imaging with MR imaging or CT should be obtained and a neurology or neurosurgery consultation considered to exclude surgically treatable conditions such as subdural hematoma, normal pressure hydrocephalus, or mass lesions.[76]

The clinician should also assess for correctable conditions that may contribute to cognitive symptoms, including depression, substance use, medication effects or interactions, and metabolic derangements. Recommended laboratory studies include vitamin B12, folate, thyroid-stimulating hormone, calcium, complete blood count, renal function, and liver function tests.[76,77] If a correctable condition is identified, it should be treated and the patient reassessed. If deficits persist following appropriate treatment, further evaluation with neuroimaging biomarkers is warranted.

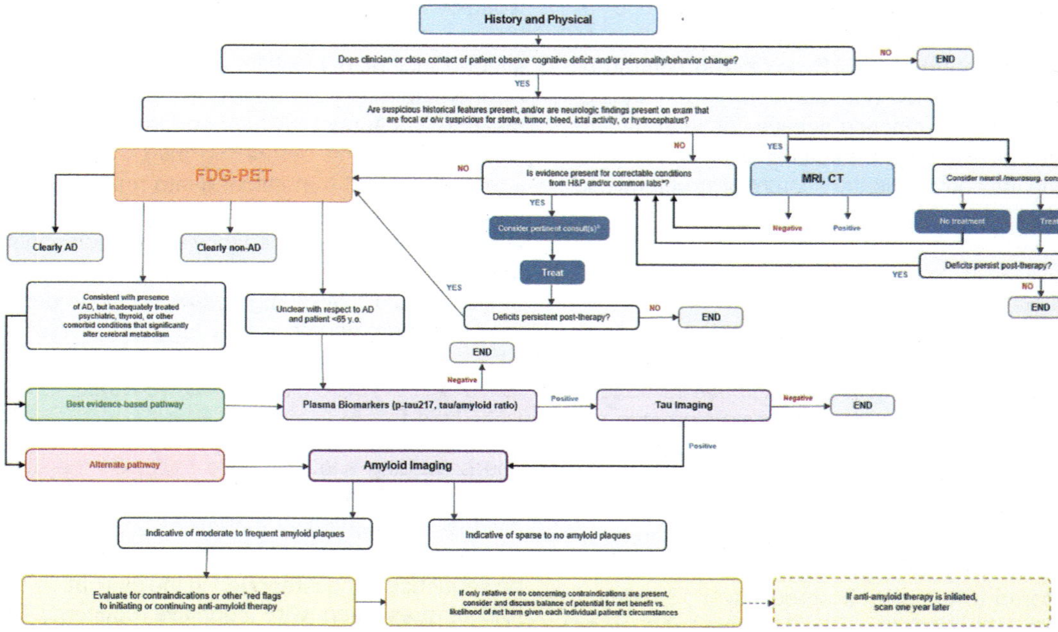

Fig. 3. Algorithm for diagnostic and image-guided therapeutic workup for patients experiencing cognitive decline and/or behavioral symptoms for which an underlying neurodegenerative process is being evaluated, including appropriate use of traditional blood labs and fluid biomarkers, as well as structural and molecular neuroimaging modalities. (Note: for patients with FDG-PET clearly consistent with AD as the condition primarily underlying the symptoms for which they are being evaluated, and having MR imaging and other clinical data that are supportive of candidacy for antiamyloid therapy, workup can then proceed with obtaining amyloid PET.) [a]Common History and Physical (H&P) items: depression, substance abuse, malnourishment, medication effects or interactions, cardiopulmonary compromise. Common labs: electrolyte/calcium imbalance, anemia, hypoxemia, infection, thyroid, renal, or hepatic dysfunction, glucose dysregulation. [b]Consults: Cardiology, Infectious Disease, Endocrine, Psych, Pulmonary, Renal.

2-[F-18]fluoro-2-deoxy-d-glucose-PET for Differential Diagnosis

When functional neuroimaging is indicated, FDG-PET should be considered as the initial study. Its established accuracy for differential diagnosis among neurodegenerative dementias provides the clinician with information about the specific pattern and severity of neurodegeneration before molecular pathology is assessed. This sequencing is supported by the European intersocietal consensus, which prioritizes FDG-PET early in the workup for nonamnestic, dysexecutive, atypical, and early-onset presentations.[39] The metabolic pattern observed on FDG-PET then directs subsequent testing along the appropriate branch of the algorithm.

Blood-Based Biomarker Screening

A development that has only recently become established is the option of blood-based biomarker screening as an early molecular step in the diagnostic pathway. As plasma p-tau217 assays have achieved diagnostic accuracy approaching that of amyloid PET and CSF measures for detecting AD pathology, with AUC values of 0.95 to 0.97 for amyloid PET status,[53] a two-step workflow using plasma p-tau217 as an initial screen, with confirmatory PET or CSF reserved for cases with intermediate results (approximately 20% of those tested), is suggested.[51]

Molecular Biomarker Confirmation and Dopaminergic Imaging

If the FDG-PET pattern is consistent with AD and antiamyloid therapy is being considered, confirmation of amyloid status is required. This can be obtained through amyloid PET or through CSF confirmation. In younger patients (under age 60), where age-related incidental amyloid positivity is lower, amyloid PET may be warranted earlier in the workup. If amyloid status is confirmed, tau PET may provide additional prognostic information for staging disease severity and informing treatment decisions, particularly in the context of therapies where tau burden has been shown to influence treatment response.[58]

If the FDG-PET pattern suggests DLB, as characterized by occipital hypometabolism with relative preservation of the posterior cingulate, but diagnosis remains uncertain, dopaminergic imaging may be considered. DaTscan (^{123}I-ioflupane Single Photon Emission Computed Tomography (SPECT)) received an expanded FDA indication in 2022 specifically for the evaluation of suspected DLB, in addition to its prior approval for differentiating parkinsonian syndromes from essential tremor.[78] [^{18}F]FDOPA PET is an FDA-approved alternative for evaluating dopaminergic function. Emerging α-synuclein PET tracers are under development though remain investigational.

If the FDG-PET findings are unclear with respect to AD, or if the metabolic pattern may reflect inadequately treated comorbid conditions that can alter cerebral metabolism, amyloid imaging can help clarify whether amyloid pathology is present. If FDG-PET indicates a non-AD pattern such as FTLD underlies a patient's cognitive decline, the evaluation can proceed along the appropriate clinical pathway without amyloid testing.

Treatment Initiation and Monitoring

For patients confirmed to have amyloid-positive AD who meet clinical criteria for antiamyloid therapy, APOE genotyping and baseline MR imaging are recommended before treatment initiation.[73] Serial MR imaging is then required during the first year of therapy for ARIA surveillance, as discussed in the Structural MR imaging section, and patients who are homozygous for the epsilon4 allele of APOE are at greater risk for such complications. Repeat amyloid imaging at approximately 1 year may be considered to assess plaque reduction, particularly in the context of treatment protocols that use amyloid clearance as a criterion for discontinuation, as demonstrated in the donanemab program.[58]

Quantification Tools Supporting Clinical Interpretation

Quantitative analysis software supports reproducible interpretation of PET imaging across clinical settings. For FDG-PET, both region-of-interest-based and voxel-based statistical methods are widely used. Several FDA-cleared software platforms are available for display and analysis of brain PET data, including NeuroQ (Syntermed Inc.), syngo. PET Cortical Analysis (Siemens Healthineers), MIMneuro (MIM Software Inc.), and CortexID (GE HealthCare). For amyloid PET, the Centiloid scale provides a standardized quantitative metric that enables comparison across different amyloid tracers and clinical sites.[79] For tau PET, the CenTauR scale has been proposed as an analogous standardization framework.[80] The integration of these quantification tools into clinical workflows facilitates more consistent interpretation, supports serial comparison of scans over time, and aids in communicating findings across institutions.

CONCLUSION AND FUTURE DIRECTIONS

The neuroimaging landscape for evaluating AD and related disorders has changed substantially since previous reviews of this topic. The core imaging science described in earlier work—which includes characteristic FDG-PET metabolic patterns for differential diagnosis, the diagnostic utility of amyloid PET, disease-specific atrophy signatures on MR imaging—remains well-supported by current evidence. What has changed is the clinical context in which these tools are applied.

Three developments have reshaped the field. First, the approval of antiamyloid immunotherapies has transformed neuroimaging from a diagnostic endeavor into an integrated component of treatment selection, eligibility confirmation, and safety monitoring. Cerebral amyloid determination is now required for treatment eligibility assessment, MR imaging has acquired a new mandatory role in ARIA surveillance, and tau PET staging has begun to inform stratified therapeutic decision-making. Second, blood-based biomarkers, particularly plasma p-tau217, have introduced a screening layer upstream of imaging that may reduce the need for amyloid PET in straightforward cases while preserving imaging resources for diagnostically more complex patients. Third, the application of DL to neuroimaging data has demonstrated the capacity to extract additional diagnostic information beyond conventional interpretation, though prospective validation in diverse clinical populations remains an important next step.

FDG-PET continues to occupy a central role in this evolving landscape. The differential diagnostic value of FDG-PET and its ability to distinguish AD from DLB, FTLD, LATE-NC, and vascular dementia based on regional metabolic patterns is not replicated by any fluid biomarker or molecular tracer currently available. The identification of LATE-NC as a distinct metabolic entity affecting approximately 10% of clinically diagnosed AD patients further underscores the importance of functional imaging in an era where treatment decisions may increasingly depend on accurate etiologic classification.

Several areas of active development are likely to influence clinical practice in the coming years. For example, α-synuclein PET tracers, if successfully developed for clinical use, could enable direct visualization of Lewy body pathology and transform the diagnosis of DLB and Parkinson's disease dementia. The role of FDG-PET as a measure of therapeutic response, such as metabolic stabilization during antiamyloid treatment representing clinical neuroprotection, has been proposed but requires prospective validation. Continued refinement of automated quantification tools, including standardized scales such as Centiloid for amyloid and CenTauR for tau, will support reproducible interpretation across clinical sites and facilitate multicenter therapeutic trials. The integration of artificial intelligence into routine clinical workflows, once validated beyond research cohorts, has the potential to extend the diagnostic reach of neuroimaging to settings where subspecialty expertise is limited.

SUMMARY

As the neuroimaging field moves increasingly from roles of primarily diagnosis toward image-guided therapies, the optimal use of neuroimaging will depend on thoughtful integration of complementary modalities at appropriate stages of the clinical evaluation. The algorithm presented in this article reflects this integration, positioning each imaging tool where its contribution to clinical decision-making is the most helpful.

CLINICS CARE POINTS

- For the purpose of establishing differential diagnosis for cognitive decline across neurodegenerative entities, FDG is the PET radiotracer with the greatest proven overall accuracy relative to the reference standard of autopsy confirmation.
- For patients with Alzheimer's disease as the diagnosis confirmed to be underlying their cognitive decline, and in whom anti-amyloid immunotherapy is to be initiated, amyloid PET imaging provides the best demonstrated quantitative assessment to follow longitudinally from before to after initiation of therapy.
- For patients in whom FDG-PET is consistent with Alzheimer's disease as the diagnostic entity underlying their cognitive decline and for whom anti-amyloid therapy is being considered based on fluid biomarker and/or amyloid PET results, semi-quantification of Tau-PET may provide additional prognostic value with respect to likely response to those treatments available currently, and confirm presence of appropriate molecular targets for anti-tau therapies now under development.

DISCLOSURES

Authors have nothing to disclose.

REFERENCES

1. GBD 2019. Dementia Forecasting Collaborators. Estimation of the global prevalence of dementia in 2019 and forecasted prevalence in 2050: an analysis for the Global Burden of Disease Study 2019. Lancet Public Health 2022;7:e105–25.
2. Braak H, Braak E. Neuropathological stageing of Alzheimer-related changes. Acta Neuropathol 1991; 82:239–59.
3. Hardy J, Selkoe DJ. The amyloid hypothesis of Alzheimer's disease: progress and problems on the road to therapeutics. Science 2002;297:353–6.
4. Heneka MT, Carson MJ, El Khoury J, et al. Neuroinflammation in Alzheimer's disease. Lancet Neurol 2015;14:388–405.
5. Livingston G, Huntley J, Liu KY, et al. Dementia prevention, intervention, and care: 2024 report of the Lancet standing Commission. Lancet 2024;404: 572–628.
6. Liscic RM, Storandt M, Cairns NJ, et al. Clinical and psychometric distinction of frontotemporal and Alzheimer dementias. Arch Neurol 2007;64:535.
7. Mrak RE, Griffin WST. Dementia with Lewy bodies: definition, diagnosis, and pathogenic relationship to Alzheimer's disease. Neuropsychiatric Dis Treat 2007;3:619.
8. Nelson PT, Dickson DW, Trojanowski JQ, et al. Limbic-predominant age-related TDP-43 encephalopathy (LATE): consensus working group report. Brain 2019;142:1503–27.
9. Grothe MJ, Silva-Rodríguez J, Desseigneur E, et al. In vivo FDG-PET metabolic signature of limbic-predominant age-related TDP-43 encephalopathy neuropathologic change. Alzheimer's Dement 2023; 19:4250–61.
10. Echavarri C, Burgmans S, Caballero MC, et al. Co-occurrence of different pathologies in dementia: implications for dementia diagnosis. J Alzheimers Dis 2012;30:909–17.
11. Sperling RA, Aisen PS, Beckett LA, et al. Toward defining the preclinical stages of Alzheimer's disease: recommendations from the NIA-AA workgroups. Alzheimer's Dement 2011;7:280–92.
12. Jack CR Jr, Bennett DA, Blennow K, et al. NIA-AA research framework: toward a biological definition of Alzheimer's disease. Alzheimer's Dement 2018; 14:535–62.
13. Jia J, Ning Y, Chen M, et al. Biomarker changes during 20 years preceding Alzheimer's disease. N Engl J Med 2024;390:712–22.
14. Jack CR Jr, Andrews JS, Beach TG, et al. Revised criteria for diagnosis and staging of Alzheimer's

disease: Alzheimer's Association Workgroup. Alzheimer's Dement 2024;20:5143–69.
15. Dubois B, Villain N, Frisoni GB, et al. Clinical diagnosis of Alzheimer's disease: recommendations of the International Working Group. Lancet Neurol 2021;20:484–96.
16. Dubois B, von Arnim CAF, Burnie N, et al. Alzheimer disease as a clinical-biological construct—an International Working Group recommendation. JAMA Neurol 2024;81:1304–11.
17. Silverman DH, Small GW, Chang CY, et al. Positron emission tomography in evaluation of dementia: regional brain metabolism and long-term outcome. JAMA 2001;286:2120–7.
18. Silverman DH. Brain 18F-FDG PET in the diagnosis of neurodegenerative dementias: comparison with perfusion SPECT and with clinical evaluation. J Nucl Med 2004;45:594–607.
19. Lesman-Segev OH, La Joie R, Stephens ML, et al. Diagnostic accuracy of amyloid versus 18F-fluorodeoxyglucose positron emission tomography in autopsy-confirmed dementia. Ann Neurol 2021;89:389–401.
20. Minoshima S, Cross D, Thientunyakit T, et al. 18F-FDG PET imaging in neurodegenerative dementing disorders: insights into subtype classification, emerging disease categories, and mixed dementia with copathologies. J Nucl Med 2022;63(Suppl 1):2S–12S.
21. Radmard M, McGirr A, Bhatt P, et al. Functional imaging in Alzheimer's disease: a systematic review and meta-analysis of ASL-MRI and FDG-PET. J Neuroimaging 2025;35:e70080.
22. Minoshima S, Giordani B, Berent S, et al. Metabolic reduction in the posterior cingulate cortex in very early Alzheimer's disease. Ann Neurol 1997;42:85–94.
23. Albert MS, DeKosky ST, Dickson D, et al. The diagnosis of mild cognitive impairment due to Alzheimer's disease: recommendations from the NIA-AA workgroups. Alzheimer's Dement 2011;7:270–9.
24. Torosyan N, Mason K, Dahlbom M, et al. Value of FDG-PET scans of non-demented patients in predicting rates of future cognitive and functional decline. Eur J Nucl Med Mol Imag 2017;44:1355–63.
25. Chiaravalloti A, Koch G, Toniolo S, et al. Comparison between early-onset and late-onset Alzheimer's disease patients with amnestic presentation: CSF and 18F-FDG PET study. Dement Geriatr Cogn Disord Extra 2016;6:108–19.
26. Graff-Radford J, Murray ME, Lowe VJ, et al. Dementia with Lewy bodies: basis of cingulate island sign. Neurology 2014;83:801–9.
27. Minoshima S, Frey KA, Koeppe RA, et al. A diagnostic approach in Alzheimer's disease using three-dimensional stereotactic surface projections of fluorine-18-FDG PET. J Nucl Med 2001;36:1238–48.
28. Nedelska Z, Schwarz CG, Lesnick TG, et al. FDG PET metabolic signatures distinguishing prodromal DLB from prodromal AD. Neurology 2021;97:e1774–84.
29. Foster NL, Heidebrink JL, Clark CM, et al. FDG-PET improves accuracy in distinguishing frontotemporal dementia and Alzheimer's disease. Brain 2007;130:2616–35.
30. Jeong Y, Cho SS, Park JM, et al. 18F-FDG PET findings in frontotemporal dementia: an SPM analysis of 29 patients. J Nucl Med 2005;46:233–9.
31. Jagust WJ, Gitcho A, Sun F, et al. Brain imaging evidence of preclinical Alzheimer's disease in normal aging. Ann Neurol 2006;59:673–81.
32. Cotta Ramusino M, Massa F, Festari C, et al. Molecular imaging for predicting conversion from mild cognitive impairment to dementia: an updated systematic review. Eur J Nucl Med Mol Imag 2024;51:2451–76.
33. Alexander GE, Furey ML, Grady CL, et al. Association of premorbid intellectual function with cerebral metabolism in Alzheimer's disease: implications for the cognitive reserve hypothesis. Am J Psychiatry 1997;154:165–72.
34. Perani D, Caminiti SP, Carli G, et al. Biological and clinical heterogeneity of amnestic mild cognitive impairment revealed by FDG-PET metabolic subtypes. Alzheimer's Dement 2023;19(Suppl):e077901.
35. Perani D, Caminiti SP, Carli G, et al. FDG-PET metabolic phenotypes of amnestic MCI: implications for prognosis and clinical trial design. Alzheimer's Dement 2024;20:1254–68.
36. Sun Y, Chen C, Liu X, et al. Diagnostic performance of deep learning-assisted [18F]FDG PET imaging for Alzheimer's disease: a systematic review and meta-analysis. Eur J Nucl Med Mol Imag 2025;52:1680–95.
37. Etminani K, Soliman A, Davidsson A, et al. A 3D deep learning model to predict the diagnosis of dementia with lewy bodies, Alzheimer's disease, and mild cognitive impairment using brain 18F-FDG PET. Eur J Nucl Med Mol Imag 2022;49:563–84.
38. Guedj E, Varrone A, Boellaard R, et al. EANM procedure guidelines for brain PET imaging using [18F]FDG, version 3. Eur J Nucl Med Mol Imag 2022;49:632–51.
39. Frisoni GB, Festari C, Cappa SF, et al. European intersocietal recommendations for the biomarker-based diagnosis of neurocognitive disorders. Lancet Neurol 2024;23:302–12.
40. Arbizu J, Festari C, Altomare D, et al. SNMMI/EANM practice guideline for brain FDG PET, version 2.0. J Nucl Med 2024;65:1810–22.
41. Johnson KA, Fox NC, Sperling RA, et al. Brain imaging in Alzheimer disease. Cold Spring Harb Perspect Med 2012;2:a006213.
42. Wilkins CH, Windon CC, Engelman CD, et al. Racial and ethnic differences in amyloid PET positivity in individuals with mild cognitive impairment or dementia: a secondary analysis of the IDEAS study. JAMA Neurol 2022;79:1139–47.

43. Mallik A, Drzezga A, Minoshima S. Clinical amyloid imaging. Semin Nucl Med 2017;47:31–43.
44. Sarro L, Senjem ML, Lundt ES, et al. Amyloid-β deposition and regional grey matter atrophy rates in dementia with lewy bodies. Brain 2016;139:2740–50.
45. Martorana A, Di Lorenzo F, Belli L, et al. Cerebrospinal fluid Aβ42 levels: when physiological become pathological state. CNS Neurosci Ther 2015;21: 921–5.
46. Rabinovici GD, Gatsonis C, Apgar C, et al. Association of amyloid positron emission tomography with subsequent change in clinical management among Medicare beneficiaries with mild cognitive impairment or dementia. JAMA 2019;321: 1286–94.
47. Rabinovici GD, Knopman DS, Arbizu J, et al. Amyloid PET and subsequent health care use among Medicare beneficiaries with mild cognitive impairment or dementia (IDEAS study, aim 2). JAMA Neurol 2023;80:1028–39.
48. Windon CC, Rabinovici GD, Engelman CD, et al. New IDEAS study: amyloid PET in a racially and ethnically diverse population. Alzheimer's Dement 2025;21:e70504.
49. Centers for Medicare and Medicaid Services. Retirement of National Coverage Determination 220.6.20 for beta amyloid positron emission tomography in dementia and neurodegenerative disease. 2023.
50. Rabinovici GD, Apostolova LG, Engber T, et al. Updated appropriate use criteria for amyloid and tau PET. Alzheimer's Dement 2025;21:e14338.
51. Brum WS, Cullen NC, Janelidze S, et al. A two-step workflow based on plasma p-tau217 to screen for amyloid β positivity with further confirmatory testing only in uncertain cases. Nat Aging 2023;3:940–52.
52. Palmqvist S, Tideman P, Cullen N, et al. Blood biomarkers to detect Alzheimer disease in primary care and secondary care. JAMA 2024;332:1245–57.
53. Barthélemy NR, Horie K, Sato C, et al. Highly accurate blood test for Alzheimer's disease is similar or superior to clinical cerebrospinal fluid tests. Nat Med 2024;30:326–33.
54. Chetelat G, Villemagne VL, Bourgeat P, et al. Relationship between atrophy and β-amyloid deposition in Alzheimer disease. Ann Neurol 2010;67:317–24.
55. Engler H, Forsberg A, Almkvist O, et al. Two-year follow-up of amyloid deposition in patients with Alzheimer's disease. Brain 2006;129:2856–66.
56. Høilund-Carlsen PF, Alavi A, Barrio JR. FDG PET for monitoring immunotherapy in Alzheimer's disease. Diagnostics 2023;13:2254.
57. van Dyck CH, Swanson CJ, Aisen P, et al. Lecanemab in early Alzheimer's disease. N Engl J Med 2023;388:9–21.
58. Sims JR, Zimmer JA, Evans CD, et al. Donanemab in early symptomatic Alzheimer disease: the TRAILBLAZER-ALZ 2 randomized clinical trial. JAMA 2023;330:512–27.
59. Musiek ES, Holtzman DM. Three dimensions of the amyloid hypothesis: time, space and "wingmen." Nat Neurosci 2015;18:800–6.
60. Desikan RS, Rafii MS, Brewer JB, et al. An expanded role for neuroimaging in the evaluation of memory impairment. AJNR Am J Neuroradiol 2013;34: 2075–82.
61. Bejanin A, Schonhaut DR, La Joie R, et al. Tau pathology and neurodegeneration contribute to cognitive impairment in Alzheimer's disease. Brain 2017; 140:3286–300.
62. Guo T, Therriault J, Bhatt P, et al. Tau pathology is associated with synaptic density and longitudinal synaptic loss in Alzheimer's disease. Mol Psychiatr 2024;29:1786–97.
63. Ossenkoppele R, Smith R, Mattsson-Carlgren N, et al. Accuracy of tau positron emission tomography as a prognostic marker in preclinical and prodromal Alzheimer disease. JAMA Neurol 2021;78:961–71.
64. Ossenkoppele R, Pichet Binette A, Groot C, et al. Amyloid- and tau-PET-positive cognitively unimpaired individuals are at high risk for future cognitive decline. Nat Med 2022;28:2381–7.
65. Ossenkoppele R, Groot C, Smith R, et al. Tau PET positivity varies with age, amyloid status, APOE genotype, and sex across the Alzheimer's disease spectrum. Nat Neurosci 2025;28:625–35.
66. Therriault J, Pascoal TA, Lussier FZ, et al. Biomarker modeling of Alzheimer's disease using PET-based Braak staging. Nat Aging 2022;2:526–35.
67. Fernandez-Arias J, Therriault J, Bhatt P, et al. Comparison of tau-PET tracers for in vivo Braak staging: the HEAD study. Alzheimer's Dement 2024;20: e14591.
68. Gogola A, Pascoal TA, Bhatt P, et al. Direct comparison of the tau PET tracers [18F]flortaucipir and [18F]MK-6240 in human subjects. J Nucl Med 2022;63:108–16.
69. Vemuri P, Simon G, Kantarci K, et al. Antemortem differential diagnosis of dementia pathology using structural MRI: differential-STAND. Neuroimage 2011;55:522–31.
70. Qiu S, Miller MI, Joshi PS, et al. Multimodal deep learning for Alzheimer's disease dementia assessment. Nat Commun 2022;13:3404.
71. Feng X, Provenzano FA, Small SA, Alzheimer's Disease Neuroimaging Initiative. A deep learning MRI approach outperforms other biomarkers of prodromal Alzheimer's disease. Alzheimers Res Ther 2022;14:45.
72. Cogswell PM, Barakos JA, Barkhof F, et al. Amyloid-related imaging abnormalities with emerging Alzheimer disease therapeutics: detection and reporting recommendations for clinical practice. AJNR Am J Neuroradiol 2022;43:E19–35.

73. Cummings J, Apostolova L, Rabinovici GD, et al. Lecanemab: appropriate use recommendations. J Prev Alzheimers Dis 2023;10:362–77.
74. Cogswell PM, Serfaty CA, Engbersen ME, et al. ARIA monitoring in clinical practice: updated considerations for anti-amyloid immunotherapy. AJNR Am J Neuroradiol 2025;46:123–31.
75. Raji CA, Torosyan N, Silverman DHS. Optimizing use of neuroimaging tools in evaluation of Alzheimer's disease and related dementias. J Alzheimers Dis 2020;77:1–13.
76. Waldemar G, Dubois B, Emre M, et al. Recommendations for the diagnosis and management of Alzheimer's disease and other disorders associated with dementia: EFNS guideline. Eur J Neurol 2007;14:e1–26.
77. Hort J, O'Brien JT, Gainotti G, et al. EFNS guidelines for the diagnosis and management of Alzheimer's disease. Eur J Neurol 2010;17:1236–48.
78. O'Shea DM, Revesz D, Davis SE, et al. Practical use of DAT SPECT in diagnosing dementia with Lewy bodies: a US perspective. Front Neurol 2024;15:1395413.
79. Klunk WE, Koeppe RA, Price JC, et al. The Centiloid Project: standardizing quantitative amyloid plaque estimation by PET. Alzheimer's Dement 2015;11:1–15.
80. Villemagne VL, Leuzy A, Bohorquez SS, et al. CenTauR: toward a universal scale and masks for standardizing tau imaging studies. Alzheimers Dement Diagn Assess Dis Monit 2023;15:e12454.

FDG-PET in Movement Disorders and Parkinsonian Syndromes

Satoshi Minoshima, MD, PhD[a,b,*], Thilo van Eimeren, MD[c,d], Alexander Drzezga, MD[c]

KEYWORDS

• FDG PET • Parkinson disease • Progressive supranuclear palsy • Corticobasal syndrome • Corticobasal degeneration • Multiple system atrophy • Dementia with Lewy bodies

KEY POINTS

- FDG PET is useful for differentiating among degenerative parkinsonian syndromes because it reflects the full network level distribution of neurodegeneration.
- Parkinson disease (PD) typically shows a reproducible metabolic network with relative hypermetabolism in pallidothalamic, pontine, cerebellar, and sensorimotor regions together with parieto-occipital cortical hypometabolism.
- Progressive supranuclear palsy, corticobasal degeneration or corticobasal syndrome, and multiple system atrophy each have recognizable FDG PET signatures, respectively centered on medial frontal, midbrain, asymmetric para-central, frontoparietal, and putaminal and or cerebellar-pontine involvement.
- Posterior cortical and occipital hypometabolism are important markers of cognitive vulnerability in PD and are especially characteristic of dementia with Lewy bodies and Parkinson disease dementia within the appropriate clinical context.
- The highest diagnostic accuracy is achieved when FDG PET is interpreted together with clinical syndrome analysis, MR imaging, dopamine transporter imaging, and selected ancillary biomarkers such as cardiac metaiodobenzylguanidine (MIBG) or amyloid PET.

INTRODUCTION

The differential diagnosis of parkinsonism remains one of the most consequential and difficult tasks in clinical neurology and nuclear medicine. Idiopathic Parkinson disease (PD) is common, but a proportion of patients presenting with parkinsonian features ultimately prove to have atypical parkinsonian syndromes such as progressive supranuclear palsy (PSP), corticobasal degeneration or corticobasal syndrome (CBD/CBS), multiple system atrophy (MSA), Parkinson disease dementia (PDD), or dementia with Lewy bodies (DLB). Clinical criteria continue to improve, yet diagnostic uncertainty is still common during the early symptomatic phase, when phenotypic overlap is greatest and disease specific therapies or prognostic counseling are most needed.[1] In this setting, imaging is used not as a substitute for expert clinical examination, but as a biologically informed extension of it.

Among molecular imaging techniques, FDG PET serves for a distinctive role because it reflects the functional consequences of neurodegeneration at

[a] Department of Radiology and Imaging Sciences, University of Utah, Salt Lake City, UT, USA; [b] Department of Nuclear Medicine, University of Cologne, Cologne, Germany; [c] Department of Nuclear Medicine, University Hospital Cologne, University of Cologne, Cologne, Germany; [d] Department of Neurology, University Hospital Cologne, University of Cologne, Cologne, Germany
* Corresponding author.
E-mail address: sminoshima@hsc.utah.edu

PET Clin 21 (2026) 499–509
https://doi.org/10.1016/j.cpet.2026.05.002
1556-8598/26/

Abbreviations	
AD	Alzheimer disease
CBD/CBS	corticobasal degeneration or corticobasal syndrome
DAT	dopamine transporter
DLB	dementia with Lewy bodies
LBD	Lewy body disease
MSA	multiple system atrophy
MSA-C	MSA, cerebellar type
PD	Parkinson disease
PDD	Parkinson disease dementia
PDRP	Parkinson disease related pattern
PSP	progressive supranuclear palsy

the systems level. Rather than depicting a single neurotransmitter pathway, FDG PET captures regional and network level alterations in synaptic activity and neuronal integrity. This is especially valuable in parkinsonian syndromes, where different diseases can produce similar motor signs through different combinations of nigrostriatal, brainstem, cerebellar, limbic, and cortical degeneration. Consensus and guideline documents now recognize FDG PET as a useful adjunct in the assessment of neurodegenerative parkinsonism, particularly when the clinical picture is atypical or when differentiation among degenerative syndromes is the main problem.[2–5]

PD itself is pathologically defined by loss of pigmented neurons in the substantia nigra pars compacta and alpha-synuclein pathology, but its metabolic phenotype extends beyond the nigrostriatal system. FDG PET studies have demonstrated posterior cortical reductions, especially in parieto-occipital regions, together with network level relative increases in pallidothalamic, pontine, cerebellar, and sensorimotor territories.[6–11] These abnormalities become especially relevant when cognition declines, because posterior cortical and visual association hypometabolism predict progression toward PDD.[12–14] By contrast, PSP and CBD are 4-repeat tauopathies, but their topographies differ. PSP most often affects brainstem, basal ganglia, diencephalic, and medial frontal systems, whereas CBD preferentially involves asymmetric frontoparietal cortex with associated basal ganglia and thalamic degeneration.[15–24] MSA is an alpha-synucleinopathy characterized by oligodendroglial cytoplasmic inclusions and degeneration of the striatonigral, olivopontocerebellar, and autonomic systems, resulting in somewhat different FDG PET signatures in the parkinsonian-predominant (MSA-P) and cerebellar-predominant (MSA-C) forms.[25–29] DLB and PDD belong to the Lewy body disease (LBD) spectrum, but DLB is operationally defined by the presence of cognitive decline before or within 1 year of parkinsonism, whereas PDD emerges after established PD. Their FDG patterns overlap, especially in posterior associative and occipital cortex, and the occipital signature has strong clinicopathologic support.[30–34]

This review summarizes the literature on FDG PET in movement disorders and parkinsonian syndromes, with an emphasis on the limited differential capability of dopamine transporter imaging, characteristic FDG PET findings in PD, PSP, CBD/CBS, MSA, and PDD/DLB, and the practical role of multimodal clinical and imaging integration in everyday differential diagnosis.[2–5,35–40]

LIMITED DIFFERENTIAL CAPABILITY OF DOPAMINE TRANSPORTER IMAGING

Clinical availability of dopamine transporter (DAT) imaging has transformed the evaluation of tremor and parkinsonism by allowing in vivo assessment of presynaptic nigrostriatal terminal integrity. In patients whose main differential diagnosis is degenerative parkinsonism versus essential tremor, drug induced parkinsonism, psychogenic parkinsonism, or some forms of vascular parkinsonism, an abnormal DAT scan is highly informative because it indicates presynaptic dopaminergic degeneration.[2–4] For this reason, DAT imaging is now well established as a tool for distinguishing neurodegenerative nigrostriatal disease from nondegenerative mimics.

Its main limitation, however, is that abnormal DAT binding is shared by most neurodegenerative parkinsonian disorders. PD, PSP, CBD/CBS, MSA-P, MSA-C with striatonigral involvement, and DLB can all show reduced striatal uptake, often before the full clinical phenotype is apparent.[2–4] Therefore, DAT imaging usually confirms that the patient belongs somewhere within the degenerative parkinsonian spectrum, but it often cannot specify which disorder is present. Guidelines explicitly note that presynaptic dopaminergic imaging is unable to reliably distinguish idiopathic PD and DLB from PSP, CBD, or putaminal variant MSA.[2] Reviews of DAT imaging similarly conclude that its value is strongest for separating degenerative from nondegenerative causes, not for resolving the internal differential diagnosis among degenerative syndromes.[3,4]

This biological limitation is not necessarily surprising. DAT tracers interrogate one shared downstream pathway, loss of nigrostriatal terminals, whereas the diseases of interest differ most in extranigral distribution. PSP is marked by 4R tau pathology in the midbrain, globus pallidus, subthalamic nucleus, and frontal systems. CBD is another 4R tauopathy, but with more asymmetric cortical and subcortical involvement. MSA is an oligodendroglial synucleinopathy affecting striatonigral and olivopontocerebellar systems. DLB and PDD are cortical and limbic Lewy body disorders superimposed on variable nigrostriatal degeneration. Because DAT imaging is relatively blind to these broader network level differences, a normal or abnormal result only partially addresses the actual clinicopathologic question.[16,21,26,30]

By contrast, FDG PET samples the downstream functional consequences of the entire disease network. This is one reason why FDG PET and metabolic pattern analysis outperform DAT imaging for differentiating PD from atypical parkinsonism and for distinguishing one atypical syndrome from another.[5,18,35–40] In practical terms, DAT imaging answers the question, *Is there degenerative nigrostriatal dysfunction*? FDG PET is more helpful for the next question, *What pattern of neurodegeneration best explains the patient's syndrome?*

FDG PET FINDINGS IN PARKINSON DISEASE

PD is an alpha-synucleinopathy characterized by degeneration of dopaminergic neurons in the substantia nigra and progressive spread of Lewy related pathology through brainstem, limbic, and neocortical regions.[1,6,30] Clinically, PD is defined by bradykinesia plus rest tremor and/or rigidity, often accompanied over time by gait impairment, nonmotor symptoms, autonomic dysfunction, sleep disorders, mood symptoms, and cognitive decline.[1] Although the motor syndrome is the diagnostic anchor, PD is clinically heterogeneous. Tremor dominant, akinetic-rigid, postural instability gait difficulty, and cognitively vulnerable phenotypes may exhibit differing rates of progression and cortical involvement.

Early regional FDG PET studies showed that even nondemented PD can be associated with cortical hypometabolism, especially in posterior regions. Eberling and colleagues reported neocortical metabolic reductions, with greatest differences in posterior brain regions despite preserved cognition.[7] Pappatà and colleagues also found temporoparietal cortical hypometabolism in nondemented PD, suggesting that posterior cortical dysfunction can precede overt dementia.[13] A particularly important observation was made by Bohnen and colleagues, who demonstrated prominent occipital metabolic reduction, especially in the primary visual cortex, in PD without dementia. Notably, the occipital reduction was greater contralateral to the more affected body side, supporting a pathophysiologic link with asymmetric nigrostriatal dysfunction rather than a purely retinal explanation.[6] This article remains highly relevant because it established that occipital involvement is not exclusive to DLB and may already be present in PD, although usually less extensive and less diagnostically dominant than in Lewy body dementia.

A major conceptual advance came from spatial covariance analysis, which identified a reproducible Parkinson disease related pattern (PDRP). This motor symptom-related network is characterized by relative hypermetabolism in pallidothalamic circuits, pons, cerebellum, and sensorimotor cortex, with relative hypometabolism in lateral premotor and parieto-occipital association cortex.[8–11] Expression of this pattern correlates with motor severity, progresses over time, and decreases with effective symptomatic treatment such as levodopa or subthalamic stimulation.[8,10] The reproducibility of the PDRP across centers and scanners has strengthened the notion that PD is associated with a network level metabolic signature, not merely isolated regional deficits.[11]

A second important PD network, the Parkinson disease cognition symptom-related pattern, is characterized by reductions in frontal and parietal association cortex and precuneus with relative increases in cerebellar vermis and dentate nuclei.[9] Unlike the motor pattern, this cognitive pattern is less responsive to standard dopaminergic therapy and appears more closely linked to executive and memory dysfunction.[9,10] As cognitive impairment emerges, posterior cortical hypometabolism becomes more extensive. Drug naive PD with mild cognitive impairment already shows posterior cortical reductions, supporting the idea that FDG PET can detect early cortical vulnerability before dementia develops.[12] Longitudinal work by Bohnen and colleagues showed that incident dementia in PD is heralded by decreased metabolism in visual association cortex and posterior cingulate, with later extension into mesiofrontal regions.[12] Garcia-Garcia and colleagues further reported that posterior parieto-occipital hypometabolism may differentiate mild cognitive impairment from PDD, emphasizing the continuum from posterior cortical dysfunction to frank dementia.[14]

For differential diagnosis, the FDG pattern in PD is often subtler than the more dramatic patterns of atypical parkinsonism. Relative preservation of striatum, pons, cerebellum, and brainstem compared with MSA or PSP is often diagnostically helpful. Posterior cortical and occipital reductions may overlap with DLB or PDD, but in clinically typical PD without early dementia the overall metabolic picture usually lacks the severe occipital dominance of DLB and the marked medial frontal or brainstem deficits of PSP.[5,35–40] Thus,

FDG PET in PD is best understood as a dynamic pattern that combines network hypermetabolism related to abnormal basal ganglia-thalamo-cortical physiology with regional posterior cortical hypometabolism that becomes more clinically salient as cognition worsens.

FDG PET FINDINGS IN PROGRESSIVE SUPRANUCLEAR PALSY

PSP is a primary 4-repeat tauopathy characterized pathologically by neuronal loss, gliosis, neurofibrillary tangles, tufted astrocytes, and coiled bodies, with predilection for the midbrain, globus pallidus, subthalamic nucleus, dentate nucleus, and frontal systems.[15,16] The classic clinical phenotype, PSP-Richardson syndrome, includes early falls, vertical supranuclear gaze palsy, axial rigidity, bradykinesia, dysarthria, dysphagia, and frontal dysexecutive dysfunction. However, the 2017 MDS criteria formalized several PSP subtypes, including PSP-parkinsonism, PSP with predominant gait freezing, PSP-frontal, PSP-speech/language, and corticobasal syndrome presentations.[15] This phenotypic diversity is one reason imaging support is valuable.

FDG PET in PSP has shown a relatively stereotyped pattern centered on midline and subcortical structures. Early comparative studies demonstrated hypometabolism in the caudate nuclei, thalamus, midbrain, and cingulate or frontal cortices, helping differentiate PSP from PD and MSA.[17] Eckert and colleagues subsequently identified a PSP related metabolic pattern characterized by metabolic decreases in the brainstem and medial frontal cortex, clearly distinct from the MSA pattern of putaminal and cerebellar hypometabolism.[18] More recent network work confirmed a PSP related pattern involving bilateral middle and medial prefrontal cortex, cingulate cortex, striatum, thalamus, and midbrain.[19]

From a visual interpretation standpoint, the most useful FDG PET clues in PSP are hypometabolism in the medial and superior frontal cortex, anterior cingulate, lateral premotor cortex, caudate, thalamus, and midbrain. Brainstem involvement, particularly the midbrain, is one of the strongest differentiators from PD, though the findings are confined in the small area, and it requires careful inspection of the images with statistical mapping. When FDG PET is read together with MR imaging evidence of midbrain atrophy or an increased magnetic resonance parkinsonism index, diagnostic confidence increases considerably.[7,39] Relative symmetry also helps—PSP usually lacks the marked hemispheric asymmetry typical of CBS, although variants can blur this rule.

Clinically, FDG PET is most valuable when PSP presents as parkinsonism without the full Richardson phenotype. PSP-parkinsonism can initially mimic PD because it may show asymmetry, tremor, and modest levodopa responsiveness. In such cases, pronounced medial superior frontal and midbrain hypometabolism, together with caudate and thalamic involvement, strongly argues against idiopathic PD and toward PSP.[18,19,35] When dementia or behavioral change is prominent, frontal hypometabolism can overlap with frontotemporal degeneration, but the combination of ocular motor dysfunction, axial syndrome, and subcortical-midbrain FDG abnormalities remains highly suggestive of PSP.

FDG PET FINDINGS IN CORTICOBASAL DEGENERATION AND CORTICOBASAL SYNDROME

CBD is also a 4-repeat tauopathy, pathologically distinguished by neuronal and glial tau inclusions, astrocytic plaques, ballooned neurons, and degeneration affecting frontoparietal cortex, basal ganglia, and related white matter tracts.[20,21] Clinically, however, the term CBS is often more useful than CBD because the corticobasal syndrome can be caused by CBD, PSP, Alzheimer disease (AD), Lewy body disease, or other pathologies.[20,24] The classic CBS phenotype at its core combines asymmetric akinetic-rigid parkinsonism and limb apraxia, while cortical sensory loss, dystonia, myoclonus, alien limb phenomena, and language or behavioral deficits are often present as well. The Armstrong criteria emphasized this clinicopathologic complexity and recognized several phenotypes that can reflect CBD pathology, not just classic CBS.[20]

FDG PET in CBD/CBS is notable for its asymmetry. Comparative studies have consistently shown marked unilateral or markedly asymmetric hypometabolism involving posterior frontal, inferior and superior parietal, sensorimotor, and sometimes temporal or occipital cortex, together with ipsilateral or contralateral basal ganglia and thalamic abnormalities depending on image orientation and side of clinical involvement.[22–24,40] Juh and colleagues found that CBD showed asymmetric cortical hypometabolism, in contrast to the more symmetric frontal-subcortical pattern of PSP.[22] Niethammer and colleagues defined a CBD related pattern characterized by bilateral but clearly asymmetric reductions in frontal and parietal cortex, thalamus, and caudate nucleus, with greater changes in the hemisphere opposite the more affected body side.[23]

This asymmetry is diagnostically important. In a patient with progressive asymmetric rigidity, apraxia, cortical sensory loss, or alien limb, a corresponding asymmetric frontoparietal hypometabolic pattern on FDG PET strongly supports CBS. Moreover, the precise distribution of cortical involvement may provide clues to the underlying pathology. Pardini and colleagues showed that different CBS pathologies are associated with different FDG patterns, suggesting that FDG PET may not only support the syndrome level diagnosis of CBS but also help infer whether the underlying disease is more likely CBD, PSP, or Alzheimer related.[24] For example, temporoparietal and posterior cingulate involvement may point more toward Alzheimer related CBS or Alzheimer copathology, whereas more dorsal frontoparietal and perirolandic asymmetry with subcortical extension is often considered more compatible with CBD pathology.

The main limitation is that FDG PET in CBS is not fully pathology specific. CBS is a syndrome, not a single disease. Even so, FDG PET remains clinically useful because it demonstrates the cortical component and because it often narrows the likely pathology better than clinical examination alone. When asymmetric frontoparietal hypometabolism is combined with corresponding asymmetric cortical atrophy on MR imaging and a compatible clinical syndrome, the diagnostic argument for CBS becomes much stronger. When the pattern is more symmetric and frontal-subcortical with prominent midbrain involvement, PSP should be reconsidered.

FDG PET FINDINGS IN MULTIPLE SYSTEM ATROPHY

MSA is a rapidly progressive alpha-synucleinopathy characterized by glial cytoplasmic inclusions and degeneration of striatonigral, olivopontocerebellar, and autonomic systems.[25,26] Clinically, MSA can be divided into MSA-P, with predominant parkinsonism, and MSA-C, with predominant cerebellar ataxia, although initial presentation can be mixed, and most patients eventually show mixed features. Autonomic failure, including orthostatic hypotension, urinary dysfunction, erectile dysfunction, and anhidrosis, is central to the diagnosis.[25] Poor levodopa response, rapid progression, stridor, pyramidal signs, and cerebellar signs also support MSA.

FDG PET in MSA is among the most distinctive in parkinsonian disorders because it reflects the major anatomic systems affected. In MSA-P, the hallmark is hypometabolism in the putamen, often with extension into other striatal regions and sometimes pons or cerebellum.[17,18,27–29,40] Ghaemi and colleagues showed that MSA-P differed from PD by reduced putaminal volume and glucose metabolism, even though striatal FDOPA uptake impairment was similar in both disorders.[28] This observation illustrates why FDG PET can differentiate PD from MSA-P when DAT imaging cannot. Kwon and colleagues reported high specificity of visual and SPM-supported FDG PET analysis for differentiating MSA from PD, with a tendency toward higher sensitivity than MR imaging.[27]

In MSA-C, FDG PET typically shows bilateral cerebellar hypometabolism, often involving cerebellar hemispheres and vermis, with pontine or brainstem extension reflecting olivopontocerebellar degeneration.[17,18,27,29,40] In mixed or advanced disease, both striatal and cerebellar systems may be involved. From a pattern analysis perspective, Eckert and colleagues identified an MSA related pattern characterized by decreased metabolism in putamen and cerebellum, a signature that was distinct from PSP and PD.[18] Visual reading often leverages the relative predominance of putaminal deficits in MSA-P and cerebellar deficits in MSA-C, though overlap is common in later stages.

The value of FDG PET in MSA lies not merely in recognition of individual regions, but in disease specific combinations. Severe bilateral putaminal hypometabolism argues strongly for MSA-P when the clinical differential diagnosis includes PD and PSP. Dominant cerebellar and pontine hypometabolism argues for MSA-C over spinocerebellar ataxias with parkinsonism or over PSP with gait dysfunction. In clinically uncertain cases, the combination of autonomic failure, MR imaging findings such as putaminal rim signal or hot cross bun sign, and FDG PET evidence of putaminal and or cerebellar hypometabolism can be highly persuasive.[25–29,37,39]

FDG PET FINDINGS IN PARKINSON DISEASE DEMENTIA AND DEMENTIA WITH LEWY BODIES

PDD and DLB are closely related alpha-synuclein disorders on the LBD spectrum that differ clinically by the timing of dementia relative to parkinsonism. PDD and DLB are operationally defined by the timing of parkinsonism and cognitive decline in the course of illness. In DLB, dementia precedes or occurs within 1 year of parkinsonism. In PDD, dementia develops after established PD. Both conditions may show fluctuating cognition, visual hallucinations, rapid eye movement (REM) sleep behavior disorder, attention-executive dysfunction, visuospatial impairment, and variable autonomic features.[30] Pathologically, both are characterized by cortical and subcortical Lewy related pathology, often with varying degrees of concomitant Alzheimer type changes.[30,31]

FDG PET has been especially influential in this part of the spectrum. Albin and colleagues reported in 1996 that pathologically verified diffuse Lewy body disease showed marked reductions in occipital glucose metabolism, helping distinguish it from other dementing illnesses.[31] This foundational study established that occipital dysfunction is not an incidental epiphenomenon, but a recurring metabolic signature of diffuse Lewy body pathology. Minoshima and colleagues then strengthened the clinicopathologic basis in 2001 by comparing autopsy confirmed AD and DLB. They found that only DLB showed significant occipital metabolic reduction, particularly in the primary visual cortex in the medial occipital lobe, and that this feature distinguished DLB from AD with high sensitivity and specificity.[32] This remains one of the most important FDG PET article in Lewy body dementia.

In visual terms, DLB typically shows hypometabolism in the primary visual cortex in the medial occipital lobe in addition to hypometabolism in the lateral occipital lobe, together with parietotemporal and often frontal associative deficits.[31–34,40] Relative preservation of posterior cingulate metabolism compared with precuneus and cuneus, the so-called cingulate island sign, may improve specificity for DLB versus AD,[33,34] however, this sign does not exist in all DLB patients. Lim and colleagues showed that occipital hypometabolism had high sensitivity, whereas the cingulate island sign had particularly high specificity.[33] Graff-Radford and colleagues subsequently linked the cingulate island sign to lower neurofibrillary tangle burden, explaining why the sign is more conspicuous when concomitant Alzheimer pathology is limited.[34] When quantitative statistical mapping analysis is applied, however, many DLB patients show decreased uptake in the posterior cingulate cortex, but the findings are relatively mild when compared to hypometabolism in the adjacent medial parietal and occipital hypometabolism, contributing to the impression of the cingulate island sign.

PDD shows substantial overlap with DLB but often appears as a continuum from PD-associated posterior cortical dysfunction to more extensive associative cortical hypometabolism.[12–14] Posterior parietal, temporal, occipital, posterior cingulate, and sometimes frontal deficits are common. The degree of occipital hypometabolism can be less striking than in classic DLB, but the distinction is not absolute. In practice, the clinical timeline remains essential. FDG PET is most helpful when the question is DLB versus AD,[41] DLB versus frontotemporal dementia, or PDD/DLB versus nondemented PD, rather than when one is trying to separate DLB from PDD purely on imaging grounds.

DIAGNOSTIC PATHWAY INCLUDING MULTIMODAL CLINICAL AND IMAGING APPROACHES FOR DIFFERENTIAL DIAGNOSIS

No single imaging test is sufficient for the full differential diagnosis of parkinsonian syndromes. The most effective diagnostic pathway begins with careful syndromic clinical classification. One first establishes whether the patient has true parkinsonism, then looks for red flags and positive features such as early falls, vertical gaze limitation, disproportionate antecollis, cerebellar signs, severe autonomic failure, alien limb phenomena, cortical sensory deficits, hallucinations, or early cognitive fluctuations.[1,15,20,25,30] This step often narrows the field even before imaging is obtained.[42]

Structural MR imaging is usually the first imaging companion because it excludes mimics and can contribute specific clues as well as excluding other structural abnormalities. Midbrain atrophy and elevated MR imaging parkinsonism index support PSP. Putaminal atrophy or rim hyperintensity and the hot cross bun sign support MSA. Asymmetric frontoparietal atrophy may support CBS, while marked hippocampal atrophy may suggest Alzheimer copathology in a cognitive syndrome.[37,39] However, structural changes associated with specific neurodegeneration typically occur in the relatively late stage, often after functional PET/SPECT imaging shows abnormal findings. Following MR imaging evaluation to exclude apparent structural abnormality, DAT imaging is then useful when the main uncertainty is degenerative versus nondegenerative parkinsonism, or DLB versus non-Lewy dementia. Its value is greatest at this gateway stage, not at the later stage of resolving PD versus PSP versus MSA versus CBS.[2–4]

FDG PET becomes especially valuable once degenerative parkinsonism is established or strongly suspected, but the exact syndrome remains uncertain. Pattern recognition at this stage is often decisive (**Fig. 1**, **Table1**). Relative preservation of striatum and cerebellum with posterior cortical abnormalities favors PD. Relatively symmetric medial superior frontal, lateral premotor, caudate, thalamic, and midbrain hypometabolism favors PSP. Markedly asymmetric frontoparietal cortical hypometabolism favors CBS. Putaminal hypometabolism with or without cerebellar and pontine deficits favors MSA-P. Dominant cerebellar and pontine hypometabolism favors MSA-C. Occipital hypometabolism, especially with or

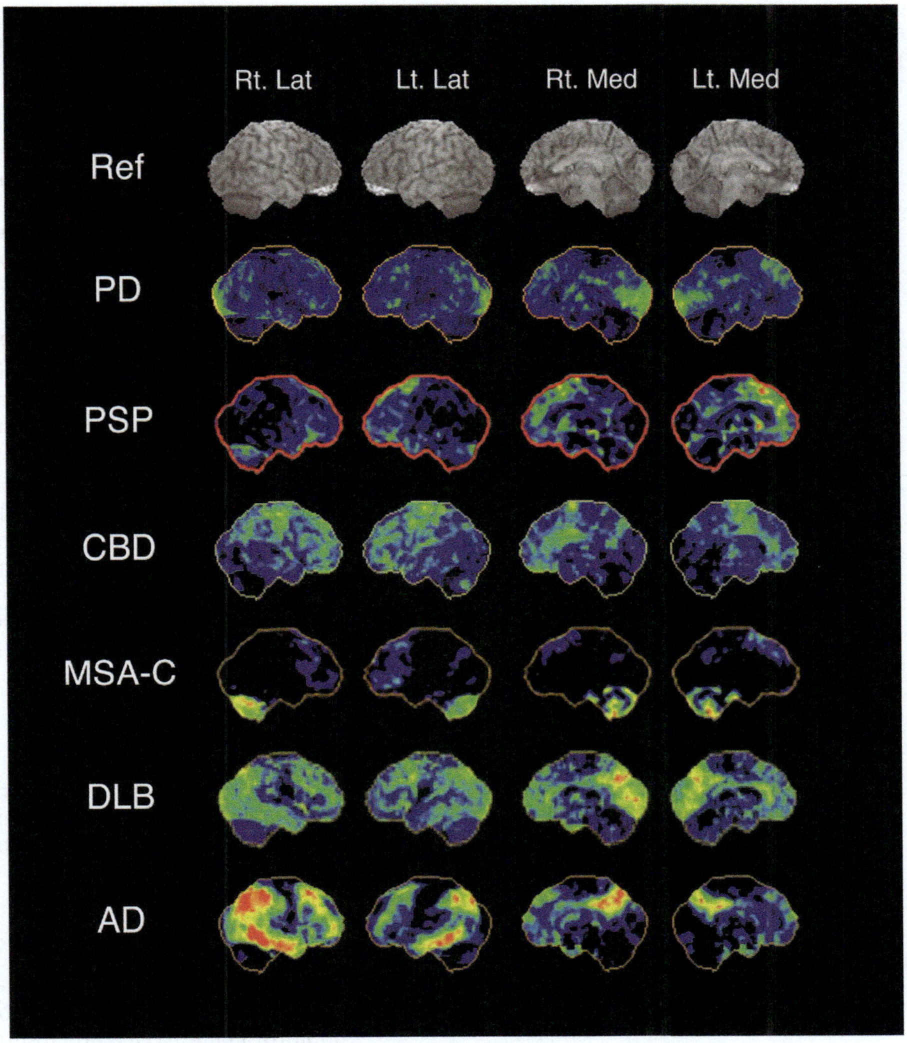

Fig. 1. FDG PET Z-score Maps (3D-SSP) in Various Parkinsonian Disorders. Color-coded areas indicate reduced FDG uptake relative to the normal database. Right lateral (Rt Lat), left lateral (Lt Lat), right medial (Rt Med), and left medial (Lt Med) brain views are shown. Cases include idiopathic PD, MSA-C, and DLB. AD is included for comparison.

without a cingulate island sign, favors DLB or PDD within the proper clinical context.[5,18,23,31–40]

Metabolic pattern analysis can further improve reproducibility by quantifying expression of validated disease related networks. Statistical mapping analysis has become a routine procedure for clinical interpretation of brain FDG PET,[43] which has been shown to improve intraobserver and interobserver diagnostic accuracy. Automated classification based on FDG PET patterns has shown high accuracy for distinguishing PD, MSA, and PSP, and meta-analytic data support strong overall diagnostic performance for FDG PET in differentiating PD from atypical parkinsonian disorders.[35,38]

Additional modalities can be layered onto this framework.[44] Cardiac MIBG scintigraphy may help separate PD or DLB from MSA and some tauopathies because postganglionic sympathetic denervation is more typical of Lewy body disease. Amyloid PET may clarify whether CBS or DLB carries substantial Alzheimer copathology. Tau PET remains investigational and is not yet a robust standalone discriminator for these syndromes, but has a promise in detecting 4-repeat tauopathies. In selected centers, dual phase FP-CIT PET or combined perfusion and DAT approaches may provide FDG-like information plus nigrostriatal assessment in a single tracer session, but dedicated FDG PET remains the more established metabolic reference standard.[39]

The practical lesson is that multimodal diagnosis should be question driven. If the question

Table 1
Summary of FDG PET findings in Parkinsonian syndromes

Disorder	Typical Pathology and Key Clinical Context	Characteristic FDG PET Findings
PD	Alpha-synuclein related Lewy pathology. Bradykinesia plus tremor, and/or rigidity, usually without early falls, gaze palsy, severe dysautonomia, or early dementia.	Relative preservation or perceived hypermetabolism in pallidothalamic circuits, pons, cerebellum, and sensorimotor cortex with relative hypometabolism in parieto-occipital and premotor association cortex. Posterior cortical and occipital reductions more evident with cognitive impairment.
PSP	4R tauopathy. Early falls, vertical gaze limitation, axial akinesia-rigidity, frontal dysexecutive syndrome.	Relatively symmetric hypometabolism in medial superior frontal cortex, lateral premotor cortex, anterior cingulate, caudate nuclei, thalamus, and midbrain.
CBD or CBS	CBD is a 4R tauopathy, but CBS may reflect CBD, PSP, AD, or other pathology. Asymmetric parkinsonism with apraxia, sometimes cortical sensory loss, dystonia, myoclonus, alien limb, or language deficits.	Markedly asymmetric hypometabolism in posterior frontal, perirolandic, and anterior parietal cortex, often extending to temporal cortex, thalamus, and basal ganglia. Greater abnormalities usually contralateral to the more affected limbs.
MSA-P	Alpha-synuclein oligodendroglial cytoplasmic inclusions with striatonigral degeneration. Parkinsonism with autonomic failure, poor levodopa response.	Putaminal hypometabolism, often with additional caudate, pontine, or cerebellar involvement.
MSA-C	Alpha-synuclein oligodendroglial cytoplasmic inclusions with olivopontocerebellar degeneration. Cerebellar ataxia plus autonomic failure, often later mixed with parkinsonism.	Bilateral cerebellar hypometabolism, frequently with pontine and brainstem extension. Striatal deficits may appear in mixed or advanced disease.
PDD	LBD Dementia arising after established PD, often with mixed Alzheimer copathology.	Posterior temporoparietal, parieto-occipital, primary visual, visual association, posterior cingulate, and later frontal hypometabolism. The findings similar to DLB and interpreted in light of temporal sequence.
DLB	Cortical and subcortical Lewy related pathology, often with variable Alzheimer copathology. Dementia before or within 1 year of parkinsonism, fluctuating cognition, and hallucinations.	Occipital hypometabolism, especially primary visual cortex in the medial occipital lobe, with parietotemporal and frontal associative deficits. Relative preservation of posterior cingulate metabolism. Hypometabolism in the primary visual cortex in the occipital lobe and the cingulate island sign support DLB over AD.

is *degenerative or not*, DAT imaging is often enough. If the question is *which degenerative parkinsonian syndrome*, FDG PET is usually more informative. If the question is *what pathology underlies this CBS or dementia syndrome*, FDG PET should be interpreted together with MR imaging, clinical phenotype, timing of cognitive symptoms, and where relevant DAT, MIBG, or amyloid biomarkers. The highest diagnostic confidence comes from concordance across clinical examination and complementary imaging, rather than from any isolated test.[2–5,35–40]

SUMMARY

FDG PET provides a systems level view of neurodegeneration that is uniquely suited to the differential diagnosis of movement disorders and parkinsonian syndromes. Its major clinical advantage over dopamine transporter imaging is that it captures the broader anatomic distribution of disease, not merely the shared endpoint of nigrostriatal loss. PD shows a characteristic combination of pallidothalamic, pontocerebellar, and sensorimotor relative hypermetabolism with posterior cortical hypometabolism that becomes more relevant as cognition declines. PSP is dominated by symmetric medial frontal, caudate, thalamic, and midbrain deficits. CBD/CBS shows striking asymmetry with frontoparietal cortical and subcortical involvement. MSA displays putaminal and or cerebellar-pontine hypometabolism depending on subtype. PDD and DLB involve posterior associative cortex, with occipital deficits and the cingulate island sign particularly useful in Lewy body dementia. Used within a multimodal clinical pathway, FDG PET can substantially improve diagnostic precision, prognostic counseling, and phenotypic stratification for research and clinical care.

CLINICS CARE POINTS

- FDG PET is useful for differentiating among degenerative parkinsonian syndromes because it reflects the full network level distribution of neurodegeneration.
- PD typically shows a reproducible metabolic network with relative hypermetabolism in pallidothalamic, pontine, cerebellar, and sensorimotor regions together with parieto-occipital cortical hypometabolism.
- PSP, CBD/CBS, and MSA each have recognizable FDG PET signatures, respectively centered on medial frontal, midbrain, asymmetric para-central, frontoparietal, and putaminal and or cerebellar-pontine involvement.
- Posterior cortical and occipital hypometabolism are important markers of cognitive vulnerability in PD and are especially characteristic of DLB and PDD within the appropriate clinical context.
- The highest diagnostic accuracy is achieved when FDG PET is interpreted together with clinical syndrome analysis, MRI, DAT imaging, and selected ancillary biomarkers such as cardiac MIBG or amyloid PET.

DECLARATION OF AI AND AI-ASSISTED TECHNOLOGIES IN THE WRITING PROCESS

This article was developed through a combination of author input and AI-assisted support. The authors used ChatGPT Atlas (OpenAI) to help identify relevant evidence, ChatGPT (OpenAI) and Copilot (Microsoft) to assist in organizing and synthesizing the collected material, and ChatGPT (OpenAI) to improve language, clarity, and overall readability. The authors critically evaluated and edited all AI-assisted output for accuracy, relevance, and suitability, and they assume full responsibility for the final content.

DISCLOSURE

None of the authors have any conflict of interest regarding the contents of this paper.

REFERENCES

1. Postuma RB, Berg D, Stern M, et al. MDS clinical diagnostic criteria for Parkinson's disease. Mov Disord 2015;30(12):1591–601. PMID: 26474316.
2. Morbelli S, Esposito G, Arbizu J, et al. EANM practice guideline/SNMMI procedure standard for dopaminergic imaging in Parkinsonian syndromes 1.0. Eur J Nucl Med Mol Imag 2020;47(8):1885–912. PMID: 32388612.
3. Ba F, Martin WRW. Dopamine transporter imaging as a diagnostic tool for parkinsonism and related disorders in clinical practice. Parkinsonism Relat Disorders 2015;21(2):87–94. PMID: 25487733.
4. Cummings JL, Henchcliffe C, Schaier S, et al. The role of dopaminergic imaging in patients with symptoms of dopaminergic system neurodegeneration. Brain 2011;134(Pt 11):3146–66. PMID: 21810889.
5. Walker Z, Gandolfo F, Orini S, et al. Clinical utility of FDG PET in Parkinson's disease and atypical parkinsonism associated with dementia. Eur J Nucl Med Mol Imag 2018;45(9):1534–45. PMID: 29779045.
6. Bohnen NI, Minoshima S, Giordani B, et al. Motor correlates of occipital glucose hypometabolism in Parkinson's disease without dementia. Neurology 1999;52(3):541–6. PMID: 10025784.
7. Eberling JL, Richardson BC, Reed BR, et al. Cortical glucose metabolism in Parkinson's disease without dementia. Neurobiol Aging 1994;15(3):329–35. PMID: 7936057.
8. Asanuma K, Tang C, Ma Y, et al. Network modulation in the treatment of Parkinson's disease. Brain 2006; 129(Pt 10):2667–78. PMID: 16844713.
9. Huang C, Mattis P, Perrine K, et al. Metabolic brain networks associated with cognitive function in Parkinson's disease. Neuroimage 2007;34(2):714–23. PMID: 17113310.
10. Huang C, Tang C, Feigin A, et al. Changes in network activity with the progression of Parkinson's disease. Brain 2007;130(Pt 7):1834–46. PMID: 17470495.
11. Meles SK, Renken RJ, Janzen A, et al. Abnormal pattern of brain glucose metabolism in Parkinson's disease: replication in three European cohorts. Eur J Nucl Med Mol Imag 2020;47(2):437–50. PMID: 31768600.
12. Bohnen NI, Koeppe RA, Minoshima S, et al. Cerebral metabolic features of Parkinson disease and

incident dementia: longitudinal study. J Nucl Med 2011;52(6):848–55. PMID: 21571793.
13. Pappata S, Santangelo G, Aarsland D, et al. Mild cognitive impairment in drug-naive patients with Parkinson's disease is associated with regional cerebral hypometabolism. Neurology 2011;77(14):1357–62. PMID: 21940621.
14. Garcia-Garcia D, Clavero P, Gasca Salas C, et al. Posterior parietooccipital hypometabolism may differentiate mild cognitive impairment from dementia in Parkinson's disease. Eur J Nucl Med Mol Imag 2012;39(11):1767–77. PMID: 22872307.
15. Höglinger GU, Respondek G, Stamelou M, et al. Clinical diagnosis of progressive supranuclear palsy: the movement disorder society criteria. Mov Disord 2017;32(6):853–64. PMID: 28467028.
16. Dickson DW, Ahmed Z, Algom AA, et al. Neuropathology of variants of progressive supranuclear palsy. Curr Opin Neurol 2010;23(4):394–400. PMID: 206 10990.
17. Juh R, Pae CU, Lee CU, et al. Different metabolic patterns analysis of Parkinsonism on the 18F-FDG PET. Eur J Radiol 2004;51(3):223–33. PMID: 15294329.
18. Eckert T, Barnes A, Dhawan V, et al. Abnormal metabolic networks in atypical parkinsonism. Mov Disord 2008;23(5):727–33. PMID: 18186116.
19. Ge J, Wu P, Peng S, et al. Reproducible network and regional topographies of abnormal glucose metabolism associated with progressive supranuclear palsy: multivariate and univariate analyses in American and Chinese patient cohorts. Hum Brain Mapp 2018;39(7):2842–58. PMID: 29536636.
20. Armstrong MJ, Litvan I, Lang AE, et al. Criteria for the diagnosis of corticobasal degeneration. Neurology 2013;80(5):496–503. PMID: 23359374.
21. Kouri N, Whitwell JL, Josephs KA, et al. Corticobasal degeneration: a pathologically distinct 4R tauopathy. Nat Rev Neurol 2011;7(5):263–72. PMID: 21487420.
22. Juh R, Pae CU, Kim TS, et al. Cerebral glucose metabolism in corticobasal degeneration: comparison with progressive supranuclear palsy using statistical mapping analysis. Neurosci Lett 2005; 383(1–2):22–7. PMID: 15936506.
23. Niethammer M, Tang CC, Feigin A, et al. A disease-specific metabolic brain network associated with corticobasal degeneration. Brain 2014;137(Pt 11): 3036–46. PMID: 25208922.
24. Pardini M, Huey ED, Spina S, et al. FDG-PET patterns associated with underlying pathology in corticobasal syndrome. Neurology 2019;92(10):e1121–35. PMID: 30700592.
25. Wenning GK, Stankovic I, Vignatelli L, et al. The movement disorder society criteria for the diagnosis of multiple system atrophy. Mov Disord 2022;37(6): 1131–48. PMID: 35445419.
26. Jellinger KA. Multiple system atrophy: an oligodendroglioneural synucleinopathy. J Alzheimers Dis 2018;62(3):1141–79. PMID: 28984582.
27. Kwon KY, Choi CG, Kim JS, et al. Comparison of brain MRI and 18F-FDG PET in the differential diagnosis of multiple system atrophy from Parkinson's disease. Mov Disord 2007;22(16):2352–8. PMID: 17894342.
28. Ghaemi M, Hilker R, Rudolf J, et al. Differentiating multiple system atrophy from Parkinson's disease: contribution of striatal and midbrain MRI volumetry and multi-tracer PET imaging. J Neurol Neurosurg Psychiatry 2002;73(5):517–23. PMID: 12397143.
29. Baudrexel S, Seifried C, Penndorf B, et al. The value of putaminal diffusion imaging versus 18F-FDG PET in the diagnosis of the Parkinson variant of multiple system atrophy. Mov Disord 2014;29(3):380–7. PMID: 24243813.
30. McKeith IG, Boeve BF, Dickson DW, et al. Diagnosis and management of dementia with Lewy bodies: fourth consensus report of the DLB consortium. Neurology 2017;89(1):88–100. PMID: 28592453.
31. Albin RL, Minoshima S, D'Amato CJ, et al. Fluoro-deoxyglucose positron emission tomography in diffuse Lewy body disease. Neurology 1996;47(2):462–6. PMID: 8757021.
32. Minoshima S, Foster NL, Sima AAF, et al. Alzheimer's disease versus dementia with Lewy bodies: cerebral metabolic distinction with autopsy confirmation. Ann Neurol 2001;50(3):358–65. PMID: 11558792.
33. Lim SM, Katsifis A, Villemagne VL, et al. The 18F-FDG PET cingulate island sign and comparison to 123I-beta-CIT SPECT for diagnosis of dementia with lewy bodies. J Nucl Med 2009;50(10):1638–45. PMID: 19759102.
34. Graff-Radford J, Murray ME, Lowe VJ, et al. Dementia with Lewy bodies: basis of cingulate island sign. Neurology 2014;83(9):801–9. PMID: 25056580.
35. Teune LK, Bartels AL, de Jong BM, et al. Typical cerebral metabolic patterns in neurodegenerative brain diseases. Mov Disord 2010;25(14):2395–404. PMID: 20669302.
36. Pagano G, Niccolini F, Politis M. Imaging in Parkinson's disease. Clin Med 2016;16(4):371–5. PMID: 27481384.
37. Broski SM, Hunt CH, Johnson GB, et al. Structural and functional imaging in parkinsonian syndromes. Radiographics 2014;34(5):1273–92. PMID: 25208280.
38. Gu SC, Yang ZH, Pan SS, et al. Metabolic pattern analysis of 18F-FDG PET as a marker for the differential diagnosis of parkinsonism: a systematic review and meta-analysis. Rev Neurosci 2019;30(7): 743–56. PMID: 31050657.
39. Hong CM, Choi SJ, Oh JS, et al. Early perfusion and dopamine transporter imaging using 18F-FP-CIT PET/CT in patients with parkinsonism. Am J Nucl Med Mol Imaging 2018;8(6):360–72. PMID: 30697456.
40. Zhao P, Zhang B, Gao S. 18F-FDG PET study on the idiopathic Parkinson's disease and multiple system atrophy, progressive supranuclear palsy, corticobasal degeneration, and dementia with lewy bodies.

Parkinsonism Relat Disorders 2012;18(Suppl 1): S60–2. PMID: 22166456.

41. Vander Borght T, Minoshima S, Giordani B, et al. Cerebral metabolic differences in Parkinson's and Alzheimer's diseases matched for dementia severity. J Nucl Med 1997;38(5):797–802. PMID: 9170449.
42. Peralta C, Strafella AP, van Eimeren T, et al, International Parkinson Movement Disorders Society-Neuroimaging Study Group. Pragmatic approach on neuroimaging techniques for the differential diagnosis of parkinsonisms. Mov Disord Clin Pract 2021;9(1): 6–19. PMID: 35005060.
43. Minoshima S, Frey KA, Koeppe RA, et al. A diagnostic approach in Alzheimer's disease using three-dimensional stereotactic surface projections of F-18-FDG PET. J Nucl Med 1995;36(7):1238–48. PMID: 7790950.
44. Höglinger G, German Parkinson's Guidelines Committee, Trenkwalder C. Diagnosis and treatment of parkinson's disease (guideline of the German Society for Neurology). Neurol Res Pract 2024;6(1):30. PMID: 38845028; PMCID: PMC11157782.

2-[^{18}F]fluoro-2-deoxy-D-glucose PET in Brain Tumors

Camille Steenhout, MD[a], Roland Hustinx, MD, PhD[b],
Andrew B. Newberg, MD[c,d], Abass Alavi, MD[e], Nadia Withofs, MD, PhD[b,*]

KEYWORDS

• [^{18}F]FDG • PET • Brain tumors • Neuro-oncology

KEY POINTS

- In gliomas, [^{18}F]FDG PET can help assess tumor aggressiveness, guide biopsy, and evaluate residual or recurrent disease, although its value is limited by high physiologic brain uptake and lower accuracy than other PET tracers.
- In brain metastases, [^{18}F]FDG PET may assist in differentiating tumor recurrence from treatment-related changes, although other PET tracers show higher diagnostic accuracy.
- In lymphomas, [^{18}F]FDG PET plays a well-established role in initial diagnosis and may also provide significant value in treatment monitoring and management.
- In meningiomas, [^{18}F]FDG PET has limited clinical value. Instead, PET imaging using somatostatin receptor ligands is preferred for tumor characterization.
- [^{18}F]FDG PET can provide useful diagnostic information in pediatric central nervous system malignancies, although interpretation may be limited by high physiologic uptake.

INTRODUCTION

Brain tumors represent a major public health concern, as they constitute a significant cause of morbidity and mortality.[1] They encompass a broad spectrum of primary and secondary neoplasms involving the central nervous system (CNS).

Among primary brain tumors in adults, glioblastoma is the most common malignant tumor, whereas meningioma represents the most frequently diagnosed nonmalignant intracranial tumor.[2] Brain metastases occur approximately 10 times more frequently than primary brain tumors and account for 9% to 10% of all cancer diagnoses.[3]

MR imaging is the main imaging modality for the diagnosis and follow-up of brain tumors,[4] due to its high sensitivity and specificity, excellent soft-tissue contrast, and relatively wide availability. However, PET provides complementary information by enabling the in vivo assessment of tumor biology beyond the structural information obtained with MR imaging. PET then can be used for differential diagnosis, tumor grading, delineation of tumor extent, surgical and radiotherapy planning, as well as posttreatment monitoring and prognostic assessment. A key advantage of PET compared with conventional MR imaging is that tracer uptake reflects specific pathophysiological

[a] Division of Nuclear Medicine and Oncological Imaging, University Hospital of Liège, Avenue de l'Hôpital, Liège, Belgium; [b] Faculty of Medicine, Division of Nuclear Medicine and Oncological Imaging, University Hospital of Liège, Avenue de l'Hôpital, Liège, Belgium; [c] Department of Radiology, Sidney Kimmel Medical College, Thomas Jefferson University, Philadelphia, PA, USA; [d] Department of Integrative Medicine and Nutritional Sciences, Sidney Kimmel Medical College, Thomas Jefferson University, Philadelphia, PA, USA; [e] Division of Nuclear Medicine, Department of Radiology, Hospital of the University of Pennsylvania, University of Pennsylvania Perelman School of Medicine, Philadelphia, PA, USA
* Corresponding author.
E-mail address: nwithofs@chuliege.be

PET Clin 21 (2026) 511–520
https://doi.org/10.1016/j.cpet.2026.05.005

Abbreviations

[18F]FDG	2-[18F]fluoro-2-deoxy-D-glucose
BBB	blood–brain barrier
CNS	central nervous system
FDA	Food and Drug Administration
GLUTs	glucose transporters
HD-MTX	high-dose methotrexate-based chemotherapy
IDH	isocitrate dehydrogenase
PCNSL	primary central nervous system lymphomas
SSTR	somatostatin receptors
TBRs	tumor-to-contralateral-normal-brain SUV ratios
WHO	World Health Organization
WHO CNS5	fifth edition of the World Health Organization Classification of Tumors of the Central Nervous System

processes and, in most cases, is largely independent of disruption of the blood–brain barrier (BBB), whereas contrast-enhanced MR imaging sequences rely on BBB breakdown.[5] Among PET radiotracers, 2-[18F]fluoro-2-deoxy-D-glucose ([18F]FDG) is the most widely used, but many other tracers are clinically available such as amino acid analogs (AA PET) or radiolabeled somatostatin receptor (SSTR) ligands.[5–7] However, it is also important to note that in the United States, no AA radiopharmaceuticals are Food and Drug Administration (FDA)-approved for clinical use. Thus, [18F]FDG is still the primary radiopharmaceutical for brain imaging, including for tumors.

Notably, a recent survey conducted by the European Organisation for Research and Treatment of Cancer–Brain Tumor Group reported that only 35% of participating centers used [18F]FDG PET in neuro-oncology, mainly for the evaluation of lymphoma and extracranial disease in patients with brain metastases. Nevertheless, in certain settings, [18F]FDG PET continues to be used because of the limited availability of AA PET, particularly in the United States.[8,9]

Management of brain tumors is multimodal, with treatment strategies guided by tumor histology and preoperative clinical considerations.[4] Therapeutic options include surgery, which remains the cornerstone of management, as well as radiation therapy, including stereotactic radiosurgery and conventional fractionated approaches. Additional treatments may involve corticosteroids, intravenous chemotherapy, or intrathecal chemotherapeutic agents, while novel therapies, including chemotherapy and immunotherapy agents, are continuously developed. Importantly, these therapeutic interventions can induce posttreatment changes within the tumor and surrounding brain parenchyma that must be carefully considered during neuroimaging assessment.[10]

Among brain tumors, the clinical role of [18F]FDG PET is not uniform. Although its value is well established in primary central nervous system lymphoma (PCNSL), its application in other brain tumors remains more selective and is generally complementary to MR imaging and other PET radiotracers. This review, therefore, provides an overview of the current role of [18F]FDG PET in the evaluation of brain tumors.

BIOLOGICAL BASIS OF [18F]FDG PET IN BRAIN TUMORS

[18F]FDG PET imaging is based on the increased glycolytic activity of tumor cells, a phenomenon known as the Warburg effect. Malignant cells preferentially use glycolysis rather than oxidative phosphorylation for energy production, even in the presence of oxygen.[11] [18F]FDG is a glucose analog transported across the BBB by glucose transporters (GLUTs), mainly GLUT1 and GLUT3, independent of BBB disruption. Once inside the cell, [18F]FDG is phosphorylated by hexokinase and then trapped intracellularly, allowing visualization with PET imaging.[12]

The main limitation of [18F]FDG PET in brain tumors assessment is the high physiologic uptake in normal gray matter, which can reduce lesion contrast and may make difficult to detect tumors with moderate metabolic activity, particularly low-grade gliomas.[5] In addition, [18F]FDG uptake is not tumor-specific: inflammatory or infectious processes may also show increased uptake, while necrotic regions in high-grade tumors may exhibit reduced uptake.[10] As [18F]FDG PET reflects glucose metabolism, it requires a fasting period of 4 to 6 hours, and factors such as hyperglycemia or insufficient fasting period can decrease the sensitivity of the examination.[13,14]

[18F]FDG PET IN GLIOMAS

In 2021, the fifth edition of the World Health Organization Classification of Tumors of the Central Nervous System (WHO CNS5) was published. This updated classification introduced major changes, emphasizing the growing role of molecular diagnostic markers alongside histology and immunohistochemistry in CNS tumor classification.[15]

Adult-type diffuse gliomas are currently classified into 3 main entities: astrocytoma isocitrate dehydrogenase (IDH) mutant; oligodendroglioma IDH-mutant and 1p/19q-codeleted; and glioblastoma IDH-wildtype. Accurate molecular characterization of these tumors is essential, as prognosis and therapeutic strategies are strongly influenced by their genetic profile.[15]

Whenever available, amino acid PET tracers are generally preferred over [^{18}F]FDG PET because of their superior tumor-to-background contrast and higher diagnostic accuracy, particularly for tumor delineation and treatment response assessment.[16] Nevertheless, [^{18}F]FDG PET remains clinically useful because of its wide availability and its ability to distinguish high-grade (WHO grade III/IV) gliomas from other malignant brain tumors. However, its specificity remains limited due to overlapping SUV_{max} values across tumor types and its reduced ability to differentiate gliomas from nonmalignant conditions, such as inflammatory or infectious diseases.[17] In the United States, [^{18}F]FDG PET is currently the only FDA-approved radiotracer for the diagnosis of brain tumors.

High-grade gliomas generally demonstrate greater [^{18}F]FDG uptake than low-grade gliomas (WHO grade I/II),[17] as illustrated in **Fig. 1**. Moreover, increased [^{18}F]FDG uptake has been identified as an independent prognostic factor in WHO grade IV gliomas, both at diagnosis and after treatment initiation.[18]

Tumor-to-contralateral-normal-brain SUV ratios (TBRs) may further improve tumor grading. However, no clear threshold has been consistently established in the literature. A commonly proposed cutoff is a TBR_{max} of 0.6, although higher thresholds, such as 0.9, have also been suggested.[19–21] Nevertheless, some low-grade gliomas may exhibit elevated TBR values, limiting the accuracy of [^{18}F]FDG PET for tumor grading at diagnosis.

Delayed imaging, performed more than 3 hours after tracer injection, has been suggested to improve the specificity of [^{18}F]FDG PET, as tracer uptake tends to decrease slightly over time in normal brain tissue while remaining stable or increasing in malignant lesions.[5,22] However, the implementation of such delayed protocols remains challenging in the routine clinical setting.

[^{18}F]FDG PET can be a valuable tool for guiding stereotactic brain biopsies by identifying regions with the highest uptake, which often correspond to higher grade tumor areas. AA PET tracers typically provide superior contrast between tumor and normal brain tissue; however, a small proportion of gliomas may show little to no amino acid uptake.[5,23] In such cases, [^{18}F]FDG PET can be used to identify suitable biopsy targets.

Pseudoprogression and radionecrosis are recognized as treatment-related changes occurring within the first 3 months after treatment and beyond 3 months, respectively, with pseudoprogression potentially extending up to 6 months in

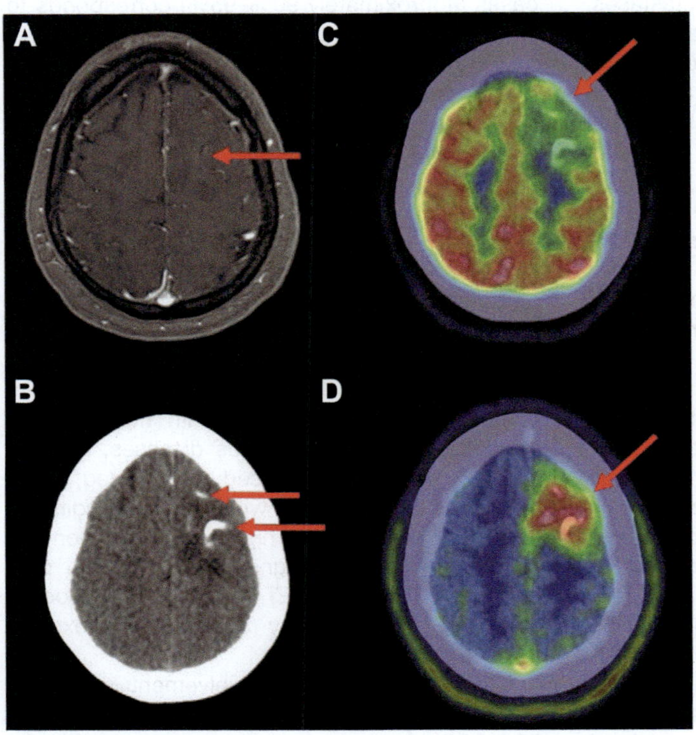

Fig. 1. (*A–D*) Brain images of a 39 year old patient with a left frontal lesion. (*A*) Postgadolinium T1-weighted MR imaging shows mild enhancement after gadolinium injection (*red arrow*). (*B*) CT scan of the PET/CT scan shows calcifications (*red arrows*), characteristic of oligodendroglial tumors. (*C*) [^{18}F]FDG PET/CT scan shows a hypometabolic lesion, with a SUV_{max} 5.6 slightly higher than white matter and lower than gray matter. TBR_{max} was estimated at 0.5 suggesting a low-grade glioma. (*D*) [^{18}F]FET PET/CT scan allowed to better estimate the extent of the lesion. TBR_{max} was estimated at 4.5, suggesting a high-grade glioma. The pathologic diagnosis was an oligodendroglioma WHO grade 2, IDH-mutant (IDH1 p.R132 mutation), and 1p/19q-codeleted. The [^{18}F]FDG PET TBR_{max} correctly predicted the low-grade glioma whereas [^{18}F]FET TBR_{max} overestimated it. (Nadia Withofs et al., Facts and Fictions About [18F]FDG versus Other Tracers in Managing Patients with Brain Tumors: It Is Time to Rectify the Ongoing Misconceptions, PET Clinics, 17 (3), 2022, 327-342, https://doi.org/10.1016/j.cpet.2022.03.004.)

patients receiving immunotherapy.[24] Differentiating tumor recurrence or progression from treatment-related changes remains challenging. The reported sensitivity and specificity of [^{18}F]FDG PET for distinguishing high-grade glioma progression from treatment-related changes vary widely in the literature.[13] Specificity may be limited by inflammatory processes, particularly in the early period following surgery and/or radiation therapy.[19] Whenever available, previous PET examinations should be used for comparison during interpretation. In the absence of treatment, tumor uptake is expected to increase between 2 PET scans, whereas lesion uptake is expected to decrease after treatment.[13]

[^{18}F]FDG PET IN BRAIN METASTASES

The differential diagnosis between brain metastases and other malignant brain tumors remains challenging with PET imaging, as [^{18}F]FDG PET typically demonstrates high uptake in both brain metastases and gliomas.[5] Moreover, brain metastases arising from primary tumors with typically low [^{18}F]FDG uptake are not optimally evaluated with this tracer. In such cases, the presence of a focal "cold spot," reflecting central necrosis and/or extensive surrounding edema, particularly in larger lesions, may nonetheless suggest a metastatic lesion.

Consequently, [^{18}F]FDG PET is not recommended for the initial diagnosis of brain metastases, for which MR imaging remains the reference technique.[25] Similarly, systematic brain acquisition for the detection of unsuspected brain metastases in patients with cancer undergoing whole-body [^{18}F]FDG PET provides only limited additional value.[26]

Assessment of treatment response in brain metastases must consider the status of the primary extra-CNS disease. Management decisions should, therefore, consider systemic tumor burden before any modification of treatment strategies is implemented.[5]

Radionecrosis following irradiation of brain metastases is relatively common, occurring in 25% of cases.[5] In this context, contrast-enhanced MR imaging does not always reliably differentiate radiation-induced changes from recurrent brain metastases. The diagnostic performance of [^{18}F]FDG PET for differentiating recurrent brain metastases from treatment-related changes varies substantially across studies. Overall, [^{18}F]FDG PET demonstrates lower diagnostic accuracy than AA PET in this setting but also than MR imaging-based perfusion imaging using arterial spin labeling, MR spectroscopy, and diffusion-weighted imaging.[25]

Nevertheless, [^{18}F]FDG PET may still be considered when amino acid radiotracers are unavailable. This could be particularly useful when recurrence is suspected within a previously irradiated field, where reduced uptake in surrounding brain tissue can increase the tumor-to-background ratio, or in tumors known to exhibit high [^{18}F]FDG avidity.[26]

As reported for gliomas, delayed [^{18}F]FDG PET acquisitions may improve diagnostic performance.[5,27]

[^{68}Ga]Ga-FAPI (fibroblast activation protein inhibitor) PET is an emerging imaging approach currently under investigation. Because BBB disruption is common in brain metastases and fibroblast activation protein expression is frequently increased in these lesions, preliminary studies suggest that [^{68}Ga]Ga-FAPI PET may provide higher lesion-to-background contrast than [^{18}F]FDG PET, as illustrated in **Fig. 2**. However, its role remains investigational and requires further validation.[28–30]

[^{18}F]FDG PET IN PRIMARY CENTRAL NERVOUS SYSTEM LYMPHOMA

PCNSL is an uncommon extranodal form of non-Hodgkin's lymphoma that involves the brain, spinal cord, leptomeninges, and/or eyes, in absence of systemic disease. The vast majority of PCNSL cases (approximately 90%–95%) corresponds to diffuse large B-cell lymphoma. Overall, PCNSL remains a rare malignancy, accounting for approximately 5% of all primary brain tumors, but its incidence has increased over the past 2 decades, most notably in the elderly.[31–33]

MR imaging remains the modality of choice for the evaluation of PCNSL.[33] Nevertheless, [^{18}F]FDG PET plays an important role in the diagnostic evaluation of PCNSL, as these lesions typically demonstrate intense and homogenous [^{18}F]FDG uptake due to very high cellular density with an accelerated glycolytic metabolism, as illustrated in **Fig. 3**. [^{18}F]FDG PET can assist in the differential diagnosis with gliomas and with nonmalignant conditions such as infectious diseases, particularly in immunocompromised patients (eg, toxoplasmosis). Compared with these conditions, PCNSL generally shows higher and more homogenous uptake. The diagnostic accuracy of pretreatment [^{18}F]FDG PET is high, with pooled sensitivity and specificity reported to be exceed 84%.[5,13,14,33,34]

Although extracerebral involvement is uncommon (approximately 4%–7%), whole-body [^{18}F]FDG PET is recommended in patient with PCNSL for initial staging and to exclude systemic

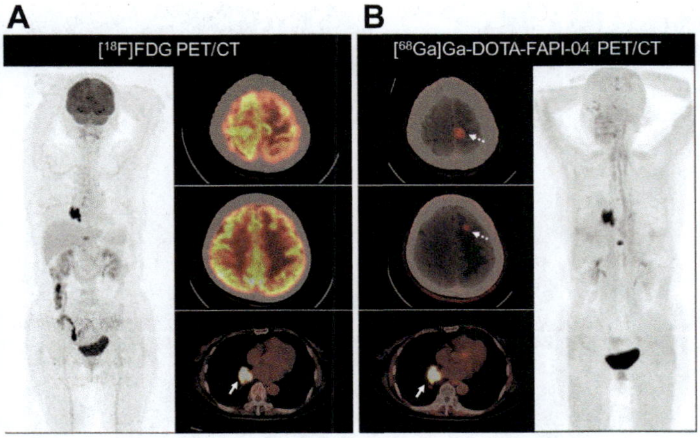

Fig. 2. (*A*, *B*) PET/CT scans of a 76 year old female patient diagnosed with non-small cell lung cancer (adenocarcinoma). (*A*) [^{18}F]FDG PET/CT shows a ring-like accumulation with a perifocal hypometabolic area relative to the gray matter in the left parietal lobe (*upper row*) and frontal lobe (*middle row*), respectively. (*B*) [^{68}Ga]Ga-DOTA-FAPI-04 PET/CT shows clearer borders of the 2 lesions. One of the lesions is only 8 to 9 mm in diameter (*dotted arrow*), which was further confirmed by a cerebral MR imaging. The primary tumor in the right upper lobe revealed intense uptake of both [^{18}F]FDG and [^{68}Ga]Ga-DOTA-FAPI-04 (*solid arrow, lower row*). (Chen, H., Pang, Y., Wu, J. et al. Comparison of [^{68}Ga]Ga-DOTA-FAPI-04 and [^{18}F] FDG PET/CT for the diagnosis of primary and metastatic lesions in patients with various types of cancer. Eur J Nucl Med Mol Imaging 47, 1820–1832 (2020). https://doi.org/10.1007/s00259-020-04769-z.)

involvement, which is a key determinant in therapeutic management.[33–36]

Notably, amino-acid PET has not demonstrated an additional diagnostic value compared with [^{18}F] FDG PET in the evaluation of PCNSL.[14]

PCNSL is associated with a generally poor prognosis. Age and functional status at diagnosis are well-established prognostic factors. Additional prognostic indicators have been proposed, including biological markers and imaging features derived from MR imaging. On [^{18}F]FDG PET, high tracer uptake and a large metabolic tumor volume have been identified as predictors of poor prognosis.[33,36]

The treatment of PCNSL is primarily based on high-dose methotrexate-based chemotherapy (HD-MTX). In elderly patients, HD-MTX-based regimens are generally used alone, whereas in younger and fit patients, they may be combined with consolidation using autologous stem cell transplantation.[37]

The International Primary CNS Lymphoma Collaborative Group recommend response assessment based mainly on MR imaging criteria. However, several studies have reported early relapse in patients considered to be in complete response on end-of-treatment MR imaging, raising concerns about the ability of MR imaging to reliably detect residual disease.[32]

Interim [^{18}F]FDG PET performed after 2 cycles of methotrexate-based chemotherapy has emerged as a robust early predictor of treatment response, particularly in patients with partial or unconfirmed responses on MR imaging.[38] The prospective

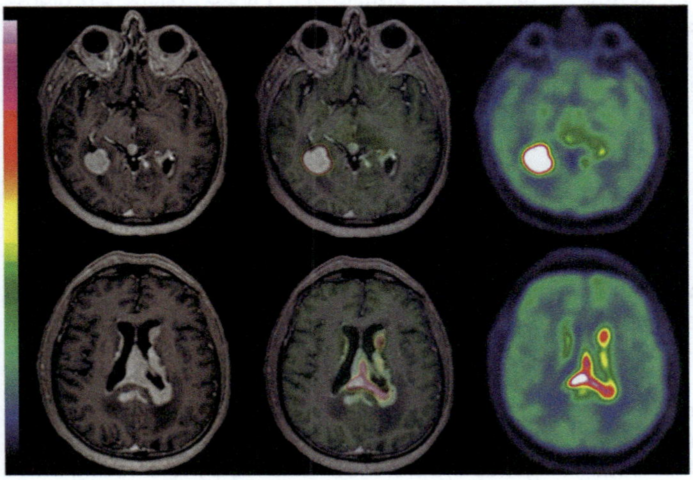

Fig. 3. Images of a 64 year old woman with PCNS lymphoma. Axial T1-weighted MR imaging shows enhanced periventricular lesions (*left*), with a corresponding intense hypermetabolism on [^{18}F]FDG PET (*right*) and fused MR imaging/PET (*middle*), and a relative extinction of cortical metabolism. (Reproduced from Horowitz T, Tabouret E, Graillon T, et al. Contribution of nuclear medicine to the diagnosis and management of primary brain tumours. Rev Neurol (Paris). 2023;179(5):394-404.13.)

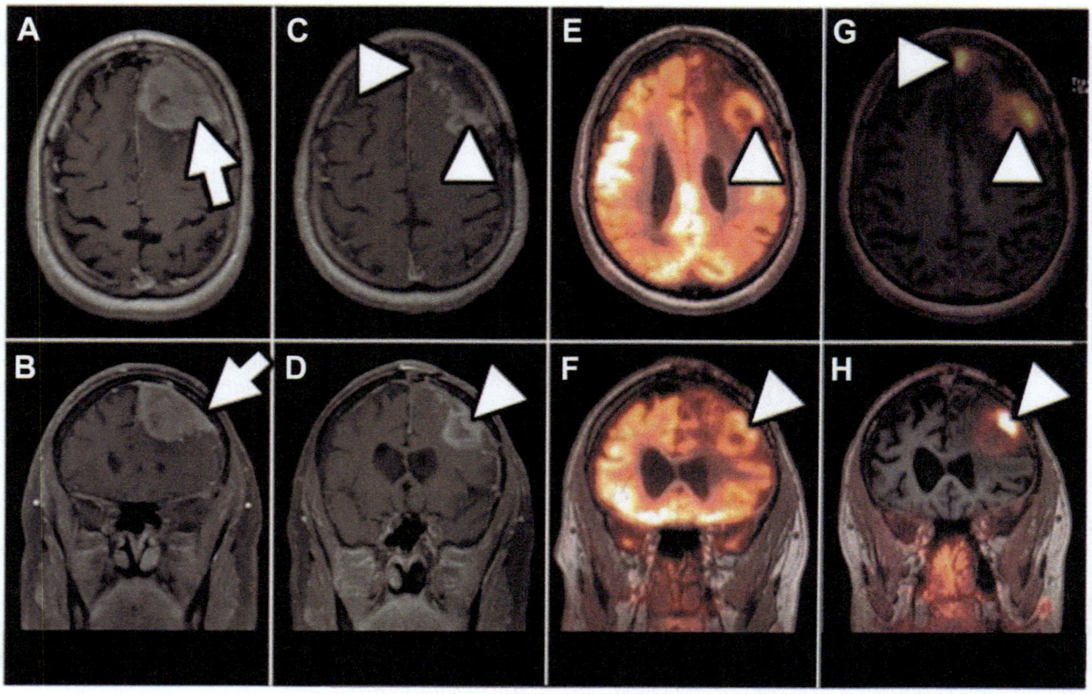

Fig. 4. Recurrent anaplastic meningioma on [^{18}F]FDG and [^{68} Ga]Ga-DOTATATE PET. Axial (*A*) and coronal (*B*) postcontrast T1-weighted MR imaging shows a large enhancing left frontal WHO grade 3 anaplastic meningioma (*white arrows*). After stereotactic radiosurgery, axial (*C*) and coronal (*D*) postcontrast T1-weighted MR imaging show persistent enhancement in the treatment bed (*white arrowheads*). There is corresponding focal increased uptake (*white arrowheads*) on fused axial (*E*) and coronal (*F*) [^{18}F]FDG PET/MR imaging, indicating viable high-grade tumor. Subsequently performed axial (*G*) and coronal (*H*) fused-[^{68}Ga]Ga-DOTATATE PET/MR images show intense uptake (*white arrowheads*) in the left frontal region, corresponding to the previously documented regions of elevated [^{18}F]FDG uptake and MR imaging enhancement. This indicates SSTRs within the residual anaplastic meningioma, therefore potential benefit in SSTRs radionuclide therapies. (Jessica Zhang, Katie Suzanne Traylor, James M. Mountz, PET and SPECT Imaging of Brain Tumors, Seminars in Ultrasound, CT and MRI, 41 (6), 2020, 530-540, https://doi.org/10.1053/j.sult.2020.08.007.)

LOCALYSE study, including 65 patients, demonstrated that persistent residual uptake on interim [^{18}F]FDG PET, defined as tracer uptake higher than that of the contralateral normal brain, was associated with a suboptimal response at the end of therapy and with poorer prognosis. These findings highlight the potential value of interim [^{18}F]FDG PET for early therapeutic stratification in patient with PCNSL.[32]

[^{18}F]FDG PET IN MENINGIOMAS

Meningiomas are the most common intracranial tumors in adults. Although most are WHO grade I, approximately 15% are grade II and around 5% are grade III.[39] PET imaging can be valuable in several clinical scenarios, including lesions located in complex anatomic regions, or when evaluating suspected recurrence of previously treated meningioma. Standard management relies on surgery and/or radiotherapy. When these treatments are not feasible or when the disease progresses despite therapy, meningiomas are considered refractory, and target radionuclide therapy may be considered.[34]

Because of the increased glycolytic activity of tumor cells, uptake of [^{18}F]FDG is generally higher in tumoral than in nontumoral tissue.[11] However, [^{18}F]FDG is not considered as the optimal tracer for the evaluation of meningiomas.

Meningiomas are typically slow-growing tumors, and their glucose metabolism may be only moderately increased. In addition, the high physiologic uptake of [^{18}F]FDG in the cerebral cortex results in a low tumor-to-background ratio, thereby limiting the sensitivity for both detection and accurate delineation of meningiomas. Furthermore, [^{18}F]FDG uptake may also be increased in inflammatory tissue, which can further reduce specificity.[40]

Meningiomas characteristically express somatostatin receptors subtype 2,[41] making SSTR ligands the preferred radiotracers for imaging these tumors, as illustrated in **Fig. 4**.[5,40,42]

AA PET may also be used in meningiomas. Compared to [^{18}F]FDG PET, it provides a higher tumor-to-background contrast. However, the availability of SSTR ligands with even greater contrast has limited its use in meningioma imaging. Notably, O-(2-[^{18}F]-fluoroethyl)-L-tyrosine ([^{18}F] FET) does not accumulate in the pituitary gland, unlike L-methyl-[^{11}C]methionine ([^{11}C]MET) and SSTR ligands, which may facilitate the detection of intrasellar invasion.[40,43]

[^{18}F]FDG IN PEDIATRIC BRAIN TUMORS

Brain tumors are the second most common malignancy after leukemia and represent the most frequent solid tumor in the pediatric population, accounting for 20% to 25% of all childhood cancers. They remain the leading cause of cancer-related mortality in children.[44]

Pediatric-type gliomas were recognized as a distinct entity in the 2021 WHO CNS5, reflecting their unique molecular features that distinguish them from adult-type gliomas.[45]

The main therapeutic approach in pediatric gliomas is surgery in association with chemotherapy and/or radiotherapy.[46]

Conventional MR imaging remains the gold standard for assessing tumor location and characteristics, although it has recognized limitations, including difficulty in differentiating tumors from tumor mimics and in accurately defining tumor type and grade. Pseudoprogression may also occur in pediatric-type gliomas, whereas pseudoresponse is less commonly observed compared with adult-type gliomas.[46]

[^{18}F]FDG PET can be used in pediatric brain tumors, exploiting the increased glucose metabolism of malignant gliomas. However, as in adults, the high physiologic glucose uptake in normal brain parenchyma results in a low tumor-to-background contrast, making it challenging to distinguish intracerebral malignancies from normal tissue or nonneoplastic lesions. This limitation is particularly pronounced in low-grade tumors, where [^{18}F]FDG uptake often approximates that of normal white matter.[46]

Consequently, the main clinical application of [^{18}F]FDG PET in pediatric brain tumors is the assessment of tumor biological behavior. Gliomas exhibiting markedly increased [^{18}F]FDG uptake are often associated with more aggressive and malignant phenotype, as illustrated in **Fig. 5**. [^{18}F]FDG PET also provides valuable information in low-grade gliomas, where higher uptake is generally correlated with an increased risk of disease progression. However, no universally accepted

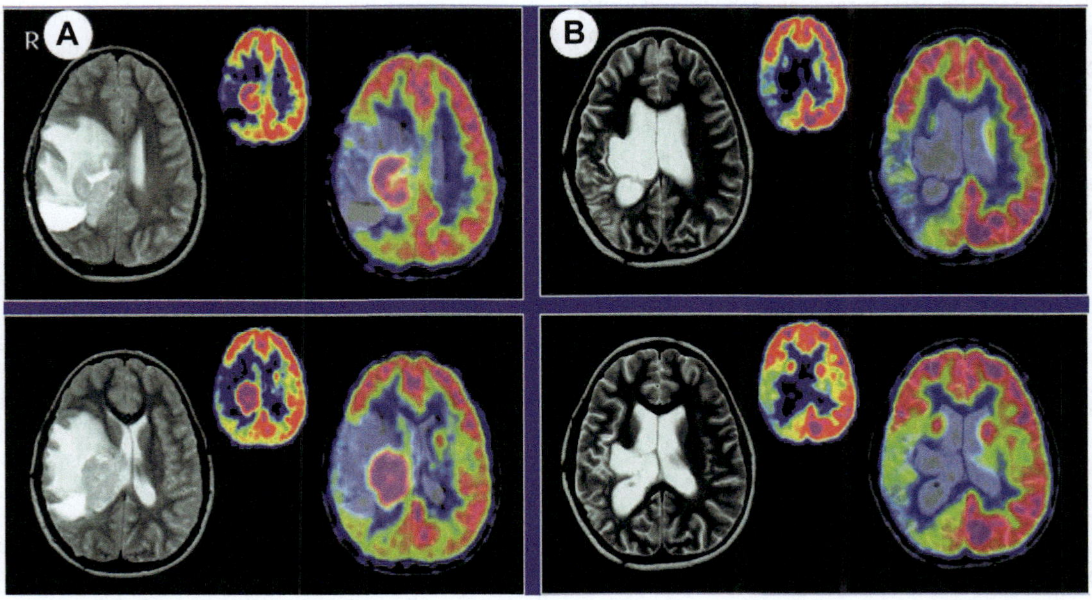

Fig. 5. (*A, B*) 11 year old boy with an anaplastic ganglioglioma in the right frontal region close to the lateral ventricle. (*A*) [^{18}F]FDG-PET scan with MR imaging coregistration (T2) at diagnosis (after biopsy) and (*B*) [^{18}F] FDG-PET with MR imaging coregistration (T2) at follow-up when a recurrence was suspected. The T2-weighted MR imaging scan at follow-up (*B*) shows contrast enhancement in the lateral posterior periphery of the surgical cavity, but the [^{18}F]FDG-PET scan with MR imaging coregistration (*B*) shows no sign of local recurrence. The boy was disease free at 2 year follow-up. (PET and MRI images courtesy of Dr. Lise Borgwardt, Rigshospitalet, Copenhagen, Denmark.)

threshold has been established to reliably identify patients at higher risk. A hotspot/brain index, calculated as $2 + 2 \times (ROI_{tumor} - ROI_{white\ matter}/[ROI_{gray\ matter} - ROI_{white\ matter}])$, of 1.83 has been proposed as the optimal cutoff to distinguish low-grade from high-grade tumors.[46,47]

[^{18}F]FDG PET can also be used to guide biopsy when coregistered with MR imaging, enabling precise identification of anaplastic regions, which often correspond to areas of highest tracer uptake. This strategy can reduce the frequency of nondiagnostic or noncontributory biopsies.[46–48]

[^{18}F]FDG PET may also be used to detect residual or recurrent disease and to differentiate it from posttherapeutic changes, such as necrosis.[46,47]

When available, PET/MR imaging systems are preferred in the pediatric population, as they substantially reduce scanning time, minimize the need for sedation or anesthesia, and also lower patient radiation exposure.[46,49,50]

In recent years, a growing body of evidence has demonstrated the amino acid PET radiotracers offer several diagnostic advantages over [^{18}F] FDG PET.[23,46,51]

SUMMARY

[^{18}F]FDG PET remains an important and widely available molecular imaging tool in neuro-oncology despite the availability of alternative PET tracers. Its widespread availability and ability to evaluate both primary brain involvement and systemic disease make it particularly valuable in the assessment of PCNSL, as well as in selected cases of gliomas, brain metastases, and pediatric brain tumors. In contrast, its role in meningiomas remains limited. Future developments, including artificial intelligence-based imaging analyses, may further enhance the role of molecular imaging in brain tumors, including the role of [^{18}F]FDG PET.[52]

DISCLOSURE

The authors have nothing to disclose.

REFERENCES

1. McNeill KA. Epidemiology of brain tumors. Neurol Clin 2016;34(4):981–98.
2. Ostrom QT, Cioffi G, Gittleman H, et al. CBTRUS statistical report: primary brain and other central nervous system tumors diagnosed in the United States in 2012–2016. Neuro Oncol 2019;21(Supplement_5): v1–100.
3. Ostrom QT, Wright CH, Barnholtz-Sloan JS. Brain metastases: epidemiology. Handb Clin Neurol 2018;149:27–42. Elsevier.
4. Weller M, Van Den Bent M, Preusser M, et al. EANO guidelines on the diagnosis and treatment of diffuse gliomas of adulthood. Nat Rev Clin Oncol 2021; 18(3):170–86.
5. Verger A, Kas A, Darcourt J, et al. PET imaging in neuro-oncology: an update and overview of a rapidly growing area. Cancers 2022;14(5):1103.
6. Chen W, Silverman DHS. Advances in evaluation of primary brain tumors. Semin Nucl Med 2008;38(4): 240–50.
7. Lewis DY, Soloviev D, Brindle KM. Imaging tumor metabolism using positron emission tomography. Cancer J 2015;21(2):129–36.
8. Mair MJ, Lohmann P, Galldiks N, et al. Availability and use of PET in patients with brain tumours – a European Organisation for Research and Treatment of Cancer - Brain Tumour Group (EORTC-BTG) survey. Eur J Nucl Med Mol Imag 2025;52(12):4627–38.
9. Galldiks N, Tonn JC, Preusser M, et al. Update to the RANO working group and EANO recommendations for the clinical use of PET imaging in gliomas. Neuro Oncol 2025;27(10):2492–3.
10. Zhang J, Traylor KS, Mountz JM. PET and SPECT imaging of brain tumors. Semin Ultrasound CT MRI 2020;41(6):530–40.
11. Warburg O. On the origin of cancer cells. Science 1956;309–14.
12. Kilbourn MR. Small molecule PET tracers for transporter imaging. Semin Nucl Med 2017;47(5): 536–52.
13. Horowitz T, Tabouret E, Graillon T, et al. Contribution of nuclear medicine to the diagnosis and management of primary brain tumours. Rev Neurol (Paris) 2023;179(5):394–404.
14. Arbizu J, Morbelli S, Minoshima S, et al. SNMMI procedure Standard/EANM practice guideline for brain [^{18}F]FDG PET Imaging, Version 2.0. J Nucl Med 2025;66(Supplement 2):S45–60.
15. Louis DN, Perry A, Wesseling P, et al. The 2021 WHO classification of tumors of the central nervous system: a summary. Neuro Oncol 2021;23(8): 1231–51.
16. Dunet V, Pomoni A, Hottinger A, et al. Performance of ^{18}F-FET versus ^{18}F-FDG-PET for the diagnosis and grading of brain tumors: systematic review and meta-analysis. Neuro Oncol 2016;18(3):426–34.
17. Albert NL, Weller M, Suchorska B, et al. Response assessment in neuro-oncology working group and European Association for Neuro-Oncology recommendations for the clinical use of PET imaging in gliomas. Neuro Oncol 2016;18(9):1199–208.
18. Colavolpe C, Metellus P, Mancini J, et al. Independent prognostic value of pre-treatment 18-FDG-PET in high-grade gliomas. J Neuro Oncol 2012; 107(3):527–35.
19. Withofs N, Kumar R, Alavi A, et al. Facts and fictions about [18F]FDG versus other tracers in managing

patients with brain tumors. Pet Clin 2022;17(3): 327–42.
20. Delbeke D, Meyerowitz C, Lapidus RL, et al. Optimal cutoff levels of F-18 fluorodeoxyglucose uptake in the differentiation of low-grade from high-grade brain tumors with PET. Radiology 1995;195(1): 47–52.
21. Takahashi M, Soma T, Mukasa A, et al. Pattern of FDG and MET distribution in High- and low-grade gliomas on PET images. Clin Nucl Med 2019;44(4): 265–71.
22. Özütemiz C, Neil EC, Tanwar M, et al. The role of dual-phase FDG PET/CT in the diagnosis and follow-up of brain tumors. Am J Roentgenol 2020; 215(4):985–96.
23. Galldiks N, Lohmann P, Aboian M, et al. Update to the RANO working group and EANO recommendations for the clinical use of PET imaging in gliomas. Lancet Oncol 2025;26(8):e436–47.
24. Okada H, Weller M, Huang R, et al. Immunotherapy response assessment in neuro-oncology: a report of the RANO working group. Lancet Oncol 2015;16-(15):e534–42.
25. Galldiks N, Langen KJ, Albert NL, et al. PET imaging in patients with brain metastasis—report of the RANO/PET group. Neuro Oncol 2019;21(5):585–95.
26. Verger A, Tolboom N, Cicone F, et al. Joint EANM/EANO/RANO/SNMMI practice guideline/procedure standard for PET imaging of brain metastases: version 1.0. Eur J Nucl Med Mol Imag 2025;52(5): 1822–39.
27. Horky LL, Hsiao EM, Weiss SE, et al. Dual phase FDG-PET imaging of brain metastases provides superior assessment of recurrence versus post-treatment necrosis. J Neuro Oncol 2011;103(1): 137–46.
28. Liu Y, Ding H, Cao J, et al. [68Ga]Ga-FAPI PET/CT in brain tumors: comparison with [18F]F-FDG PET/CT. Front Oncol 2024;14:1436009.
29. Sadeghpour S, Aghaee A, Ahmadzadehfar H, et al. Revealing the hidden: a systematic review and meta-analysis of FAPI-based tracers imaging for brain metastatic lesions. Eur J Nucl Med Mol Imag 2026;53(3):1419–33.
30. Chen H, Pang Y, Wu J, et al. Comparison of [68Ga] Ga-DOTA-FAPI-04 and [18F] FDG PET/CT for the diagnosis of primary and metastatic lesions in patients with various types of cancer. Eur J Nucl Med Mol Imag 2020;47(8):1820–32.
31. Lauw MIS, Lucas CHG, Ohgami RS, et al. Primary central nervous system lymphomas: a diagnostic overview of key histomorphologic, immunophenotypic, and genetic features. Diagnostics 2020;10-(12):1076.
32. Rozenblum L, Houillier C, Baptiste A, et al. Interim FDG-PET improves treatment failure prediction in primary central nervous system lymphoma: an LOC network prospective multicentric study. Neuro Oncol 2024;26(7):1292–301.
33. Rozenblum L, Houillier C, Soussain C, et al. Role of positron emission tomography in primary central nervous system lymphoma. Cancers 2022;14(17): 4071.
34. Verger A, Couturier O. Rôle de la TEP en neuro-oncologie : apport des traceurs FDG, aux acides aminés et des récepteurs de la somatostatine dans la prise en charge des tumeurs cérébrales. Med Nucl 2025;49(6):325–9.
35. Rozenblum L, Galanaud D, Houillier C, et al. [18F] FDG PET-MRI provides survival biomarkers in primary central nervous system lymphoma in the elderly: an ancillary study from the BLOCAGE trial of the LOC network. Eur J Nucl Med Mol Imag 2023;50(12):3684–96.
36. Barajas RF, Politi LS, Anzalone N, et al. Consensus recommendations for MRI and PET imaging of primary central nervous system lymphoma: guideline statement from the International Primary CNS Lymphoma Collaborative Group (IPCG). Neuro Oncol 2021;23(7):1056–71.
37. Rachdi A, Hernandez-Tost H, Herzi D, et al. Recent advances in the diagnosis and the treatment of primary CNS lymphoma. Rev Neurol (Paris) 2023; 179(5):481–9.
38. Verger A, Albert NL, Brendel M, et al. EANM insights on PET-based response assessment in neuro-oncology: things are moving forward! EANM J 2025;1:100008.
39. Yarabarla V, Mylarapu A, Han TJ, et al. Intracranial meningiomas: an update of the 2021 World Health Organization classifications and review of management with a focus on radiation therapy. Front Oncol 2023;13:1137849.
40. Galldiks N, Albert NL, Sommerauer M, et al. PET imaging in patients with meningioma—report of the RANO/PET group. Neuro Oncol 2017;19(12): 1576–87.
41. Dutour A, Kumar U, Panetta R, et al. Expression of somatostatin receptor subtypes in human brain tumors. Int J Cancer 1998;76(5):620–7.
42. Albert NL, Preusser M, Traub-Weidinger T, et al. Joint EANM/EANO/RANO/SNMMI practice guideline/procedure standards for diagnostics and therapy (theranostics) of meningiomas using radiolabeled somatostatin receptor ligands: version 1.0. Eur J Nucl Med Mol Imag 2024;51(12):3662–79.
43. Galldiks N, Lohmann P, Albert NL, et al. Current status of PET imaging in neuro-oncology. Neuro-Oncol Adv 2019;1(1):vdz010.
44. Uslu L, Donig J, Link M, et al. Value of ^{18}F-FDG PET and PET/CT for Evaluationeof Pediatric palignancims. J Nucl Med 2015;56(2):274–86.
45. d'Amati A, Bargiacchi L, Rossi S, et al. Pediatric CNS tumors and 2021 WHO classification: what do

oncologists need from pathologists? Front Mol Neurosci 2024;17:1268038.
46. Piccardo A, Albert NL, Borgwardt L, et al. Joint EANM/SIOPE/RAPNO practice guidelines/SNMMI procedure standards for imaging of paediatric gliomas using PET with radiolabelled amino acids and [18F]FDG: version 1.0. Eur J Nucl Med Mol Imag 2022;49(11):3852–69.
47. Stanescu L, Ishak GE, Khanna PC, et al. FDG PET of the brain in pediatric patients: imaging spectrum with MR imaging correlation. Radiographics 2013; 33(5):1279–303.
48. Patil S, Biassoni L, Borgwardt L. Nuclear medicine in pediatric neurology and neurosurgery: Epilepsy and brain tumors. Semin Nucl Med 2007;37(5):357–81.
49. Sager G, Akgun E, Abuqbeitah M, et al. Comparison of brain F-18 FDG PET/MRI with PET/CT imaging in pediatric patients. Clin Neurol Neurosurg 2021;206:106669.
50. Aboian MS, ReisTeixeira S, Zhuang H, et al. Management of pediatric brain tumors with the aid of PET/MR imaging. Pet Clin 2026;21(2):229–43.
51. Antonevskaya TL, Yadgarov MYA, Likar YUN. Diagnostic and prognostic value of [18F] FET PET imaging in pediatric and adolescent brain tumors: a systematic review and meta-analysis. Clin Transl Imaging 2025;13(3):283–301.
52. Safarian A, Mirshahvalad SA, Farbod A, et al. Artificial intelligence for tumor [18F]FDG PET imaging: advancements and future trends - part II. Semin Nucl Med 2025;55(5):856–68.

FDG-PET in Traumatic Brain Injury and Postconcussive Sequelae

Rizwan Naseer, MD[a], Melika Mirbod, MD[b], Yousr Hassan, MD[b], Abass Alavi, MD[c], Cyrus Ayubcha, MD, PhD[d,*]

KEYWORDS

• Traumatic brain injury • FDG PET • Brain metabolism • Chronic traumatic encephalopathy • Concussion • Neuroimaging • Tau PET • Amyloid PET

KEY POINTS

- Fluoro-D-glucose (FDG) PET reveals dynamic metabolic changes in traumatic brain injury (TBI), with early hypermetabolism followed by persistent hypometabolism.
- The extent and distribution of hypometabolism correlate with injury severity, repetition, and clinical outcomes.
- Repetitive TBI is associated with widespread metabolic dysfunction in frontal, temporal, limbic, and cerebellar regions.
- FDG remains the most validated PET tracer for TBI, while tau and amyloid imaging presently lack consistency for clinical use.
- Standardization of imaging protocols and longitudinal studies are needed to improve diagnostic and prognostic utility.

INTRODUCTION

Traumatic brain injury (TBI) affects millions of people worldwide and can lead to a wide range of outcomes, from subtle cognitive deficits to coma or a persistent vegetative state. TBIs are a leading cause of disorders of consciousness (DOC); recent advances in neuroimaging and refined clinical assessment tools are driving targeted therapies aimed at accelerating recovery and improving functional outcomes.[1]

TBI affects all populations, but certain groups have disproportionately high rates of mild TBI (mTBI), including military personnel, athletes, and individuals involved in road traffic accidents.[2] Military service members have a higher prevalence of mTBI than civilians, with injuries resulting from both blast and nonblast mechanisms.[3] In sports, concussions contribute substantially to the overall TBI burden, particularly in contact sports such as football, ice hockey, and soccer, which have the highest incidence per exposure. Millions of sport-related concussions occur annually in the United States, and repetitive head impacts increase the risk of subsequent injury.[4] Athletes with prior concussions are more likely to sustain additional ones, and evidence also indicates sex differences in sports-related concussion, with female athletes demonstrating a higher incidence and, in some cases, prolonged symptoms.[5] Beyond military and athletic contexts, road traffic collisions remain a leading global cause of TBIs.

TBI typically results from heterogeneous, multifocal damage affecting the cerebral hemispheres

[a] Department of Medicine, Trinity Health System, Steubenville, OH, USA; [b] Department of Radiology, Hospital of the University of Pennsylvania, Philadelphia, PA, USA; [c] Division of Nuclear Medicine, Department of Radiology, Hospital of the University of Pennsylvania, University of Pennsylvania Perelman School of Medicine, Philadelphia, PA, USA; [d] Department of Neurosurgery, University of California San Diego, San Diego, CA, USA
* Corresponding author. 9500 Hilman Drive, La Jolla, CA 92093.
E-mail address: CyrusAyubcha@hms.harvard.edu

PET Clin 21 (2026) 521–531
https://doi.org/10.1016/j.cpet.2026.05.006

Abbreviations

[18F]FDG	2-deoxy2-(18F)fluoro-D-glucose
ADNI	Alzheimer's disease Neuroimaging Initiative
Aβ	amyloid-beta
CTE	chronic traumatic encephalopathy
DAI	diffuse axonal injury
FDG	fluoro-D-glucose
FIM	Functional Independence Measure
FIM-c	the cognitive component of the FIM
FIM-m	the motor component of the FIM
GCS	Glasgow Coma Scale
GOS-E	Glasgow Outcome Scale–Extended
mTBI	mild TBI
sTBI	severe TBI
TBI	traumatic brain injury

and brainstem. Biomechanically, rapid head movements generate inertial forces that produce strain and deformation throughout brain tissue. Rotational motion, in particular, induces shear deformation that strongly correlates with injury risk.[6] The brain is more sensitive to rotational than linear acceleration, as rotational forces create widespread tissue strain extending beyond the site of impact.[7] Evidence from sports and other impact settings shows that rotational acceleration frequently exceeds thresholds associated with mTBI, reinforcing its role in diffuse tissue deformation and clinical symptoms. Although linear acceleration contributes to head kinematics, rotational acceleration generates greater shear strain within the brain parenchyma, underlying many of the structural and neurophysiological changes observed after mTBI.[5]

Accordingly, TBI is broadly divided into primary and secondary injury phases based on timing and mechanisms.[7] Primary brain injury occurs at the moment of impact and involves direct mechanical damage, such as contusions, vascular disruption, and diffuse axonal injury (DAI) from rotational shearing, that cannot be reversed. These acceleration–deceleration injuries can also lead to intracranial hemorrhages.[1] The first 60 minutes after injury are especially critical, as prompt medical intervention during this period can significantly influence survival and recovery outcomes.[8] Secondary brain injury develops hours to days later, driven by biochemical cascades such as neuroinflammation, cerebral edema, increased intracranial pressure, ischemia, or hemorrhage, which can further exacerbate neurologic outcomes.[9]

The Glasgow Coma Scale (GCS) remains the standard clinical tool for assessing consciousness after trauma and classifies TBI severity as mild, moderate, or severe based on neurologic responsiveness.[10] Most TBIs, specifically those with a GCS score between 13 and 15, are considered mild and represent the majority of clinical cases.[10] Still, individuals may experience persistent concussive symptoms such as cognitive impairments, fatigue, headaches, and mood disturbances like depression or irritability.[11] However, the GCS has limitations. It does not stratify underlying biomechanical or pathophysiological processes well and can be unreliable in sedated or intubated patients.[12]

TBI is associated with significant long-term neurologic consequences. Posttraumatic epilepsy accounts for approximately 10% to 20% of acquired epilepsy cases, most commonly emerging within 2 years of injury.[13] Disruption of the blood–brain barrier and persistent neuroinflammatory responses contribute to heightened neuronal excitability and seizure susceptibility, though the precise mechanisms remain incompletely defined.[14] Another common complication is posttraumatic headache, which can be acute or chronic and is among the most prevalent and persistent symptoms following injury, often leading to pain, functional impairment, and decreased quality of life.[15] Repetitive head impacts or severe TBI (sTBI) is also linked to chronic traumatic encephalopathy (CTE), a progressive neurodegenerative condition thought to involve abnormal tau protein accumulation, neuroinflammation, and axonal injury.[15] The high prevalence of these outcomes underscores the importance of early recognition, mechanistic understanding, and targeted therapy in TBI care.

Brain imaging plays a critical role in evaluating TBI, providing objective data that complements clinical assessment. Beyond standard structural imaging, molecular imaging, particularly PET, is being increasingly used to study injury mechanisms and guide prognosis. PET imaging employs 3 main categories of radiotracers in this context: [18F]FDG tracers assess cerebral glucose metabolism, identifying regions of altered neuronal activity after injury; tau-specific tracers visualize neurofibrillary tangles associated with chronic neurodegeneration linked with CTE; and amyloid tracers target amyloid-beta (Aβ) plaques linked to cognitive decline and long-term neuropathology.

[18F]FDG-PET IMAGING

[18F]FDG is the most common PET tracer used in modern-day metabolic imaging. It is a glucose analog with a positron-emitting radionuclide fluorine-18 substituted for the normal hydroxyl group at the C-2 position in the glucose molecule.[16] The uptake of [18F]FDG by cells is directly associated with cellular glycolysis, and this characteristic is employed to assess metabolism. Since its development in the early 1970s, it has been verified as a tracer able to reflect metabolic activity and has been extensively used in neuroimaging.[17]

[18F]FDG-PET IMAGING IN SINGLE-EVENT TRAUMATIC BRAIN INJURY

Early PET studies of mTBI using [18F]FDG assessed regional metabolism and cerebral blood flow.[18–23] These studies demonstrate that metabolic patterns vary with time since injury and mechanism of injury.[24] In the hyperacute phase, TBI is often characterized by hypermetabolism, reflecting excitotoxic activity, followed by hypometabolism in the subacute phase, indicating functional impairment.[25–27] Interestingly, recent animal studies have shown that regional time courses may differ; for example, a single mTBI induced a transient increase in [18F]FDG uptake in the amygdala and somatosensory cortex with a gradual return to baseline within a week after injury, but a sustained elevation in uptake across the motor cortex was observed.[28] In chronic stages, hypometabolism predominates, consistent with structural damage and neurodegeneration[29–34] (**Fig. 1**).

Studies of sTBI using [18F]FDG have shown localized hypermetabolism within the first month after injury.[35] More broadly, [18F]FDG imaging identifies an acute phase of hypermetabolism lasting up to approximately 6 hours in moderate TBI and sTBI, whereas in mTBI, this hypermetabolic response appears to be limited to the immediate postinjury period.[36]

Increased [18F]FDG uptake in the days to months following sTBI has been associated with greater clinical improvement and better long-term outcomes.[37,38] Overall, [18F]FDG imaging indicates that hypometabolism is a hallmark of TBI across all severities, with both the magnitude and duration of metabolic reduction correlating with injury severity[36,39] (**Figs. 2** and **3**).

[18F]FDG-PET IMAGING IN REPEAT TRAUMATIC BRAIN INJURY AND LONG-TERM SEQUELAE

Applications of [18F]FDG imaging in repeated mTBI remain limited but provide important insights. In an animal study, Selwyn and colleagues[40] showed that shorter intervals between repeated impacts led to increased neuronal degeneration and greater microglial and astrocyte activation. In humans, Bang and colleagues[41] reported reduced [18F]FDG uptake in the bilateral dorsolateral prefrontal cortices and right middle

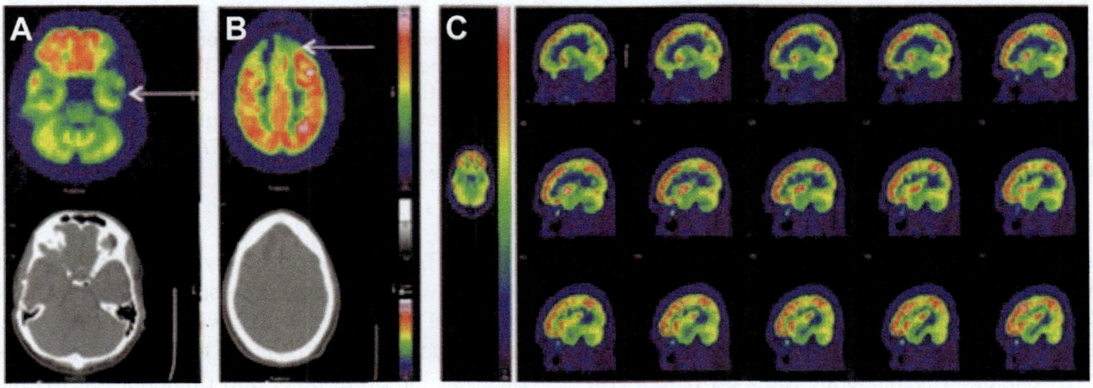

Fig. 1. (*A–C*) Clinical [18F]FDG-PET scans from 3 patients with traumatic brain injury. (*A*) A 25 year old man with one moderate, nonblast TBI underwent imaging 5 months after the event. There was no documented use of medication, sleep disturbance, headache or pain, or visual complaint. The scan demonstrates reduced metabolic activity in the left temporal region, corresponding to mild tissue loss/encephalomalacia visible on CT. (*B*) A 28 year old man with 1 severe, nonblast TBI was scanned 12.5 months after injury. No medication use, sleep disturbance, headache or pain, or visual complaint was documented. The PET study reveals more extensive trauma, with marked frontal metabolic reduction (*arrow*) corresponding to encephalomalacia. (*C*) A 35 year old man with repeated blast-related mild TBIs was imaged 43 months after injury. He was taking the pain medication Ultram and reported mild bodily pain and moderate sleep disturbance; CT showed no abnormalities. The PET scan demonstrates marked frontal metabolic elevation, which could be related to medication use. The scale shown in (*C*) applies to all panels, with red indicating higher [18F]FDG accumulation. (*From* Image reprinted without changes from Byrnes KR et al.[88] Under the Creative Commons Attribution 4.0 International License (CC BY). https://creativecommons.org/licenses/by/4.0/.)

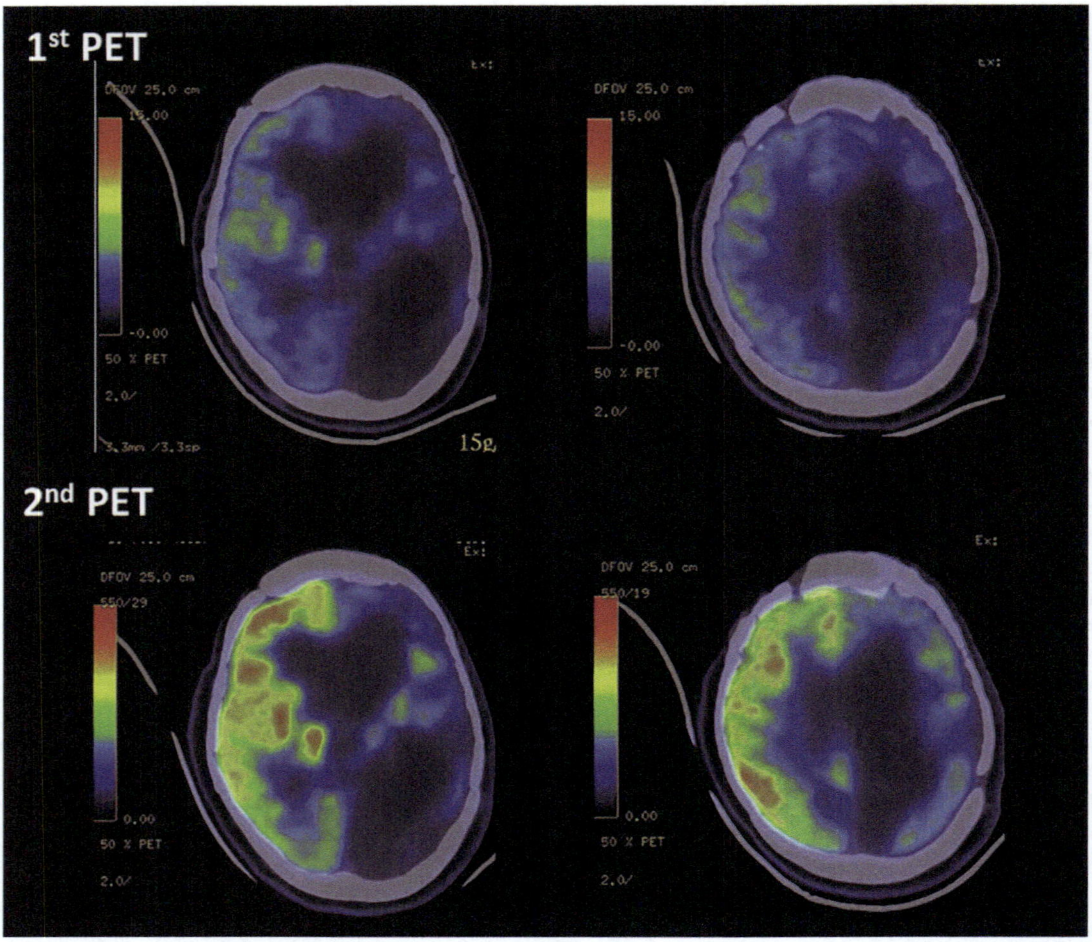

Fig. 2. At both evaluated time points, patients with moderate-to-severe TBI showed higher [18F]FDG uptake on the hemisphere corresponding to the site of injury. On average, the first [18F]FDG PET/CT scan was performed 782 days after the traumatic event during a prolonged hospitalization period. The second scan followed after a mean interval of 657 days. (*From* Yamaki T, Uchino Y, Henmi H, et al. Increased brain glucose metabolism in chronic severe traumatic brain injury as determined by longitudinal 18F-FDG PET/CT. J Clin Neurosci 2018;57:20–25. https://doi.org/10.1016/j.jocn.2018.08.052; Reproduced with permission.[89])

orbitofrontal cortex of boxers, with higher uptake in these regions correlating with better visuospatial performance. Similarly, Buchsbaum and colleagues[42] found that veterans with repeated mTBI exhibited significantly reduced global [18F] FDG uptake compared to controls. Peskind and colleagues[43] were the first to demonstrate hypometabolism in the cerebellum and medial temporal lobe in veterans exposed to repetitive blast injuries. In a recent clinicopathological series of those with repetitive mTBI, antemortem [18F] FDG-PET patients showed glucose hypometabolism that generally paralleled structural atrophy, most prominently in the thalamus (4 out of 5), medial temporal/limbic regions (4 out of 5), and left dorsal frontal cortex (3 out of 5), with no other regions consistently affected.[44] In a recent [18F] FDG-PET/MR imaging study of retired soccer players, worse performance on phonemic/semantic verbal fluency correlated with reduced regional brain glucose metabolism in the right hippocampus, left temporal pole, and posterior left middle temporal gyrus, where cognitive performance was similarly related to decreased uptake in the left temporal pole, and posterior left middle temporal gyrus.[45] Consistent with these findings, Meabon and colleagues[46] observed that increasing numbers of mTBIs were associated with greater neuronal loss, microglial activation, diffusion abnormalities, cognitive and sensorimotor impairment, and reduced cerebellar [18F] FDG uptake in the chronic phase (**Fig. 4**).

The timing of imaging also influences observed metabolic patterns. Cummins and colleagues[47]

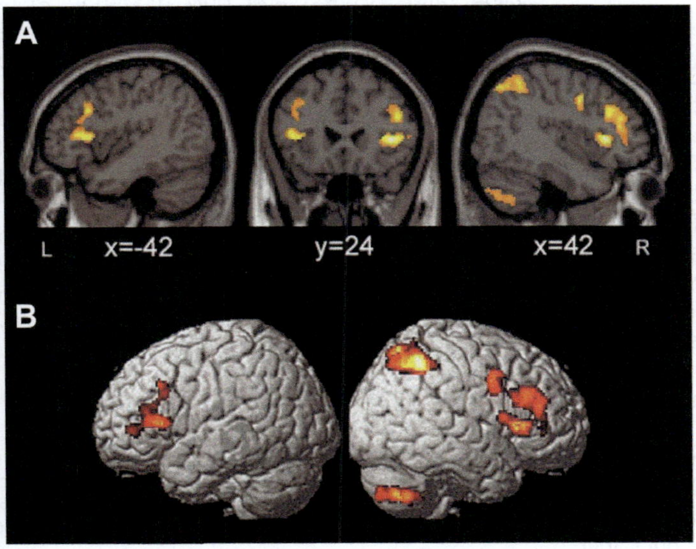

Fig. 3. (*A, B*) Areas showing elevated glucose utilization on [18F]FDG PET in individuals with traumatic brain injury following rehabilitation are presented in sagittal and coronal views (*A*) and in 3 dimensional reconstructions (*B*). (*From* Image reprinted without changes from Pingue V et al.[90] Under the Creative Commons Attribution 4.0 International License (CC BY). https://creativecommons.org/licenses/by/4.0/.)

found no significant differences in [18F]FDG uptake after adjusting for covariates in veterans with a remote history of mild-to-severe TBI. In single-event mTBI, chronic symptoms, including memory, cognitive, auditory, and sensorimotor deficits, have also been evaluated with [18F]FDG imaging. Umile and colleagues[48] reported reduced uptake in the temporal lobes and hippocampus, which correlated with poorer memory performance. In patients with persistent cognitive and psychiatric symptoms after concussion, Komura and colleagues[49] observed decreased prefrontal activity alongside increased limbic uptake, potentially linked to depressive symptoms. Finally, Kato and colleagues[50] found reduced metabolism in the bilateral frontal and temporal lobes, thalamus, and cerebellum in patients with DAI 6 months postinjury, while metabolic activity in the right cingulate gyrus and bilateral medial frontal gyrus correlated positively with intelligence scores.

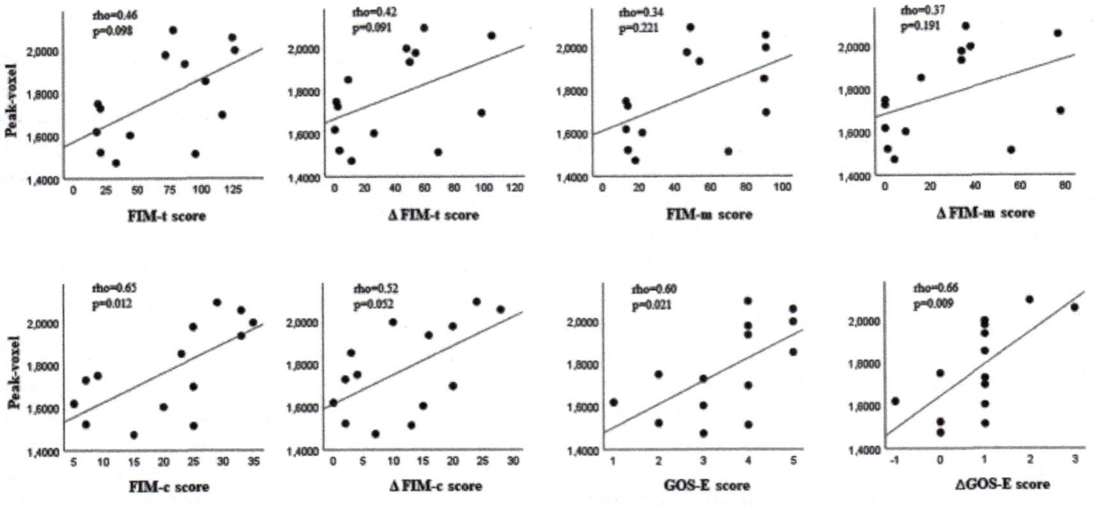

Fig. 4. Associations between resting glucose utilization in the right precentral gyrus and rehabilitation outcomes in patients with traumatic brain injury. Shown are the relationships between [18F]FDG PET measures of baseline glucose uptake in the right precentral gyrus and status at discharge, expressed both as absolute totals and as change from before to after treatment on the following measures: the Functional Independence Measure (FIM), the motor component of the FIM (FIM-m), the cognitive component of the FIM (FIM-c), and the Glasgow Outcome Scale–Extended (GOS-E). (*From* Image reprinted without changes from Pingue V et al.[90] Under the Creative Commons Attribution 4.0 International License (CC BY). https://creativecommons.org/licenses/by/4.0/.)

[18F]FDG-PET IMAGING UTILITY FOR DIAGNOSIS

CTE is rarely imaged using [18F]FDG PET. The current diagnosis of CTE requires confirmation at postmortem examination. Among the limited available studies, a comparative analysis of [18F]FDG PET imaging of 15 boxers with a history of repeated TBI when compared to 7 healthy subjects found decreased uptake in the cingulate cortex, parieto–occipital and frontal lobes bilaterally, posterior cingulate cortex, and cerebellum.[51] Despite this, [18F]FDG remains the most reliable tracer in reflecting metabolic abnormalities in TBI; however, it has the limitation of being nonspecific to various injury processes in mTBI. The inflammatory processes and cellular dysfunction in mTBI can simultaneously present in tissues due to other diseases or the normal aging process, and in these cases, [18F] FDG PET will not reflect a single process but rather the combined magnitude of such processes.[35] Moreover, the assessment of small regions of the brain is difficult to make accurate or otherwise replicate, given the fundamental resolution of PET imaging.[52] The inconsistencies in the [18F]FDG PET imaging can be due to heterogeneities among patients or possibly due to mTBI affecting different regions of the brain, leading to changes in corresponding regions only.[53]

TAU-PET IMAGING

Tau is a microtubule-associated phosphoprotein that, when hyperphosphorylated, forms neurofibrillary tangles implicated in tauopathies and mTBI-related CTE.[54] In CTE, tau deposition appears to start in the medial temporal lobe and spread along default mode cortical regions, with relatively little subcortical involvement.[55–57] Early tau-PET with fluorine-18 2-(1-{6-[(2-[F-18]fluoroethyl)(methyl) amino]-2-naphthyl}ethylidene)malononitrile ([18F] FDDNP) lacked sufficient specificity and selectivity,[58] prompting development of newer tracers (eg, 18FMK6240/florquinitau, 18FRO948, 18FPI2620, 18FGTP1, and 18FJNJ64326067), including in silico–derived candidates such as CNS4, mainly for neurodegenerative disease but now applied to TBI.[59–61] Across studies, tauPET uptake often aligns with known tau-rich regions but also shows off target or nonspecific binding, including monoamine oxidase A (MAOA) and hemorrhagic/blood product–related signal,[55,60,62–64] and CTE/mTBI results are heterogeneous: some cohorts of former football players or patients with TBI show little or no group level tau-PET elevation, while others show modest, regionally restricted increases with overlapping standardized uptake value ratio (SUVRs) and only moderate PET–pathology correlations.[56,65–70] Alzheimer's disease Neuroimaging Initiative (ADNI)-based and mixed cohort analyses further suggest that head injury or TBI history may be associated with higher tau burden and worse cognition in subsets of impaired or amyloid positive individuals, but without establishing a CTE-specific pattern.[71,72] Overall, tau is a promising biological marker to distinguish CTE from Alzheimer's disease and healthy controls, but current tau tracers remain inconsistent and incompletely validated in CTE-related tauopathies.[56,66,68]

AMYLOID-PET IMAGING

Aβ consists of 36 to 43 amino acid fragments that, when abnormally accumulated, form toxic plaques implicated in synaptic dysfunction and neuronal death.[73] Because Aβ deposition in typical mTBI and CTE is extremely low,[74] Aβ PET tracers such as Carbon-11 Pittsburgh Compound-B ([11C]PiB), [18F]florbetapir, and [18F]FDDNP (which also binds tau) have limited applicability. [11C]PiB and [18F] florbetapir show off target binding and relatively low binding efficiency at in vivo imaging concentrations.[75] Most CTE studies, including DIAGNOSE CTE, report no significant differences in [18F]florbetapir uptake between exposed and control groups, with only occasional reports of small regional increases.[76–79] Technical constraints (small target regions, partial volume effects, and short [11C] half-life) and minimal true Aβ burden further reduce sensitivity and reproducibility.[52,75] Overall, Aβ PET has not proven reliable for diagnosing or staging CTE, though larger observational and ADNI-based datasets in Veterans and older adults indicate that remote TBI or head injury history may interact with amyloid burden, when present, to confer earlier cognitive impairment, greater cortical thinning, or faster decline.[78–82]

AMYLOID-PET AND TAU-PET IMAGING IN TRAUMATIC BRAIN INJURY POPULATIONS

Recent amyloid and tau imaging studies in TBI populations suggest a unique biomarker signature in assessing long-term effects of traumatic insults. In a cross-sectional PET study of long-term survivors of a single moderate-to-severe TBI, Hicks and colleagues[83] found no significant increase in global Aβ burden or regional tau uptake compared with controls, and neither amyloid nor tau burden was associated with time since injury or age at injury. Similarly, de Bruin and colleagues[84] reported that Vietnam War veterans with prior TBI did not show higher global Aβ or tau-PET signal overall, although they demonstrated altered regional distributions, with relatively greater Aβ and tau deposition in fronto-parietal regions and altered amyloid–tau coupling patterns compared to veterans without TBI.

In a study of a younger (mean age of 40 years) cohort of 23 subjects at risk for trauma-related neurodegeneration after repeated TBIs, Eagle and colleagues[85] found no group differences in Aβ PET, tau-PET, MR imaging volumetrics, plasma biomarkers, or neurocognitive outcomes despite substantially greater symptom burden. These findings have motivated large longitudinal initiatives, including the DIAGNOSE CTE Research Project and the Boston University Alzheimer's Disease Research Center Clinical Core, which were established to refine in vivo fluid and neuroimaging biomarkers and to better characterize the clinical and biological features of posttraumatic neurodegeneration and CTE across exposed populations.[86,87]

In acute TBI settings, there is protein elevation and significant PET detectable biomarker activity, but amyloid and tau-based PET imaging in chronic TBI cases have yielded mixed results, showing limited correlation with long-term deposition or specific protein burden. The progression to chronic, PET-identifiable lesions is not yet fully understood, which highlights the necessity for more longitudinal studies. Notably, Tau-PET is emerging as a critical tool for identifying specific CTE-related tauopathy. Although the current clinical utility in TBI remains limited, both tau and amyloid-based PET imaging serve as effective research tools for developing and understanding imaging-detectable patterns of TBI (**Fig. 5**).

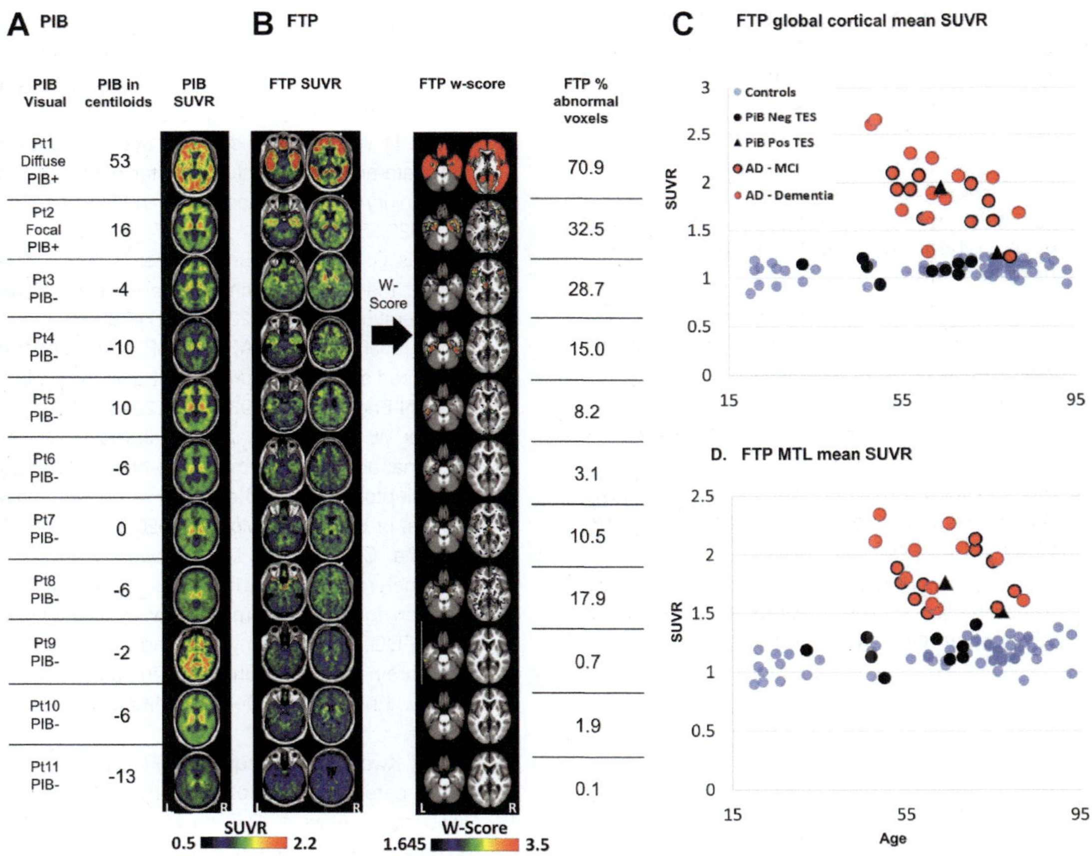

Fig. 5. (*A–C*) Panel A presents [11C]PiB amyloid scans, including qualitative readouts, Centiloid measurements, and SUVR maps. Panel B shows [18F]FTP tau data as SUVR maps, w-score maps, and the proportion of voxels exceeding a w-score threshold of 1.645. Panel C displays average FTP SUVR, and panel D shows average medial temporal lobe SUVR, for participants with TES (*black triangles* indicating PiB-positive cases; *black circles* indicating PiB-negative cases), alongside individuals with MCI (*red circles with black borders*), Alzheimer's disease dementia (*solid red circles*), and cognitively normal controls (*blue circles*). (*From* Lesman-Segev OH, La Joie R, Stephens ML, et al. Tau PET and multimodal brain imaging in patients at risk for chronic traumatic encephalopathy. NeuroImage Clin 2019;24:102025. https://doi.org/10.1016/j.nicl.2019.102025; Reproduced with permission.[91])

SUMMARY

PET imaging in TBI remains an evolving field, with significant limitations in the current literature. Most studies are observational, cross-sectional, and underpowered, with substantial heterogeneity in injury severity, mechanisms, and timing of imaging. The lack of standardized clinical and imaging timelines, along with inadequate adjustment for confounding factors such as age, sex, and comorbidities, further limits interpretation. In CTE, diagnosis still relies on postmortem histopathology, and variability in exposure to repetitive head impacts complicates study comparisons.

Overall, there is a need for standardized diagnostic criteria and larger, well-controlled studies to better define TBI and CTE. Current evidence does not yet support the widespread clinical use of tau and Aβ radiotracers, whereas [18F] FDG remains the most validated tracer for assessing metabolic changes. Development of more specific radiotracers may enable earlier detection of chronic sequelae and improve clinical management.

CLINICS CARE POINTS

- FDG PET can detect metabolic abnormalities even when structural imaging appears normal.
- Chronic hypometabolism is a hallmark of TBI and correlates with cognitive and functional impairment.
- Repetitive head trauma is associated with more widespread and persistent metabolic deficits.
- PET findings must be interpreted cautiously due to lack of specificity and overlap with other conditions.
- Tau and amyloid PET imaging are currently research tools and should not be used routinely in clinical TBI evaluation.

DISCLOSURE

No disclosures.

REFERENCES

1. Johnson-Black PH, Carlson JM, Vespa PM. Traumatic brain injury and disorders of consciousness. Handb Clin Neurol 2025;207:75–96.
2. Meshberg-Cohen S, Cook JM, Fischer IC, et al. Mild traumatic brain injury in U.S. military veterans: results from the National Health and Resilience in Veterans Study. Psychiatry 2024;87(4):314–28.
3. Phipps H, Mondello S, Wilson A, et al. Characteristics and impact of U.S. military blast-related mild traumatic brain injury: a systematic review. Front Neurol 2020;11:559318.
4. Daneshvar DH, Nowinski CJ, McKee AC, et al. The epidemiology of sport-related concussion. Clin Sports Med 2011;30(1):1–vii.
5. Tierney GJ. Concussion biomechanics, head acceleration exposure and brain injury criteria in sport: a review. Sports Biomech 2022;23(11):1888–916.
6. Lota KS, Malliaropoulos N, Blach W, et al. Rotational head acceleration and traumatic brain injury in combat sports: a systematic review. Br Med Bull 2022; 141(1):33–46.
7. Kleiven S. Why most traumatic brain injuries are not caused by linear acceleration but skull fractures are. Front Bioeng Biotechnol 2013;1:15.
8. Lerner EB, Moscati RM. The golden hour: scientific fact or medical "urban legend". Acad Emerg Med 2001;8(7):758–60.
9. Kinoshita K. Traumatic brain injury: pathophysiology for neurocritical care. J Intensiv Care 2016;4:29.
10. Ginsberg J, Smith T. Traumatic brain injury. In: StatPearls. StatPearls Publishing; 2025.
11. Hume CH, Wright BJ, Kinsella GJ. Systematic review and meta-analysis of outcome after mild traumatic brain injury in older people. J Int Neuropsychol Soc 2022;28(7):736–55.
12. Andraos C, Siddiqi A, Brazdzionis J, et al. Limitations of the Glasgow coma scale: challenges and considerations. Cureus 2025;17(2):e78900.
13. Annegers JF, Hauser WA, Coan SP, et al. A population-based study of seizures after traumatic brain injuries. N Engl J Med 1998;338(1):20–4.
14. Löscher W, Friedman A. Structural, molecular, and functional alterations of the blood-brain barrier during epileptogenesis and epilepsy: a cause, consequence, or both? Int J Mol Sci 2020;21(2):591.
15. Ayubcha C, Revheim M-E, Newberg A, et al. A critical review of radiotracers in the positron emission tomography imaging of traumatic brain injury: FDG, tau, and amyloid imaging in mild traumatic brain injury and chronic traumatic encephalopathy. Eur J Nucl Med Mol Imag 2021;48(2): 623–41.
16. Litt HK, Kwon DH, Velazquez AI. FDG PET scans in cancer care. JAMA Oncol 2023;9(9):1304.
17. Newberg A, Alavi A, Reivich M. Determination of regional cerebral function with FDG-PET imaging in neuropsychiatric disorders. Semin Nucl Med 2002; 32(1):13–34.
18. Alavi A, Alves W, Fazekas F, et al. Comparison of CT, MRI and PET brain imaging in acute head injury. J Nucl Med 1988;29:910.
19. George J, Alavi A, Zimmerman R, et al. Metabolic (PET) correlates of anatomic lesions (CT/MRI) produced by head trauma. J Nucl Med 1989;30:802.

20. Alves WM, Langfitt TW, Alavi A, et al. Sensitivity and specificity of CT, MRI and PET in head injury. J Cereb Blood Flow Metab 1987;7:629.
21. Alavi A, Uzzell BP, Kuhl DE, et al. Radionuclide and computed tomography scans in evaluation of head injury patients. J Nucl Med 1977;18:614.
22. Martinez F, Kim CK, Alavi A, et al. Cerebellar hypometabolism after head trauma: functional imaging with fluorine-18 FDG PET. J Nucl Med 1987; 28:699.
23. Fazekas F, Alavi A, Alves W, et al. Assessment of cerebral glucose metabolism in head trauma by positron emission tomography (PET). Neurology 1978;37:326.
24. Giarratana AO. From imaging to intervention: emerging potential of PET biomarkers to shape therapeutic strategies for TBI-induced neurodegeneration. Front Neurol 2025;16:1637243.
25. Marklund N, Sihver S, Hovda DA, et al. Increased cerebral uptake of [18F]fluoro- deoxyglucose but not [1-14C]glucose early following traumatic brain injury in rats. J Neurotrauma 2009;26(8):1281–93.
26. Marklund N, Sihver S, Långström B, et al. Effect of traumatic brain injury and nitrone radical scavengers on relative changes in regional cerebral blood flow and glucose uptake in rats. J Neurotrauma 2002;19(10):1139–53.
27. Langfitt TW, Obrist WD, Alavi A, et al. Computerized tomography, magnetic resonance imaging, and positron emission tomography in the study of brain trauma: preliminary observations. J Neurosurg 1986;64(5):760–7.
28. Li Y, Liu K, Li C, et al. 18F-FDG PET combined with MR spectroscopy elucidates the progressive metabolic cerebral alterations after blast-induced mild traumatic brain injury in rats. Front Neurosci 2021; 15:593723.
29. Brabazon F, Wilson CM, Shukla DK, et al. [18F]FDG-PET combined with MRI elucidates the pathophysiology of traumatic brain injury in rats. J Neurotrauma 2017;34(5):1074–85.
30. Selwyn R, Hockenbury N, Jaiswal S, et al. Mild traumatic brain injury results in depressed cerebral glucose uptake: an 18FDG PET study. J Neurotrauma 2013;30(23):1943–53.
31. Liu YR, Cardamone L, Hogan RE, et al. Progressive metabolic and structural cerebral perturbations after traumatic brain injury: an in vivo imaging study in the rat. J Nucl Med 2010;51(11):1788–95.
32. Stocker RP, Cieply MA, Paul B, et al. Combat-related blast exposure and traumatic brain injury influence brain glucose metabolism during REM sleep in military veterans. Neuroimage 2014;99:207–14.
33. Vaquero J, Zurita M, Bonilla C, et al. Progressive increase in brain glucose metabolism after intrathecal administration of autologous mesenchymal stromal cells in patients with diffuse axonal injury. Cytotherapy 2017;19(1):88–94.
34. Wu H-M, Huang S-C, Hattori N, et al. Selective metabolic reduction in gray matter acutely following human traumatic brain injury. J Neurotrauma 2004; 21(2):149–61.
35. Bergsneider M, Hovda DA, Shalmon E, et al. Cerebral hyperglycolysis following severe traumatic brain injury in humans: a positron emission tomography study. J Neurosurg 1997;86(2):241–51.
36. Byrnes KR, Wilson CM, Brabazon F, et al. FDG-PET imaging in mild traumatic brain injury: a critical review. Front Neuroenerg 2014;5:13.
37. Yamaki T, Imahori Y, Ohmori Y, et al. Cerebral hemodynamics and metabolism of severe diffuse brain injury measured by PET. J Nucl Med 1996;37(7): 1166–70.
38. Worley G, Hoffman JM, Paine SS, et al. 18-Fluorodeoxyglucose positron emission tomography in children and adolescents with traumatic brain injury. Dev Med Child Neurol 1995;37(3):213–20.
39. Bergsneider M, Hovda DA, Lee SM, et al. Dissociation of cerebral glucose metabolism and level of consciousness during the period of metabolic depression following human traumatic brain injury. J Neurotrauma 2000;17(5):389–401.
40. Selwyn RG, Cooney SJ, Khayrullina G, et al. Outcome after repetitive mild traumatic brain injury is temporally related to glucose uptake profile at time of second injury. J Neurotrauma 2016;33(15): 1479–91.
41. Bang SA, Song YS, Moon BS, et al. Neuropsychological, metabolic, and GABAA receptor studies in subjects with repetitive traumatic brain injury. J Neurotrauma 2016;33(11):1005–14.
42. Buchsbaum MS, Simmons AN, DeCastro A, et al. Clusters of low 18F-fluorodeoxyglucose uptake voxels in combat veterans with traumatic brain injury and post-traumatic stress disorder. J Neurotrauma 2015;32(22):1736–50.
43. Peskind ER, Petrie EC, Cross DJ, et al. Cerebrocerebellar hypometabolism associated with repetitive blast exposure mild traumatic brain injury in 12 Iraq war veterans with persistent post-concussive symptoms. Neuroimage 2011;54(Suppl. 1):S76–82.
44. Asken BM, Tanner JA, VandeVrede L, et al. Multimodal biomarkers of repetitive head impacts and traumatic encephalopathy syndrome: a clinicopathological case series. J Neurotrauma 2022;39(17–18):1195–213.
45. Aranha MR, Coutinho AM, Carneiro CG, et al. Brain glucose metabolism and gray matter volume in retired professional soccer players: a cross- sectional [18F] FDG-PET/MRI study. Arq Neuropsiquiatr 2023;81(5): 433–43.
46. Meabon JS, Huber BR, Cross DJ, et al. Repetitive blast exposure in mice and combat veterans causes persistent cerebellar dysfunction. Sci Transl Med 2016;8(321):321ra6.

47. Cummins TDR, Doré V, Feizpour A, et al. Tau, β-amyloid, and glucose metabolism following service-related traumatic brain injury in Vietnam war veterans: the Australian imaging biomarkers and lifestyle study of aging-veterans study (AIBL-VETS). J Neurotrauma 2023;40(11–12):1086–97.
48. Umile EM, Sandel ME, Alavi A, et al. Dynamic imaging in mild traumatic brain injury: support for the theory of medial temporal vulnerability. Arch Phys Med Rehabil 2002;83(11):1506–13.
49. Komura A, Kawasaki T, Yamada Y, et al. Cerebral glucose metabolism in patients with chronic mental and cognitive sequelae after a single blunt mild traumatic brain injury without visible brain lesions. J Neurotrauma 2019;36(5):641–9.
50. Kato T, Nakayama N, Yasokawa Y, et al. Statistical image analysis of cerebral glucose metabolism in patients with cognitive impairment following diffuse traumatic brain injury. J Neurotrauma 2007;24(6): 919–26.
51. Provenzano FA, Jordan B, Tikofsky RS, et al. F-18 FDG PET imaging of chronic traumatic brain injury in boxers: a statistical parametric analysis. Nucl Med Commun 2010;31(11):952–7.
52. Moghbel MC, Saboury B, Basu S, et al. Amyloid-β imaging with PET in Alzheimer's disease: is it feasible with current radiotracers and technologies? Eur J Nucl Med Mol Imag 2012;39(2):202–8.
53. Huang CX, Li YH, Lu W, et al. Positron emission tomography imaging for the assessment of mild traumatic brain injury and chronic traumatic encephalopathy: recent advances in radiotracers. Neural Regen Res 2022;17(1):74–81.
54. Iqbal K, Liu F, Gong C-X, et al. Tau in Alzheimer disease and related tauopathies. Curr Alzheimer Res 2010;7(8):656–64.
55. Leuzy A, Chiotis K, Lemoine L, et al. Tau PET imaging in neurodegenerative tauopathies—Still a challenge. Mol Psychiatr 2019;24:1112–34.
56. Barrio JR, Small GW, Wong K-P, et al. In vivo characterization of chronic traumatic encephalopathy using [F-18]FDDNP PET brain imaging. Proc Natl Acad Sci USA 2015;112(16):E2039–47.
57. Alosco ML, Mejía Pérez J, Culhane JE, et al. 18F-MK-6240 tau PET in patients at-risk for chronic traumatic encephalopathy. Mol Neurodegener 2025; 20(1):23.
58. Thompson PW, Ye L, Morgenstern JL, et al. Interaction of the amyloid imaging tracer FDDNP with hallmark Alzheimer's disease pathologies. J Neurochem 2009;109(2):623–30.
59. Tonietto M, Sotolongo-Grau O, Roé-Vellvé N, et al. Head-to-head comparison of tau PET tracers [18F]PI-2620 and [18F]RO948 in non-demented individuals with brain amyloid deposition: the TAU-PET FACEHBI cohort. Alzheimers Res Ther 2024; 16:257.
60. Butler T, Chiang GC, Niogi SN, et al. Tau PET following acute TBI: off-target binding to blood products, tauopathy, or both? Frontiers in Neuroimaging 2022;1:958558.
61. Qi B, Guan L, Tan J, et al. Identification of novel tau positron emission tomography tracers for chronic traumatic encephalopathy by comprehensive in silico screening and molecular dynamics simulation. Phys Chem Chem Phys 2025;27(2):754–67.
62. Villemagne VL, Furumoto S, Fodero-Tavoletti MT, et al. The challenges of tau imaging. Future Neurol 2012;7(4):409–21.
63. Villemagne VL, Okamura N. In vivo tau imaging: obstacles and progress. Alzheimer's Dement 2014; 10(3 Suppl.):S254–64.
64. Varlow C, Vasdev N. Evaluation of tau radiotracers in chronic traumatic encephalopathy. J Nucl Med 2023;64(3):460–5.
65. Dhaynaut M, Grashow R, Normandin MD, et al. Tau positron emission tomography and neurocognitive function among former professional american-style football players. J Neurotrauma 2023;40(15–16): 1614–24.
66. Su Y, Protas H, Luo J, et al. Flortaucipir tau PET findings from former professional and college American football players in the DIAGNOSE CTE research project. Alzheimer's Dement 2024;20:1827–38.
67. Vanderlinden G, Michiels L, Koole M, et al. Tau imaging in late traumatic brain injury: a [18F]MK-6240 positron emission tomography study. J Neurotrauma 2024;41(3–4):420–9.
68. Alosco ML, Su Y, Stein TD, et al, DIAGNOSE C. T. E. Research Project. Associations between near end-of-life flortaucipir PET and postmortem CTE-related tau neuropathology in six former American football players. Eur J Nucl Med Mol Imag 2023;50(2):435–52.
69. Marklund N, Vedung F, Lubberink M, et al. Tau aggregation and increased neuroinflammation in athletes after sports- related concussions and in traumatic brain injury patients: a PET/MR study. Neuroimage, Clin 2021;30:102665.
70. Krishnadas N, Doré V, Lamb F, et al. Case report: 18F-MK6240 tau positron emission tomography pattern resembling chronic traumatic encephalopathy in a retired Australian rules football player. Front Neurol 2020;11:598980.
71. Mohamed AZ, Cumming P, Nasrallah FA. Escalation of tau accumulation after a traumatic brain injury: findings from positron emission tomography. Brain Sci 2022;12(7):876.
72. Risacher SL, West JD, Deardorff R, et al. Head injury is associated with tau deposition on PET in MCI and AD patients. Alzheimer's Dement: Diagnosis, Assessment & Disease Monitoring 2021;13(1):e12230.
73. Sun X, Chen W-D, Wang Y-D. β-Amyloid: the key peptide in the pathogenesis of Alzheimer's disease. Front Pharmacol 2015;6:221.

74. Stern RA, Adler CH, Chen K, et al. Tau positron-emission tomography in former National Football League players. N Engl J Med 2019;380(18):1716–25.
75. Kepe V, Moghbel MC, Långström B, et al. Amyloid-β positron emission tomography imaging probes: a critical review. J Alzheimers Dis 2013;36(4):613–31.
76. Wang M-L, Wei X-E, Yu M-M, et al. Self-reported traumatic brain injury and in vivo measure of AD-vulnerable cortical thickness and AD- related biomarkers in the ADNI cohort. Neurosci Lett 2017; 655:115–20.
77. Mohamed AZ, Cumming P, Srour H, et al. Amyloid pathology fingerprint differentiates post-traumatic stress disorder and traumatic brain injury. Neuroimage, Clin 2018;19:716–26.
78. Stern RA, Trujillo-Rodriguez D, Tripodis Y, et al, DIAGNOSE CTE Research Project Investigators. Amyloid PET across the cognitive spectrum in former professional and college American football players: findings from the DIAGNOSE CTE research project. Alzheimers Res Ther 2023;15(1):166.
79. Leiva-Salinas C, Singh A, Layfield E, et al. Early brain amyloid accumulation at PET in military instructors exposed to subconcussive blast injuries. Radiology 2023;307(5):e221608.
80. Mohamed AZ, Nestor PJ, Cumming P, et al. Traumatic brain injury fast- forwards Alzheimer's pathology: evidence from amyloid positron emission tomography imaging. J Neurol 2022;269(2):873–84.
81. Thomas KR, Clark AL, Weigand AJ, et al. Cognition and amyloid-β in older veterans: characterization and longitudinal outcomes of data-derived phenotypes. J Alzheimers Dis 2024;99(1):417–27.
82. Turk KW, Marin A, Schiloski KA, et al. Head injury exposure in veterans presenting to memory disorders clinic: an observational study of clinical characteristics and relationship of event-related potentials and imaging markers. Front Neurol 2021;12:626767.
83. Hicks AJ, Ponsford JL, Spitz G, et al. β-Amyloid and tau imaging in chronic traumatic brain injury: a cross-sectional study. Neurology 2022;99(11):e1131–41.
84. de Bruin H, Groot C, Kamps S, et al. Amyloid-β and tau deposition in traumatic brain injury: a study of Vietnam war veterans. Brain Communications 2025; 7(1):fcaf009.
85. Eagle SR, Puccio A, Svirsky S, et al. Identifying a biological signature of trauma-related neurodegeneration following repeated traumatic brain injuries compared with healthy controls. Neurotrauma Reports 2025;6(1):560–8.
86. Alosco ML, Mariani ML, Adler CH, et al. Developing methods to detect and diagnose chronic traumatic encephalopathy during life: rationale, design, and methodology for the DIAGNOSE CTE research project. Alzheimers Res Ther 2021;13(1):136.
87. Alosco ML, Morrison M, Au R, et al. Boston University Alzheimer's Disease Research Center Clinical Core: infrastructure to facilitate research on post-traumatic Alzheimer's disease and related dementias. Alzheimer's Dement 2025;21(9):e70654.
88. Byrnes KR, Wilson CM, Brabazon F, et al. FDG-PET imaging in mild traumatic brain injury: a critical review. Front Neuroenerg 2014;5:13.
89. Yamaki T, Uchino Y, Henmi H, et al. Increased brain glucose metabolism in chronic severe traumatic brain injury as determined by longitudinal 18F-FDG PET/CT. J Clin Neurosci 2018;57:20–5.
90. Pingue V, Bossert I, D'Ambrosio D, et al. Brain glucose metabolism in patients with traumatic brain injury undergoing rehabilitation: a longitudinal 18F-FDG PET study. Front Neurol 2025;16:1556427.
91. Lesman-Segev OH, La Joie R, Stephens ML, et al. Tau PET and multimodal brain imaging in patients at risk for chronic traumatic encephalopathy. Neuroimage Clin 2019;24:102025.

Brain [18F]FDG-PET in Encephalitis and Postinfectious Neurocognitive Syndromes

Eric Guedj, MD, PhD[a,*], Tatiana Horowitz, MD, MSc[a],
Antoine Verger, MD, PhD[b]

KEYWORDS

• FDG PET • Autoimmune encephalitis • Viral encephalitis • Post-COVID condition • Long COVID • Postinfectious syndromes • Brain metabolism • Neuroinflammation

KEY POINTS

- Fluorodeoxyglucose (FDG) PET is a sensitive functional biomarker in autoimmune encephalitis and frequently detects abnormalities when MR imaging is normal or equivocal.
- In post-coronavirus infectious disease (COVID) condition and related postinfectious neurocognitive syndromes, FDG PET reveals hypometabolic patterns in selected patients, supporting objective cerebral dysfunction, differential diagnosis, and longitudinal assessment.
- Diagnostic value is highest when FDG PET is interpreted as a metabolic pattern rather than as an isolated regional abnormality.
- Interpretation requires careful consideration of clinical confounders, including age, medications, and seizure timing in encephalitis. When semiquantification is used, explicit attention should be paid to the normalization strategyand to the suitability of the normative database.
- Translocator protein (TSPO) PET provides complementary information on neuroimmune activation but currently remains a research-oriented adjunct.

INTRODUCTION

Both encephalitic disorders and post-infectious neurocognitive syndromes can present with substantial clinical impairment despite normal or equivocal structural imaging. In these settings, brain [18F]FDG PET can help bridge this gap by characterizing cerebral metabolism at regional and network levels, including functional abnormalities that may precede overt structural injury, extend beyond visible MR imaging lesions, or involve distributed patterns/networks poorly captured by routine anatomic sequences.[1–4]

The role of fluorodeoxyglucose (FDG) PET is therefore less to detect a focal lesion than to characterize a functional metabolic phenotype. FDG PET may then support the cerebral biological plausibility of a syndrome, refine differential diagnosis, and reduce uncertainty within a broader clinicobiological reasoning process.

This review focuses on 3 settings in which FDG PET has established, selective, or emerging practical relevance: autoimmune encephalitis (AE), viral encephalitis/infectious encephalopathy, and post-infectious neurocognitive syndromes, particularly post-coronavirus infectious disease (COVID)

[a] Aix-Marseille University (AMU), Department of Nuclear Medicine, Timone Hospital, IMoTheP Team, Institut Fresnel, Marseille, France; [b] Department of Nuclear Medicine, Nancyclotep Imaging Platform, IADI Laboratory, INSERM U1254, Université de Lorraine, Nancy, France
* Corresponding author. Laboratoire de Médecine Nucléaire, Hôpital de la Timone, 264 rue Saint Pierre, 13005 Marseille, France.
E-mail address: eric.guedj@univ-amu.fr

PET Clin 21 (2026) 533–540
https://doi.org/10.1016/j.cpet.2026.05.003

Abbreviation	
AE	autoimmune encephalitis

condition. The aim is deliberately pragmatic: to define where FDG PET adds value, where its role remains selective, and how results should be reported to avoid overattribution (**Table 1**). Complementary evidence from TSPO PET is also discussed, as it may help move the field from metabolic pattern recognition toward more explicit neuroimmune phenotyping.

AUTOIMMUNE ENCEPHALITIS

AE is the setting in which FDG PET currently has the strongest and most reproducible clinical rationale among inflammatory brain diseases. A systematic review and meta-analysis reported pooled sensitivity around 83%, exceeding that of MR imaging in several early or otherwise nondiagnostic presentations.[1] This is clinically relevant because AE often requires treatment decisions before structural imaging becomes unequivocal, and because antibody testing may be delayed, incomplete, or negative despite a highly compatible syndrome.[2,4] In practice, FDG PET is most valuable when AE is strongly suspected but not yet fully documented: when MR imaging is normal or equivocal, when antibody results are pending or negative, or when persistent or relapsing symptoms raise the question of active disease versus residual postinflammatory dysfunction.

The first contribution of FDG PET is increased sensitivity during the diagnostic window. Probasco and colleagues showed that abnormal brain metabolism is a common early finding in AE, supporting the use of PET when conventional investigations remain inconclusive.[5] Semiquantitative approaches may further improve reproducibility; for example, the cortex/striatum metabolic ratio proposed by De Leiris and colleagues captures one recurring AE signature.[6] Quantitative FDG PET can also support diagnostic confidence in seronegative AE when formal immunologic confirmation is missing.[7] PET should not replace clinical criteria, CSF, EEG, or antibody testing, but it may materially strengthen the probability of an autoimmune process. Of note, the Graus criteria acknowledge possible role of FDG PET for definite autoimmune limbic encephalitis, where medial temporal hypermetabolism may support the imaging criterion when MR imaging is normal.[4]

The second contribution is metabolic phenotyping. Anti-n-methyl-d-aspartate receptor (NMDAR) encephalitis has repeatedly been associated with an anteroposterior metabolic gradient, often combining relative frontotemporal hypermetabolism with posterior or occipital hypometabolism, although the balance varies with disease stage and treatment[8,9] (**Fig. 1**A). Anti-leucine-rich glioma inactivated protein 1 (LGI1) encephalitis frequently combines mesiotemporal and basal ganglia abnormalities, with a characteristic contrast between subcortical hypermetabolism and cortical hypometabolism[10,11] (**Fig. 1**B). Paraneoplastic limbic encephalitis associated with onconeural antibodies,

Table 1
Pragmatic clinical positioning of FDG PET in the main scenarios reviewed

Clinical Setting	Main Added Value	Main Limitations	Best Positioning
Autoimmune encephalitis	Early sensitivity, syndrome-oriented pattern recognition, support in seronegative cases, and selected follow-up	Limited specificity; seizure, treatment, movement-disorder, and aging-related confounding	Strongest indication; use when MR imaging is normal/equivocal, antibody status is pending/negative, or evolution remains unclear
Viral encephalitis	Functional clarification of unresolved deficits; occasional help in sequelae or subtle presentations	Sparse evidence; strong confounding in acute illness	Selective second-line adjunct, not routine
Postinfectious/post-COVID syndromes	Biological cerebral support for persistent symptoms; differential diagnosis; possible longitudinal insight	Heterogeneous phenotypes; methodological dependence; risk of false attribution	Selected patients after standard workup; not a binary confirmatory test

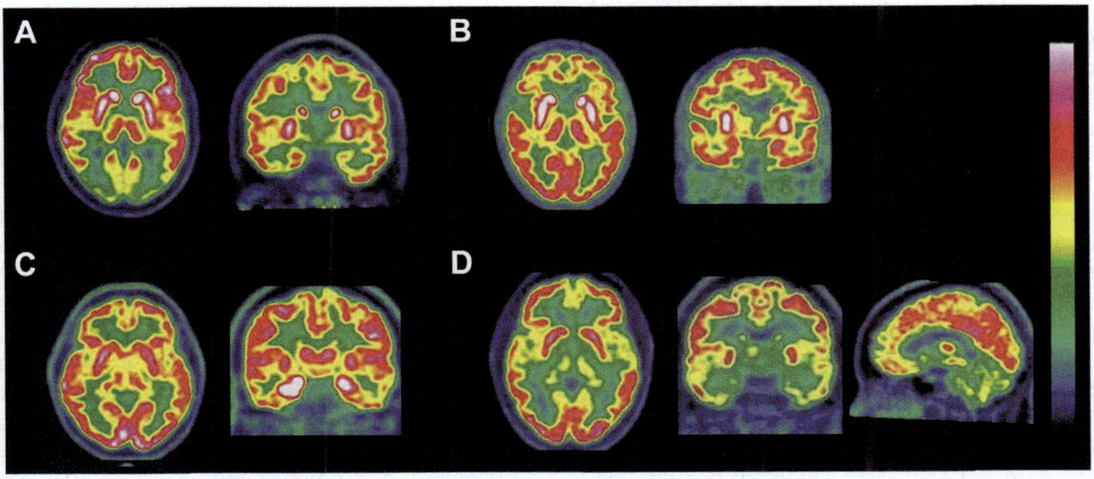

Fig. 1. Representative examples of brain [18F]FDG PET images: (*A*) a 20-year-old woman with anti-NMDAR encephalitis showing an anteroposterior metabolic gradient characterized by frontotemporal hypermetabolism coupled with posterior, predominantly occipital hypometabolism; (*B*) an 83-year-old man with anti-LGI1 encephalitis showing corticostriatal dissociation, with basal ganglia/striatal hypermetabolism coexisting with cortical hypometabolism; (*C*) a 61-year-old man with anti-Hu, onconeural antibody-associated limbic encephalitis in the context of small-cell lung cancer, showing intense medial temporal hypermetabolism; and (*D*) a 44-year-old woman with post-COVID condition showing hypometabolism in bilateral orbital gyri, medial temporal regions, brainstem, and cerebellum.

such as anti-Hu, may show intense medial temporal hypermetabolism in the active phase (**Fig. 1**C). These patterns are not pathognomonic, but they may be highly suggestive when integrated with symptoms, electroencephalogram (EEG), MR imaging, cerebrospinal fluid (CSF), and antibody profile. TSPO PET has also begun to describe complementary neuroinflammatory distributions in anti-LGI1 encephalitis, although this remains mechanistic rather than routine clinical evidence.[12]

These diagnostic and phenotyping principles also apply across the age spectrum. In pediatric AE, children may present with seizures, behavioral change, developmental regression, or mixed neuropsychiatric symptoms while MR imaging remains normal or only subtly abnormal; pediatric series support FDG PET as a useful adjunct in selected cases.[13,14] Rasmussen encephalitis remains a classic example of extensive hemispheric dysfunction on PET that may exceed early MR imaging abnormalities.[15]

Across both adult and pediatric AE, serial FDG PET may also provide additional value when clinical evolution remains difficult to interpret, particularly when persistent or recurrent symptoms raise the question of ongoing inflammatory activity, treatment response, or residual postinflammatory dysfunction. Recent longitudinal work suggests that persistent or evolving regional metabolic changes may carry prognostic information.[16]

Moreover, FDG PET may provide an etiologic opportunity beyond brain phenotyping. In selected paraneoplastic contexts, especially when limbic encephalitis, onconeural antibodies, or an otherwise suspicious clinical profile raise concern for occult malignancy, whole-body FDG PET/CT can contribute to tumor screening and etiologic clarification. This brain–body capability is particularly relevant in AE because the same examination may help characterize cerebral dysfunction while also addressing a potential systemic trigger.

The main limitation of FDG PET in AE is not low sensitivity, but limited specificity. Mesiotemporal hypermetabolism may reflect recent seizures; striatal abnormalities may be influenced by aging, movement disorders, or medication; and diffuse cortical abnormalities may mimic neurodegenerative patterns if interpreted outside the clinical context. Semiquantitative approaches may improve reproducibility, but their interpretation depends on preprocessing, normalization strategy, including reference-region selection, and the suitability of the normative database. Reports should therefore document seizure timing, relevant treatments, disease phase, age, analytical approach, normalization/reference method, and key interpretive limitations.

VIRAL ENCEPHALITIS AND INFECTIOUS ENCEPHALOPATHY

In viral encephalitis, FDG PET should not be considered a first-line examination. Acute management strongly relies on MR imaging, cerebrospinal fluid analysis, microbiological testing, EEG, and the global neurologic scenario. PET becomes relevant only in selected situations, typically when symptoms remain poorly explained by structural imaging or when functional follow-up may clarify persistent deficits.[17–20]

Most published data concern herpes simplex virus encephalitis. Acute studies have reported limbic and extralimbic hypermetabolism, whereas later examinations may show residual hypometabolism compatible with tissue injury and network disconnection.[17–19] Similar case-based observations have been reported in HHV-6 limbic encephalitis, particularly in immunocompromised settings.[20] These data support biological plausibility and occasional clinical usefulness, but they do not define a standardized diagnostic algorithm comparable to that of AE.

Accordingly, FDG PET in viral encephalitis remains adjunctive and question-driven. It may help explain ongoing cognitive or behavioral symptoms, support differential diagnosis when MR imaging findings are subtle, or document the functional aftermath of infection. Sedation, critical illness, antiseizure medication, altered consciousness, and seizure timing all complicate interpretation. PET should therefore be reserved for focused questions rather than presented as a routine test in acute viral encephalitis.

POSTINFECTIOUS NEUROCOGNITIVE SYNDROMES, WITH EMPHASIS ON POST-COVID CONDITION

Postinfectious neurocognitive syndromes pose a different problem. The issue is generally not acute diagnosis but the biological characterization of persistent cognitive, fatigue-related, autonomic, sensory, or neuropsychiatric symptoms in patients whose conventional investigations may be unrevealing. Earlier postinfectious entities such as chronic fatigue syndrome/myalgic encephalomyelitis have provided historical FDG PET reports of cortical and brainstem hypometabolism[21] and TSPO PET evidence of microglial activation,[22] anticipating the current post-COVID literature. In this area, post-COVID condition has become the dominant clinical model and the main source of FDG PET evidence.[23–34]

A key point is that postinfectious syndromes, and especially post-COVID condition, are clinically heterogeneous. This heterogeneity spans cognitive, fatigue-related, autonomic, sensory, sleep, affective, and exercise-tolerance domains, with direct implications for PET interpretation. It likely contributes to interindividual variability in the topography and magnitude of metabolic abnormalities and argues against any overly rigid expectation of a single canonical pattern.

In severe acute COVID-19 encephalopathy, FDG PET has documented fronto-cingulo-insular and broader neocortical hypometabolism in critical-care or hospitalized patients, with associations to cognitive impairment in subacute follow-up.[26,27] The present review focuses on the postacute persistent phase, where the diagnostic question shifts from acute injury to the functional characterization of persistent symptoms. Across monocentric studies, multicenter analyses, and external cohorts, FDG PET in post-COVID condition has identified in a subset of patients convergent hypometabolic patterns involving fronto-orbito-olfactory regions, limbic/paralimbic territories, brainstem, and cerebellum[23–25,28] (**Fig. 1**D). This convergence argues against a random imaging signal. At the same time, these abnormalities are not universal and should not be used as a binary diagnostic criterion for post-COVID condition. The most defensible interpretation is that FDG PET may provide biological support for persistent symptoms and identify network-level cerebral dysfunction in a subset of patients. Pediatric series have reported overlapping fronto-orbital and limbic hypometabolic patterns in children, supporting biological plausibility across age groups and across a range of initial infection severity.[29]

Longitudinal data reinforce that view. Follow-up studies show improvement in some patients and more persistent abnormalities in others, indicating heterogeneous trajectories rather than a single fixed phenotype.[30–32] Prospective work in initially hospitalized patients has also linked PET abnormalities with neuropsychological performance, suggesting meaningful cognitive correlates.[30] This longitudinal perspective moves the field beyond purely cross-sectional description and toward a more nuanced understanding of recovery, persistence, and residual disability.

Another strength of FDG PET in this setting is differential diagnosis. Clinicians may need to distinguish a postinfectious syndrome from evolving neurodegeneration, epilepsy-related dysfunction, psychiatric disease, or mixed conditions. PET can be useful when it reveals a network coherent with postinfectious patterns and inconsistent with classic Alzheimer's disease or frontotemporal dementia or AE phenotypes, or when it instead redirects attention toward another mechanism. In that sense, PET is often most useful not as a confirmatory marker but as a discriminator within a complex clinical workup.

Methodological caution is central. The apparent topography and statistical robustness of post-COVID metabolic abnormalities may vary according to normalization strategy and reference region, age distribution of controls, scanner harmonization, and clinical composition of the cohort. These issues are not secondary technical details; they directly shape interpretability. Reference datasets also deserve renewed scrutiny, because pandemic-related societal effects may have modified the notion of normal metabolism, an issue recently emphasized for FDG PET databases after the COVID-19 pandemic.[33] The main risk is therefore not merely false positivity but false attribution, namely assigning a real metabolic abnormality to a postinfectious mechanism when another explanation is more likely.

Of note, rare vaccine-associated neurologic presentations have also been explored with FDG PET. Pilot data show that functional abnormalities may be demonstrable in selected patients with neurologic symptoms after COVID-19 vaccination, but current evidence remains limited, hypothesis-generating, and insufficient to infer causality.[34]

TSPO PET AND NEUROINFLAMMATION IMAGING

TSPO PET offers a complementary perspective by targeting glial activation rather than glucose metabolism. In AE, TSPO tracers have begun to reveal in vivo inflammatory patterns that are not identical to FDG abnormalities. In broader AE cohorts, [18F]DPA-714 PET/MR imaging detected abnormalities in a substantial proportion of patients and suggested added sensitivity for inflammatory activity.[35]

The rationale for discussing TSPO PET alongside FDG PET is that the 2 modalities interrogate different but potentially complementary biological dimensions. FDG PET primarily reflects the metabolic consequences of dysfunction at regional and network levels, whereas TSPO PET is more directly oriented toward neuroimmune activation. A region showing altered FDG uptake does not necessarily indicate whether active inflammation is still present, while TSPO PET may help address that question more directly. This complementarity is particularly attractive for biological stratification and treatment monitoring in immunomodulatory settings.

Post-COVID condition has also become a key field for TSPO PET. Independent studies using different tracers have reported persistent neuroinflammation in subsets of patients with fatigue and cognitive symptoms.[36–38] Some work has additionally suggested combined brain and body inflammatory signals, reinforcing the concept of multisystem involvement in at least part of the post-COVID spectrum.[38]

However, TSPO PET remains primarily investigational. Genotype effects, tracer availability, small sample sizes, limited standardization, and unresolved specificity issues constrain immediate clinical deployment. FDG PET remains the more mature modality because it is broadly available, technically standardized, and already linked to recognized syndrome-associated patterns.[3] TSPO PET should therefore be considered a research-oriented complement with strong mechanistic value and promising future relevance for biological stratification and therapy monitoring.

CLINICAL IMPLEMENTATION

The principal operational rule is that FDG PET should be requested for a defined clinical question. In AE, that question may be whether a supportive metabolic pattern is present despite normal MR imaging, whether the distribution favors a particular syndrome, or whether persistent symptoms are more compatible with active disease than with residual injury. In postinfectious syndromes, the question is usually whether a coherent metabolic network supports the cerebral biological plausibility of symptoms and whether alternative explanations should be considered (see **Table 1**).

In clinical practice, usefulness depends less on the disease label than on the precision of the question. In AE, PET is most valuable when the clinician needs support for a strong but incompletely documented suspicion, seeks a syndrome-compatible metabolic phenotype, or wishes to interpret persistent symptoms after treatment. In viral encephalitis, PET should remain a second-line adjunct reserved for unresolved diagnostic or follow-up questions. In postinfectious syndromes, the examination should not be framed as a binary confirmatory test, but rather as a tool for biological support, differential diagnosis, and stratification in selected patients.

Interpretation should follow a structured framework. Acquisition and reconstruction should comply with current brain FDG PET guidelines.[3] Reports should document relevant confounders, especially seizure timing, glucose status, medications, sedation, and disease phase. Visual analysis should be complemented by semiquantitative tools whenever feasible, provided that the analytical pipeline, normalization strategy including reference-region selection, and suitability of the normative database are clearly specified. Semiquantification may improve consistency and pattern recognition, but it cannot replace clinical integration. The greatest interpretive risk is false attribution: a genuine metabolic abnormality read as proof of the wrong mechanism. Reports should therefore distinguish clearly between supportive compatibility, nonspecificity, and discordance with the suspected syndrome.

SUMMARY

Brain [18F]FDG PET has established a meaningful but indication-dependent role in encephalitic and postinfectious brain disorders. The strongest evidence and clearest clinical utility concern autoimmune encephalitis, where FDG PET improves sensitivity, supports syndrome-oriented pattern recognition, and may contribute to selected follow-up or prognostic stratification.[1–16] In viral encephalitis, PET should remain selective and question-driven rather than routine.[17–20] In post-COVID condition and related postinfectious syndromes, FDG PET can support cerebral biological plausibility and help with differential diagnosis in a subset of patients, but interpretation remains highly dependent on clinical context and methods.[21–34]

The field is now evolving from descriptive metabolic pattern recognition toward multimodal neuroimmune phenotyping. In that transition, TSPO PET is attractive because it may link cerebral dysfunction to inflammatory activity more directly.[12,35–38] For present-day clinical practice, however, FDG PET remains the established and useable tool. Its main strength is not to replace clinical reasoning, but rather to serve as an additional biomarker when symptoms, MR imaging findings, and biological data do not fully align.

CLINICS CARE POINTS

- In suspected autoimmune encephalitis, brain [18F]FDG PET is particularly useful when MRI is normal or equivocal, antibody results are pending or negative, or the clinical syndrome remains highly suggestive despite incomplete documentation.
- FDG PET should be interpreted as a disease-related metabolic pattern rather than as an isolated regional abnormality; syndrome-oriented patterns may support diagnostic confidence but are not pathognomonic.
- In autoimmune encephalitis, seizure timing, antiseizure medication, sedation, immunotherapy, age, and disease stage should always be considered, because they may substantially influence brain metabolism.
- Mesiotemporal hypermetabolism should not automatically be attributed to limbic encephalitis; recent seizures and peri-ictal activity are major differential considerations.
- In selected paraneoplastic autoimmune encephalitis contexts, whole-body FDG PET/CT may provide added clinical value by combining brain metabolic assessment with occult malignancy screening.
- In viral encephalitis, FDG PET is not a first-line diagnostic test; it is best reserved for focused clinical questions, such as unexplained persistent cognitive or behavioral deficits, subtle MRI findings, or follow-up of functional sequelae.
- In post-COVID condition and related post-infectious neurocognitive syndromes, FDG PET may support objective evidence of cerebral dysfunction in selected patients, but it should not be used as a binary diagnostic test.
- The main clinical value of FDG PET in post-infectious syndromes is often differential diagnosis, particularly when distinguishing post-infectious network dysfunction from neurodegenerative, epileptic, psychiatric, or mixed mechanisms.
- Semi-quantitative FDG PET analysis can improve reproducibility, but reports should explicitly state the normalization strategy, reference region, analytical pipeline, and suitability of the normative database.
- TSPO PET may provide complementary information on neuroimmune activation, but it currently remains primarily investigational and should not be considered a routine replacement for FDG PET in clinical decision-making.

REFERENCES

1. Bordonne M, Chawki MB, Doyen M, et al. Brain 18F-FDG PET for the diagnosis of autoimmune encephalitis: a systematic review and a meta-analysis. Eur J Nucl Med Mol Imaging 2021;48(12):3847–58.
2. Morbelli S, Djekidel M, Hesse S, et al. Role of 18F-FDG-PET imaging in the diagnosis of autoimmune encephalitis. Lancet Neurol 2016;15(10):1009–10.
3. Guedj E, Varrone A, Boellaard R, et al. EANM procedure guidelines for brain PET imaging using [18F]FDG, version 3. Eur J Nucl Med Mol Imaging 2022;49(2):632–51.
4. Graus F, Titulaer MJ, Balu R, et al. A clinical approach to diagnosis of autoimmune encephalitis. Lancet Neurol 2016;15(4):391–404.
5. Probasco JC, Solnes L, Nalluri A, et al. Abnormal brain metabolism on FDG-PET/CT is a common early finding in autoimmune encephalitis. Neurol Neuroimmunol Neuroinflamm 2017;4(4):e352.
6. De Leiris N, Ruel B, Vervandier J, et al. Decrease in the cortex/striatum metabolic ratio on [18F]-FDG

PET: a biomarker of autoimmune encephalitis. Eur J Nucl Med Mol Imaging 2022;49(3):921–31.
7. Roman SN, Naasan G, Lippa SM, et al. Quantitative brain FDG PET/CT in seronegative autoimmune encephalitis. Ann Clin Transl Neurol 2024;11(5):1211–23.
8. Leypoldt F, Buchert R, Kleiter I, et al. Fluorodeoxyglucose positron emission tomography in anti-N-methyl-D-aspartate receptor encephalitis: distinct pattern of disease. J Neurol Neurosurg Psychiatry 2012;83(7):681–6.
9. Probasco JC, Solnes L, Nalluri A, et al. Decreased occipital lobe metabolism by FDG-PET/CT: an anti-NMDA receptor encephalitis biomarker. Neurol Neuroimmunol Neuroinflamm 2017;4(4):e413.
10. Zhao X, Zhou C, Chen H, et al. Subcortical hypermetabolism associated with cortical hypometabolism is a common metabolic pattern in patients with anti-leucine-rich glioma-inactivated 1 antibody encephalitis. J Neurol 2020;267(6):1564–74.
11. Sadaghiani MS, Roman S, Diaz-Arias LA, et al. Comparison of quantitative FDG-PET and MRI in anti-LGI1 autoimmune encephalitis. Neuroradiology 2023;65(3):1011–21.
12. Wang J, Ge J, Jin L, et al. Characterization of neuroinflammation pattern in anti-LGI1 encephalitis based on TSPO PET and symptom clustering analysis. Eur J Nucl Med Mol Imaging 2023;50(8):2394–408.
13. Aydos U, Akdemir UO, Gokcay A, et al. Brain 18F-fluorodeoxyglucose PET in children with possible autoimmune encephalitis. Clin Nucl Med 2023; 48(4):341–7.
14. Lagarde S, Lepine A, Caietta E, et al. Cerebral (18) FluoroDeoxy-Glucose Positron Emission Tomography in paediatric anti N-methyl-D-aspartate receptor encephalitis: a case series. Brain Dev 2016;38(5): 461–70.
15. Fiorella DJ, Provenzale JM, Coleman RE, et al. 18F-fluorodeoxyglucose positron emission tomography and MR imaging findings in Rasmussen encephalitis. AJNR Am J Neuroradiol 2001;22(7):1291–9.
16. Cerne D, Raffa S, Benvenuto G, et al. Longitudinal changes in [18F]FDG PET brain metabolism as a prognostic marker in autoimmune encephalitis. Eur J Nucl Med Mol Imaging 2026;53(2):1183–97.
17. Meyer MA, Hubner KF, Raja S, et al. Sequential positron emission tomographic evaluations of brain metabolism in acute herpes encephalitis. J Neuroimaging 1994;4(2):104–5.
18. Singhal T, Cao Q, Vyas S, et al. Ventral striatal/septal hypermetabolism in HSV encephalitis. Clin Nucl Med 2019;44(3):e196–8.
19. Wong KK, Kuo PH, Frey KA. Chronic sequelae of herpes simplex encephalitis demonstrated on FDG PET/CT. Clin Nucl Med 2010;35(12):976–8.
20. Hubele F, Bilger K, Kremer S, et al. Sequential FDG PET and MRI findings in a case of human herpes virus 6 limbic encephalitis. Clin Nucl Med 2012;37(7):716–7.
21. Tirelli U, Chierichetti F, Tavio M, et al. Brain positron emission tomography (PET) in chronic fatigue syndrome: preliminary data. Am J Med 1998;105(3A): 54S–8S.
22. Nakatomi Y, Mizuno K, Ishii A, et al. Neuroinflammation in patients with chronic fatigue syndrome/myalgic encephalomyelitis: an 11C-(R)-PK11195 PET study. J Nucl Med 2014;55(6):945–50.
23. Guedj E, Campion JY, Dudouet P, et al. 18F-FDG brain PET hypometabolism in patients with long COVID. Eur J Nucl Med Mol Imaging 2021;48(9):2823–33.
24. Verger A, Barthel H, Tolboom N, et al. 2-[18F]-FDG PET for imaging brain involvement in patients with long COVID: perspective of the EANM Neuroimaging Committee. Eur J Nucl Med Mol Imaging 2022; 49(11):3599–606.
25. Verger A, Kas A, Dudouet P, et al. Visual interpretation of brain hypometabolism related to neurological long COVID: a French multicentric experience. Eur J Nucl Med Mol Imaging 2022;49(9):3197–202.
26. Hosp JA, Dressing A, Blazhenets G, et al. Cognitive impairment and altered cerebral glucose metabolism in the subacute stage of COVID-19. Brain 2021;144(4):1263–76.
27. Kas A, Soret M, Pyatigoskaya N, et al. The cerebral network of COVID-19-related encephalopathy: a longitudinal voxel-based 18F-FDG-PET study. Eur J Nucl Med Mol Imaging 2021;48(8):2543–57.
28. Goehringer F, Bruyère A, Doyen M, et al. Brain 18F-FDG PET imaging in outpatients with post-COVID-19 conditions: findings and associations with clinical characteristics. Eur J Nucl Med Mol Imaging 2023; 50(4):1084–9.
29. Cocciolillo F, Di Giuda D, Morello R, et al. Orbitofrontal cortex hypometabolism in children with post-COVID condition (long COVID): a preliminary experience. Pediatr Infect Dis J 2022;41(8):663–5.
30. Heyer S, Meyer M, Hossu G, et al. Brain 18F-FDG-PET abnormalities and their associations with neuropsychological assessment in initially hospitalized patients with post-COVID-19 conditions: a prospective and longitudinal study. Eur J Nucl Med Mol Imaging 2025;52(9):3404–11.
31. Horowitz T, Dudouet P, Campion JY, et al. Persistent brain metabolic impairment in long COVID patients with persistent clinical symptoms: a nine-month follow-up [18F]FDG-PET study. Eur J Nucl Med Mol Imaging 2024;51(11):3215–22.
32. Martini AL, Carli G, Kiferle L, et al. Time-dependent recovery of brain hypometabolism in neuro-COVID-19 patients. Eur J Nucl Med Mol Imaging 2022; 50(1):90–102.
33. Guedj E, Horowitz T, Verger A. Brain [18F]FDG-PET databases after the COVID-19 pandemic: rethinking normality. EANM J 2025;1:100009.
34. Siripongsatian D, Kunawudhi A, Promteangtrong C, et al. Alterations in 18F-FDG PET/MRI and 15O-Water

PET brain findings in patients with neurological symptoms after COVID-19 vaccination: a pilot study. Clin Nucl Med 2022;47(3):e230–9.
35. Zhang M, Meng H, Zhou Q, et al. Microglial activation imaging using 18F-DPA-714 PET/MRI for detecting autoimmune encephalitis. Radiology 2024;310(3):e230397.
36. Braga J, Lepra M, Kish SJ, et al. Neuroinflammation after COVID-19 with persistent depressive and cognitive symptoms. JAMA Psychiatry 2023;80(8):787–98.
37. VanElzakker MB, Bues HF, Brusaferri L, et al. Neuroinflammation in post-acute sequelae of COVID-19 (PASC) as assessed by [11C]PBR28 PET correlates with vascular disease measures. Brain Behav Immun 2024;119:713–23.
38. Visser D, Golla SSV, Palard-Novello X, et al. Varying levels of inflammatory activity in brain and body of patients with persistent fatigue and difficulty concentrating after COVID-19: a TSPO PET study. J Nucl Med 2025;66(11):1787–94.

[18]F-fluorodeoxyglucose PET in Major Psychiatric Disorders

Rodolfo Ferrando, MD, MSc[a,b,*], Artur Martins Coutinho, MD, PhD[c]

KEYWORDS

• Fluorodeoxyglucose F18 • Positron-emission tomography • Schizophrenia
• Substance-related disorders • Depressive disorder • Bipolar disorder • Diagnosis • Differential

KEY POINTS

- ^{18}F-fluorodeoxyglucose (FDG)-PET identifies reproducible metabolic abnormalities in major psychiatric disorders, best interpreted as distributed circuit and network dysfunction rather than as fixed disease-specific signatures.
- These abnormalities are shaped by clinical state, illness stage, treatment exposure, medication effects, recent substance use, and comorbidity.
- In schizophrenia, FDG-PET most consistently shows frontal hypometabolism, with positive symptoms linked to relative striatal and paralimbic hypermetabolism, and abnormal frontotemporal and cortical-subcortial metabolic connectivity.
- In substance use disorders, abnormalities are often state dependent, with acute drug effects superimposed on longer-term dysfunction of prefrontal control systems and mesolimbic reward pathways.
- In mood disorders, FDG-PET findings are heterogeneous, but depression often shows frontal hypometabolism and bipolar disorder may involve persistent corticolimbic dysregulation.

INTRODUCTION

As PET enters its sixth decade, this commemorative issue marks 50 years since the first human administration of ^{18}F-fluorodeoxyglucose (FDG). The earliest clinical FDG work at the University of Pennsylvania was focused on cerebral glucose metabolism and on formalizing the FDG method for quantifying local cerebral glucose utilization in humans.[1,2] This helped establish FDG-PET as a foundational tool for systems-level brain research, complementing earlier perfusion techniques.[3]

Half a century later, FDG remains the most widely used PET radiotracer worldwide and the leading technique for assessing regional cerebral glucose metabolism, a robust proxy of synaptic activity. In psychiatry, FDG-PET has primarily characterized metabolic alterations across distributed circuits and networks. Their expression is shaped by illness stage, clinical state, treatment exposure, and comorbidity, and may align more closely with symptom dimensions than with diagnostic categories.

FDG-PET studies have shown metabolic abnormalities in major psychiatric disorders such as schizophrenia and depression, often involving prefrontal regions relevant to cognition.[4] Growing interest in functional FDG-PET reflects the state-

[a] Academic Unit of Nuclear Medicine and Molecular Imaging, Hospital de Clínicas, Universidad de la República (UDELAR); [b] Department of Functional Brain Imaging, Uruguayan Center for Molecular Imaging (CUDIM), Montevideo, Uruguay; [c] Nuclear Medicine Center (LIM-43), Institute of Radiology, Hospital das Clinicas, Faculdade de Medicina da Universidade de Sao Paulo (FMUSP), Sao Paulo, Brazil
* Corresponding author. Department of Functional Brain Imaging, Uruguayan Center for Molecular Imaging (CUDIM). Av. Dr. Américo Ricaldoni 2010, Montevideo, Uruguay, 11600.
E-mail address: rodolfo.n.ferrando@gmail.com

PET Clin 21 (2026) 541–552
https://doi.org/10.1016/j.cpet.2026.05.007

Abbreviations

AUD	alcohol use disorder
BD	bipolar disorder
bvFTD	behavioral variant frontotemporal dementia
FDG	^{18}F-fluorodeoxyglucose
PPD	primary psychiatric disorder
THC	tetrahydrocannabinol

dependent nature of many clinically relevant processes.[5]

This review summarizes reproducible findings across chronic psychosis, addictions, and mood disorders, and discusses the current clinical relevance of FDG-PET in selected scenarios.

PRACTICAL CONSIDERATIONS SPECIFIC TO PSYCHIATRIC ^{18}F-FLUORODEOXYGLUCOSE-PET

General aspects of brain FDG-PET acquisition, processing, and quantification are addressed in current procedure standards.[6] In psychiatric cohorts, interpretation is particularly sensitive to uptake conditions because behavioral state, emotional activation, medication exposure, and recent substance use may influence network-level metabolism. Standardized uptake conditions and documentation of prescan factors are therefore essential (**Table 1**).

CHRONIC PSYCHOSIS AND SCHIZOPHRENIA SPECTRUM DISORDERS

Schizophrenia is a chronic psychotic disorder characterized by positive symptoms (hallucinations and delusions), negative symptoms (blunted affect, avolition, and anhedonia), and disorganized thinking. It is associated with substantial disability and increased suicide risk. FDG-PET has played a central role in investigating its pathophysiology and treatment-relevant brain dysfunction.

Hypofrontality and Prefrontal Hypometabolism

Since Ingvar and Franzén identified reduced prefrontal blood flow in schizophrenia,[7] hypofrontality has become a replicated hallmark of the disorder.[8] FDG-PET has repeatedly shown frontal hypometabolism, consistent with impaired executive control.[9] Evidence outside the frontal cortex is less consistent and may vary across illness course, partly with antipsychotic exposure.[9] Prefrontal dysfunction, however, is not always a simple resting-state reduction. Early-stage or drug-naïve patients may show increased prefrontal activity, often with prominent positive symptoms.[10] Classic activation paradigms showed absent dorsolateral prefrontal recruitment during the Wisconsin Card Sorting Test in unmedicated patients, later replicated in treated cohorts, supporting the concept of task-dependent hypofrontality across different modalities such as single-photon emission computed tomography (SPECT), PET, and functional magnetic resonance imaging (fMRI).[11–14] This distinction matters because most psychiatric FDG studies are acquired at rest, whereas many mechanistic models derive from activation paradigms.

Positive Symptoms and Auditory Verbal Hallucinations

FDG-PET findings related to positive symptoms—particularly auditory verbal hallucinations—emphasize subcortical and paralimbic engagement with reduced frontal control. In patients with active psychosis, FDG-PET linked positive symptoms to higher metabolism in medial temporal regions, basal ganglia, and thalamus.[15] In first-episode schizophrenia with prominent hallucinations, FDG abnormalities likewise highlighted paralimbic and subcortical involvement rather than a single focal cortical signature.[16] High-resolution FDG-PET further supports a frontostriatal imbalance, with hallucinating patients showing lower frontal uptake, including cingulate, and higher putaminal uptake than nonhallucinating patients.[17] During hallucination-like auditory stimulation, patients with a history of severe auditory verbal hallucinations showed exaggerated metabolic responses in limbic/paralimbic regions, including amygdala, and abnormal modulation of speech- and language-related cortical areas.[18]

Frontosubcortical Imbalance as an Integrative Framework

Beyond cortical hypofunction, FDG-PET studies also implicate basal ganglia, thalamus, and paralimbic regions, often as an elevated subcortical-to-cortical metabolic ratio.[19,20] This pattern provides a useful, though nonspecific, framework for chronic psychosis and may persist in chronic schizophrenia,[21] supporting a trait-like FDG component and aligning with current neurochemical models.

Complementary non-FDG studies support a predominantly presynaptic dopaminergic abnormality linked to reduced prefrontal regulation of striatal function,[22–24] together with glutamate–dopamine interactions supported by inverse associations between cortical glutamate and striatal dopamine synthesis and by N-methyl-D-aspartate (NMDA) blockade studies.[25,26]

Table 1
Key practical factors affecting ^{18}F-fluorodeoxyglucose-PET interpretation in psychiatric cohorts

Factor	Potential Impact	Recommendation
Behavioral/emotional activation during uptake (anxiety, panic, rumination, agitation, psychomotor activation)	State-related changes in network-level metabolism	Ensure a quiet, low-stimulation uptake environment and document relevant symptoms/ behavior
Environmental stimulation during uptake (conversation, reading, phone use, repeated interaction)	Uncontrolled modulation of regional/network activity	Standardize uptake conditions and minimize unnecessary stimulation
Acute clinical state (intoxication, withdrawal, insomnia, mania, florid psychosis)	May dominate the metabolic pattern relative to more stable abnormalities	Document current state and interpret findings cautiously
Medication and substance exposure (psychotropics, recent dose changes, caffeine, and other drugs)	May alter cerebral metabolism and affect comparability	Record treatment status, timing of last dose, recent changes, and relevant exposures
Sedation	May affect metabolism if administered during uptake	If necessary, administer late, about 30–40 min after injection, ideally just before acquisition

The Effects of Antipsychotic Treatment

Antipsychotic exposure is a major modifier of FDG-PET findings in schizophrenia, particularly prefrontal hypometabolism and cortical–subcortical imbalance. Typical antipsychotics have been associated with reduced prefrontal activity and increased basal ganglia metabolism/activity,[27,28] likely related to dopamine receptor blockade and downstream striatal adaptations; this mechanism has been discussed in relation to progressive basal ganglia enlargement in structural imaging studies.[29]

Although atypical antipsychotics may improve negative symptoms, their effects on prefrontal function remain mixed, with studies reporting either reduced prefrontal metabolism or increased perfusion after treatment.[30,31] These opposite directions likely reflect differences between metabolism and perfusion, resting versus task-based designs, and prefrontal subregional effects; improvement may also reduce compensatory demand, yielding lower prefrontal signal despite better clinical status. Treatment effects are therefore best viewed as region-specific shifts that may improve network function rather than a uniform directional change.[32,33]

Functional and Metabolic Connectivity

The concept of disrupted connectivity in schizophrenia can be traced back to Wernicke[34] and Bleuler[35] and later gained empirical support from PET/SPECT studies showing abnormal interregional coupling.[36] Additional studies reported frontotemporal, temporolimbic, and frontolimbic disconnection patterns, with partial improvement during remission,[37,38] later corroborated by fMRI.

The disconnection hypothesis posits failed functional integration across distributed neural systems in schizophrenia, potentially related to impaired synaptic plasticity.[39] Recent FDG-PET metabolic connectivity studies, particularly in treatment-resistant schizophrenia, have shown dose-related alterations in global topology and frontotemporal/cortical–subcortical organization.[40,41]

Genetic and Clinical Risk Studies

Much of the functional neuroimaging evidence in schizophrenia risk states comes from perfusion/activation studies (SPECT and $^{15}O\text{-}H_2O$ PET), supporting prefrontal dysfunction and state-dependent hypofrontality as vulnerability-related phenotypes.[42,43]

From an FDG-centered perspective, the clearest contribution has come from pharmacogenetic endophenotype studies.[44] Using FDG-PET, a D1 receptor polymorphism modulated dorsolateral prefrontal activity during clozapine treatment and predicted response,[45] while a D3 genotype linked to tardive dyskinesia risk was associated with basal ganglia hypermetabolism under haloperidol.[46] These findings show how FDG-PET can link genetic variation to regionally specific metabolic signatures relevant to both efficacy and adverse effects.

Complementary non-FDG studies in ultra-high-risk states support a dopaminergic risk framework, particularly elevated presynaptic striatal function preceding transition and predicting treatment response.[47,48]

ADDICTIONS AND SUBSTANCE USE DISORDERS

Addiction is a brain disorder driven by repeated exposure to drugs or other reinforcing stimuli and shaped by genetic and environmental factors. A shared mechanism across substances is increased extracellular dopamine in limbic regions, particularly the nucleus accumbens.[49]

A common ^{18}F-fluorodeoxyglucose-PET Framework Across Addictions

Across substances, FDG-PET findings are best interpreted within a state–trait framework. Acute drug exposure typically elevates synaptic dopamine, whereas chronic use is associated with neuroadaptive changes affecting prefrontal–striatal circuits involved in reward, cue salience, habit formation, and executive control.[50,51] Orbitofrontal dysfunction may promote compulsive drug seeking, while dorsolateral prefrontal and anterior cingulate dysfunction may weaken restraint and increase impulsivity, contributing to an imbalance between cue salience and top–down control.51 This framework helps interpret the substance-specific FDG-PET patterns summarized below.

Alcohol

Alcohol remains a major cause of preventable morbidity and mortality. FDG-PET studies have consistently shown global reductions in cerebral glucose metabolism during intoxication, most pronounced in the cerebellum and occipital cortex, with increased brain acetate uptake, supporting a shift toward acetate as an alternative energy substrate.[52]

During acute intoxication perfusion and glucose metabolism may diverge, with frontolimbic perfusion increases and metabolic decreases in occipital cortex and cerebellum.[53] Moderate alcohol exposure has also been associated with global metabolic reduction, with relative decreases in occipital cortex and cerebellum but relative increases in striatum, amygdala, insula, and midbrain, suggesting transient bias toward reward/salience circuitry during intoxication.[54]

In alcohol use disorder (AUD) and chronic heavy drinking, FDG-PET shows reduced metabolism in frontal executive regions with relative increases in striatal and cingulate regions, consistent with impaired control and altered reward processing.[55,56]

Complementary receptor PET studies support dopaminergic and opioid involvement during alcohol exposure and AUD.[57,58] In AUD, PET has reported reduced striatal D2 receptor availability, blunted dopamine release with partial recovery after abstinence, and alterations in CB1 and mGluR5,[59,60] aligning with FDG-PET evidence for a frontostriatal model of impaired control and compulsive alcohol use.

FDG-PET may help detect alcohol-related cognitive impairment, including Wernicke encephalopathy. Reported patterns include predominant prefrontal and cingulate hypometabolism, sometimes despite unremarkable MRI, supporting a clinical role in selected cases.[61]

Opioids

FDG-PET has shown that acute opioid agonism (eg, buprenorphine) can decrease brain glucose metabolism.[62] In heroin dependence, an integrated resting-state FDG-PET/fMRI study reported hypometabolism in the anterior insula and inferior parietal cortex, with decreased metabolic connectivity between the anterior insula and dorsolateral prefrontal cortex, consistent with disruption across salience and executive-control systems.[63] In remitted opioid dependence, abnormalities have also been linked to anterior cingulate, insular, and frontal regions.[64] Compared with methadone-maintained patients, individuals in protracted abstinence showed higher relative metabolism in the right supramarginal gyrus and thalamus, but sustained-attention deficits persisted, suggesting only partial recovery.[65] Overall, FDG-PET supports state-dependent network disruption involving salience/interoceptive, executive-control, and affective/limbic systems.

These findings are complemented by PET evidence of reduced dopamine signaling and by opioid receptor studies showing increased receptor binding during early abstinence.[66,67]

Cocaine and Stimulant Drugs

FDG-PET studies have demonstrated hypometabolism in prefrontal and cingulate regions in cocaine use disorder, with overlapping perfusion reductions.68·69 During early abstinence, initial reductions in anterior cortical activity may be followed by transient hypermetabolism in basal ganglia and orbitofrontal cortex within the first week, linked to heightened cue salience and compulsive seeking.[51] Thereafter, sustained metabolic reductions can persist for months, with some evidence of partial normalization with longer abstinence, supporting a state–trait framework in which early withdrawal effects are superimposed on longer-lasting circuit dysfunction.[70,71]

A meta-analysis supports dopaminergic downregulation across stimulant use disorders.[72] PET studies in cocaine dependence have shown reduced striatal D2 receptor availability associated with lower orbitofrontal and anterior cingulate metabolism, together with blunted striatal dopamine release,[73] linking dopaminergic downregulation to altered salience processing, reduced motivation, and impaired control.

PET studies also implicate glutamatergic and synaptic changes, including reduced mGluR5 availability and lower SV2A binding in anterior cingulate and prefrontal regions.[74,75]

Cannabis

Cannabis use has increased, and it remains the most widely used illicit substance worldwide.

Δ9-tetrahydrocannabinol (THC) acts primarily via CB1 receptors, which are densely expressed in frontal cortex, thalamus, hippocampus, amygdala, globus pallidus, and cerebellum. FDG-PET findings suggest a state-dependent pattern, with acute THC exposure associated with relative metabolic increases in frontal cortical and cerebellar regions, whereas chronic use has been linked to regional metabolic reductions, particularly in frontal areas.[76,77]

Fig. 1 shows bilateral mesial-predominant temporal hypometabolism in a chronic cannabis user with cognitive complaints, extending beyond a purely frontocerebellar pattern.

Dopaminergic PET studies suggest that cannabis use is characterized more by altered dopaminergic reactivity than by consistently reduced baseline striatal D2 receptor availability.[77,78] Endocannabinoid-system imaging indicates CB1 receptor downregulation in dependence, with relatively rapid normalization after abstinence and associations with withdrawal symptoms, providing molecular context for the state-dependent FDG patterns.[79]

MOOD DISORDERS

Depression

Depression is a major cause of disability, premature mortality, and reduced quality of life. Early PET perfusion studies showed reduced blood flow in prefrontal and anterior cingulate regions.[80,81] FDG-PET later demonstrated broader hypometabolism involving cortical, subcortical, and cerebellar regions, particularly within frontal and limbic systems.[81,82] In depressed patients with cognitive impairment, reduced anterior medial prefrontal flow and altered cerebellar vermis perfusion were also reported.[80]

Reduced serotonin transporter binding has been described in major depression across several regions, including putamen, thalamus, limbic structures, and raphe nuclei.[83] Reduced mu-opioid receptor availability in the amygdala and hippocampus was reported even in subclinical depression.84 Together, these findings suggest that FDG hypometabolism reflects broader monoaminergic and opioid dysfunction.

Bipolar Disorder

Bipolar disorder (BD) shares with unipolar depression a pattern of globally reduced brain metabolism during depressive episodes.85 Abnormal metabolic activity has been reported in frontal regions and the caudate nucleus in both depressive and manic phases,[81,86] and may persist beyond acute mood episodes. In older euthymic adults with BD, FDG-PET has shown bilateral hypermetabolism in the amygdala and parahippocampal regions together with bilateral hypometabolism in the dorsolateral prefrontal cortex, consistent with persistent corticolimbic dysregulation.[87] A recent multimodal meta-analysis supported state-dependent abnormalities in prefrontal, parietal, and limbic regions, particularly involving the right posterior cingulate cortex at rest and the right caudate/ventral striatum across paradigms.[88]

FDG-PET findings in mania are limited and heterogeneous, partly because full manic episodes are difficult to study and mood phase is not always stratified. Reported abnormalities include hypermetabolism in the anterior cingulate, caudate, ventral striatum, and subgenual/medial prefrontal regions, supporting frontostriatal dysfunction in reward and affect regulation.[88,89]

^{18}F-fluorodeoxyglucose-PET in Treatment Monitoring and Response Prediction

FDG-PET has been investigated for treatment monitoring and response prediction in mood disorders. In treatment-resistant depression, electroconvulsive therapy has been associated with clinical improvement and partial normalization of hypometabolism, likely through modulation of corticolimbic networks.[81]

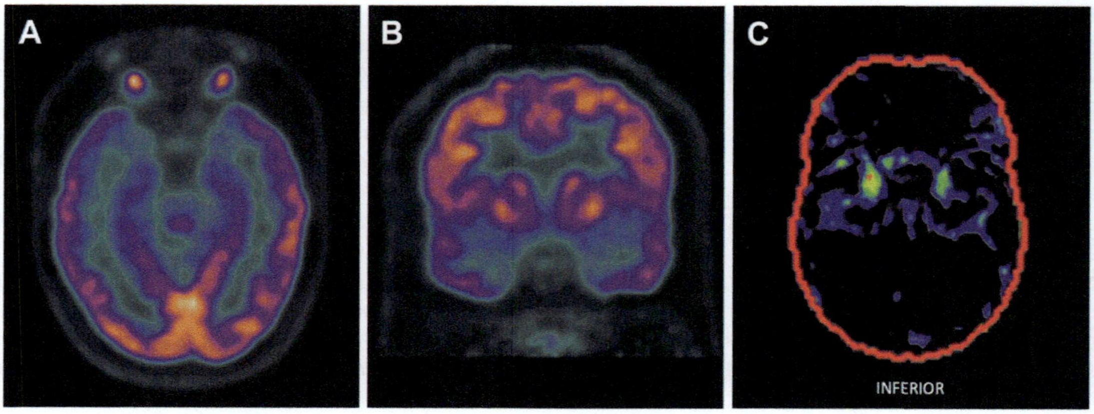

Fig. 1. (*A-C*) Brain FDG-PET in a 36-year-old man with frequent cannabis use and a 1-year history of cognitive complaints. Neuropsychological evaluation revealed dysexecutive frontosubcortical features associated with an amnestic syndrome with predominant mesiotemporal involvement. Imaging showed bilateral temporal hypometabolism, most pronounced in the mesial temporal regions. Axial image oriented along the long axis of the temporal lobes (*A*), coronal image (*B*), and inferior view of statistical surface projections (*C*).

FDG-PET has also been explored as a predictive tool for other interventions: baseline insular metabolism was proposed as a treatment-selection biomarker for cognitive-behavioral therapy versus escitalopram, but this was not supported prospectively; subgenual cingulate metabolism has also been linked to response to deep-brain stimulation.[90]

DIFFERENTIATING PSYCHIATRIC DISORDERS FROM NEURODEGENERATIVE AND OTHER BRAIN DISEASES

Neurodegenerative Mimics of Psychiatric Disorders

Behavioral variant frontotemporal dementia (bvFTD) is a major cause of early-onset dementia and frequently overlaps clinically with primary psychiatric disorders (PPDs), leading to misdiagnosis in both directions and diagnostic delays averaging 5 to 6 years from symptom onset.91

MRI and FDG-PET typically show frontotemporal atrophy or hypometabolism in bvFTD, usually with predominant frontal involvement; asymmetry may support a neurodegenerative process.91 Although structural imaging is recommended in suspected bvFTD, FDG-PET is often more sensitive, particularly in early or atypical cases and when MRI is normal. However, specificity is limited, as up to 40% of patients with PPD may also show hypometabolism, usually milder than in bvFTD, and a normal FDG-PET argues against, but does not fully exclude, bvFTD.[91,92] Follow-up FDG-PET after at least 1 year may reduce diagnostic uncertainty, and quantitative analysis may improve visual interpretation.[91,93]

Beyond bvFTD, dementia with Lewy bodies is particularly relevant in the differential diagnosis with PPD because hallucinations, delusions, affective symptoms, and cognitive fluctuations may mimic PPD. However, its FDG-PET pattern is often characteristic, typically with posterior hypometabolism involving the occipital cortex. Alzheimer's disease is also an important differential diagnosis, since psychiatric symptoms may occasionally occur in early clinical stages, although its imaging pattern is usually easier to recognize.[94] An illustrative PET case in this differential diagnostic setting is shown in **Fig. 2**.

Mood Disorders in Older Adults and Neurodegeneration

Mood disorders, particularly late-life depression and BD, may overlap clinically with neurodegenerative disease. FDG-PET can aid this distinction, with clinically normal scans reported in most patients with depression.81 Representative patterns in this differential diagnostic setting are shown in **Fig. 3**. In older adults with BD and cognitive impairment, findings have been heterogeneous, with some cases overlapping with age-related neurodegenerative phenotypes and others showing no consistent cortical metabolic pattern, arguing against a single substrate for cognitive impairment in BD (**Fig. 4**).[95,96]

Autoimmune and Encephalitic Mimics of Psychiatric Disorders

Autoimmune, infectious, and postinfectious encephalitic disorders, as well as systemic autoimmune diseases with neuropsychiatric

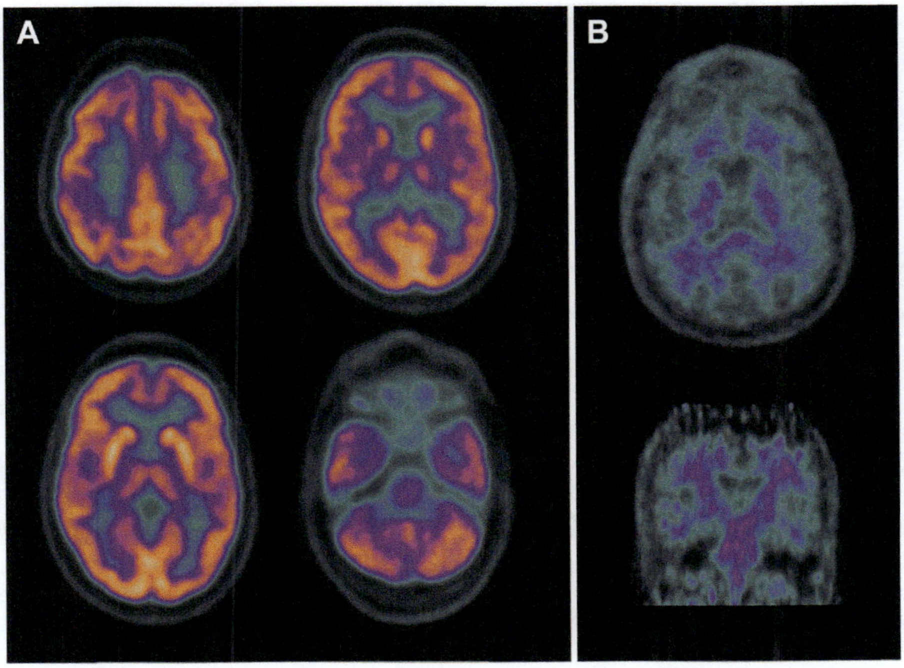

Fig. 2. (*A*, *B*) A 65-year-old woman with long-standing psychiatric disease, progressive psychotic and behavioral symptoms, cognitive decline, and Parkinsonian features, with marked worsening over the last 2 years. Frontotemporal lobar degeneration, atypical Alzheimer disease, and dementia with Lewy bodies were considered. Selected axial FDG-PET images (*A*) show preserved cortical and subcortical metabolism. ^{11}C-PiB PET (*B*) is negative for cortical amyloid deposition (top: axial; bottom: coronal). The findings favor a PPD rather than a superimposed neurodegenerative process.

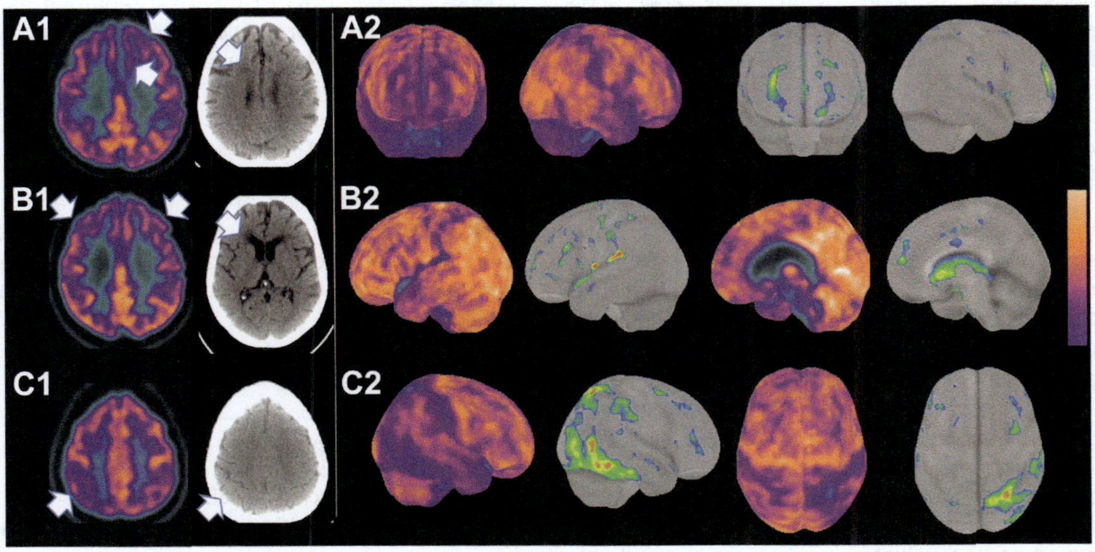

Fig. 3. (*A-C*) Brain FDG-PET/CT in 3 older women with mood disorders and cognitive complaints. In 2 cases (*A*, *B*), FDG-PET showed mild prefrontal hypometabolism, not supporting Alzheimer disease; white matter small-vessel changes were visible on computed tomography (CT). In the third case (*C*), FDG-PET showed right temporoparietal hypometabolism, consistent with a neurodegenerative pattern suggestive of Alzheimer disease. Axial PET/CT images (A1–C1) and 3D surface projections with corresponding Z-score maps (A2–C2) are shown.

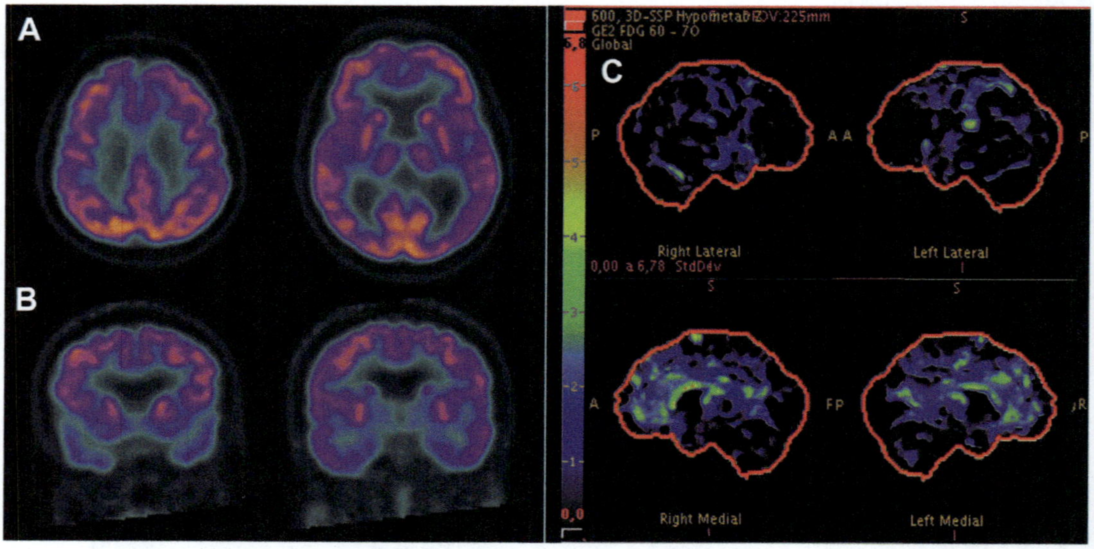

Fig. 4. (*A-C*) Brain FDG-PET in a 65-year-old woman with BD and progressive cognitive and behavioral changes suggestive of bvFTD. FDG-PET showed mild diffuse cortical and subcortical hypometabolism with mesial frontal predominance, without a pattern suggestive of neurodegeneration. Selected axial (*A*) and coronal (*B*) images and corresponding statistical surface projections (*C*) are shown.

involvement, particularly neuropsychiatric lupus, are important PPD mimics in which FDG-PET may be useful. Imaging findings include mesial temporal abnormalities, often hypermetabolic in the acute phase, in limbic encephalitis, the characteristic anti-NMDA receptor pattern of anterior hypermetabolism with posterior/occipital hypometabolism, and less specific cortical–subcortical metabolic abnormalities in neuropsychiatric lupus.[97,98] Chronic postinfectious conditions such as long COVID may also show recurrent FDG-PET abnormalities, although findings remain heterogeneous and not yet fully standardized.[99]

CONCLUSIONS AND PRACTICAL CLINICAL RELEVANCE

In routine psychiatric practice, FDG-PET is not a stand-alone diagnostic test for primary psychiatric conditions defined by the Diagnostic and Statistical Manual of Mental Disorders (DSM), and should not be used routinely. Its main value is supportive, particularly when metabolic patterns help refine biologically informed phenotypes in patients with prominent cognitive, negative, affective, or behavioral symptoms. This role is especially relevant in complex presentations—such as late-onset psychosis, catatonia, severe treatment resistance, mixed neuropsychiatric syndromes, or rapid progression—where the key question is whether cerebral metabolism supports a primary psychiatric circuit disorder or suggests an alternative brain disease.

In these settings, FDG-PET is most useful for differential diagnosis, less by confirming a specific psychiatric disorder than by showing whether the metabolic pattern suggests a neurologic or neurodegenerative condition, a nonspecific circuit-level abnormality, or the need for broader etiologic investigation. It should be interpreted with MRI, neurologic examination, medication and substance exposure, laboratory or cerebrospinal fluid studies when indicated, and longitudinal clinical course. Overall, FDG-PET is best regarded as a systems-level tool for phenotyping and diagnostic reasoning in selected complex cases.

DECLARATION OF AI AND AI-ASSISTED TECHNOLOGIES IN THE WRITING PROCESS

During the preparation of this work the authors used generative AI. After using this tool, the authors reviewed and edited the content as needed and take full responsibility for the content of the publication.

CLINICS CARE POINTS

- 18F-fluorodeoxyglucose (FDG)-PET should not be used to establish a routine diagnosis of primary psychiatric disorders; its value is supportive in selected complex cases.
- Consider FDG-PET when late-onset symptoms, rapid progression, severe treatment resistance, cognitive decline, or mixed neuropsychiatric features suggest possible brain disease.

- Interpret psychiatric FDG-PET findings with MRI, neurological examination, medication and substance exposure, laboratory/CSF data when indicated, and longitudinal clinical course.
- Standardize uptake conditions and document anxiety, agitation, insomnia, intoxication, withdrawal, recent medication changes, caffeine/drug exposure, and sedation timing.
- In complex neuropsychiatric presentations, FDG-PET can help distinguish nonspecific psychiatric circuit-level abnormalities from patterns suggesting neurodegenerative, autoimmune, encephalitic, or other brain disorders.

DISCLOSURE

R. Ferrando declares no commercial or financial conflicts of interest related to this work. A M. Coutinho has served on the scientific Advisory board of Masima and is also a cofounder and a minority shareholder at Masima.

REFERENCES

1. Hess S, Høilund-Carlsen PF, Alavi A. Historic images in nuclear medicine: 1976: the first issue of Clinical Nuclear Medicine and the first human FDG study. Clin Nucl Med 2014;39(8):701–3.
2. Reivich M, Kuhl D, Wolf A, et al. The [18F]fluorodeoxyglucose method for the measurement of local cerebral glucose utilization in man. Circ Res 1979; 44(1):127–37.
3. Ingvar DH, Lassen NA. Regional cerebral blood flow in man determined by the intra-arterial injection of an inert gas (133Xe). Circ Res 1966;18(3):237–47.
4. Schöll M, Damián A, Engler H. Fluorodeoxyglucose PET in neurology and psychiatry. Pet Clin 2014;9: 371–90.
5. Hahn A, Gryglewski G, Nics L, et al. Quantification of task-specific glucose metabolism with constant infusion of 18F-FDG. J Nucl Med 2016;57:1933–40.
6. Arbizu J, Morbelli S, Minoshima S, et al. SNMMI procedure Standard/EANM practice guideline for brain [18F]FDG PET imaging, version 2.0. J Nucl Med 2025;66(Suppl 2):S45–60.
7. Ingvar DH, Franzén G. Abnormalities of cerebral blood flow distribution in patients with chronic schizophrenia. Acta Psychiatr Scand 1974;50: 425–62.
8. Hill K, Mann L, Laws KR, et al. Hypofrontality in schizophrenia: a meta-analysis of functional imaging studies. Acta Psychiatr Scand 2004;110:243–56.
9. Townsend L, Pillinger T, Selvaggi P, et al. Brain glucose metabolism in schizophrenia: a systematic review and meta-analysis of 18FDG-PET studies in schizophrenia. Psychol Med 2023;53:4880–97.
10. Catafau A, Parellada E, Lomeña F, et al. Prefrontal and temporal blood flow in schizophrenia: resting and activation HMPAO-SPECT patterns in young neuroleptic-naive patients with acute disease. J Nucl Med 1994;35:935–41.
11. Weinberger DR, Berman KF, Zec RF. Physiological dysfunction of dorsolateral prefrontal cortex in schizophrenia: I. Regional cerebral blood flow evidence. Arch Gen Psychiatry 1986;43:114–24.
12. Berman KF, Zec RF, Weinberger DR. Physiological dysfunction of dorsolateral prefrontal cortex in schizophrenia: II. Role of medication, attention, and mental effort. Arch Gen Psychiatry 1986;43: 126–35.
13. Ragland JD, Gur RC, Glahn DC, et al. Frontotemporal cerebral blood flow change during executive and declarative memory tasks in schizophrenia: a positron emission tomography study. Neuropsychology 1998;12:399–413.
14. Riehemann S, Volz HP, Stützer P, et al. Hypofrontality in neuroleptic-naive schizophrenic patients during the Wisconsin card sorting Test–a fMRI study. Eur Arch Psychiatry Clin Neurosci 2001;251:66–71.
15. Seethalakshmi R, Parkar SR, Nair N, et al. Regional brain metabolism in schizophrenia: an FDG-PET study. Indian J Psychiatry 2006;48(3):149–53.
16. Parellada E, Lomena F, Font M, et al. Fluordeoxyglucose-PET study in first-episode schizophrenic patients during the hallucinatory state, after remission and during linguistic-auditory activation. Nucl Med Commun 2008;29(10):894–900.
17. Kim JH, Son YD, Kim JH, et al. Neural signature for auditory hallucinations in schizophrenia: a high-resolution positron emission tomography study with fludeoxyglucose (18F). Clin Psychopharmacol Neurosci 2018;16(3):324–32.
18. Horga G, Fernández-Egea E, Mané A, et al. Brain metabolism during hallucination-like auditory stimulation in schizophrenia. PLoS One 2014;9(1): e84987.
19. Resnick SM, Gur RE, Alavi A, et al. Positron emission tomography and subcortical glucose metabolism in schizophrenia. Psychiatry Res 1988;24:1–11.
20. Volkow ND, Wolf AP, Brodie JD, et al. Brain interactions in chronic schizophrenics under resting and activation conditions. Schizophr Res 1988;1:47–53.
21. Wolkin A, Jaeger J, Brodie JD, et al. Persistence of cerebral metabolic abnormalities in chronic schizophrenia as determined by positron emission tomography. Am J Psychiatry 1985;142:564–71.
22. Laruelle M, Abi-Dargham A, van Dyck CH, et al. Single photon emission computerized tomography imaging of amphetamine-induced dopamine release in drug-free schizophrenic subjects. Proc Natl Acad Sci USA 1996;93(17):9235–40.

23. Howes OD, Kambeitz J, Kim E, et al. The nature of dopamine dysfunction in schizophrenia and what this means for treatment. Arch Gen Psychiatry 2012;69(8):776–86.
24. Meyer-Lindenberg A, Miletich RS, Kohn PD, et al. Reduced prefrontal activity predicts exaggerated striatal dopaminergic function in schizophrenia. Nat Neurosci 2002;5(3):267–71.
25. Jauhar S, McCutcheon R, Borgan F, et al. The relationship between cortical glutamate and striatal dopamine in first-episode psychosis: a cross-sectional multimodal PET and magnetic resonance spectroscopy imaging study. Lancet Psychiatry 2018;5:816–23.
26. Kegeles LS, Abi-Dargham A, Zea-Ponce Y, et al. Modulation of amphetamine-induced striatal dopamine release by ketamine in humans: implications for schizophrenia. Biol Psychiatry 2000;48:627–40.
27. Holcomb HH, Cascella NG, Thaker GK, et al. Functional sites of neuroleptic drug action in the human brain: PET/FDG studies with and without haloperidol. Am J Psychiatry 1996;153:41–9.
28. DeLisi LE, Holcomb HH, Cohen RM, et al. Positron emission tomography in schizophrenic patients with and without neuroleptic medication. J Cereb Blood Flow Metab 1985;5(2):201–6.
29. Chakos MH, Lieberman JA, Bilder RM, et al. Increase in caudate nuclei volumes of first-episode schizophrenic patients taking antipsychotic drugs. Am J Psychiatry 1994;151:1430–6.
30. Molina V, Gispert JD, Reig S, et al. Cerebral metabolic changes induced by clozapine in schizophrenia and related to clinical improvement. Psychopharmacology (Berl) 2005;178(1):17–26.
31. Lahti AC, Holcomb HH, Weiler MA, et al. Functional effects of antipsychotic drugs: comparing clozapine with haloperidol. Biol Psychiatry 2003;53:601–8.
32. Davis CE, Jeste DV, Eyler LT. Review of longitudinal functional neuroimaging studies of drug treatments in patients with schizophrenia. Schizophr Res 2005;78:45–60.
33. Lahti AC, Holcomb HH, Weiler MA, et al. Clozapine but not haloperidol re-establishes normal task-activated rCBF patterns in schizophrenia within the anterior cingulate cortex. Neuropsychopharmacology 2004;29(1):171–8.
34. Wernicke C. Grundrisse der Psychiatrie. Leipzig, Germany: Thieme; 1906.
35. Bleuler E. Dementia praecox or the group of schizophrenias. New York: International Universities Press; 1911.
36. Weinberger DR, Berman KF, Suddath R, et al. Evidence of dysfunction of a prefrontal-limbic network in schizophrenia: a magnetic resonance imaging and regional cerebral blood flow study of discordant monozygotic twins. Am J Psychiatry 1992;149: 890–7.
37. Erkwoh R, Sabri O, Willmes K, et al. Aspects of cerebral connectivity in schizophrenia. A comparative CBF study on treated schizophrenics before and after medication. Fortschr Neurol Psychiatr 1999; 67(7):318–26.
38. Meyer-Lindenberg AS, Olsen RK, Kohn PD, et al. Regionally specific disturbance of dorsolateral prefrontal–hippocampal functional connectivity in schizophrenia. Arch Gen Psychiatry 2005;62: 379–86.
39. Friston KJ. The disconnection hypothesis. Schizophr Res 1998;30:115–25.
40. De Simone G, Iasevoli F, Barone A, et al. Addressing brain metabolic connectivity in treatment-resistant schizophrenia: a novel graph theory-driven application of 18F-FDG-PET with antipsychotic dose correction. Schizophr 2024;10:116.
41. de Bartolomeis A, De Simone G, Iasevoli F, et al. A novel graph theory-driven application of 18F-FDG-PET with antipsychotic dose correction and a machine learning approach to capture discrete brain metabolic connectivity in treatment-resistant schizophrenia. Int J Neuropsychopharmacol 2025;28(Suppl 2):ii74.
42. Berman KF, Torrey EF, Daniel DG, et al. Regional cerebral blood flow in monozygotic twins discordant and concordant for schizophrenia. Arch Gen Psychiatry 1992;49(12):927–34.
43. Blackwood DH, Glabus MF, Dunan J, et al. Altered cerebral perfusion measured by SPECT in relatives of patients with schizophrenia. Correlations with memory and P300. Br J Psychiatry 1999;175:357–66.
44. Basile VS, Masellis M, Potkin SK, et al. Pharmacogenomics in schizophrenia: the quest for individualized therapy. Hum Mol Genet 2002;11(20):2517–30.
45. Potkin SG, Basile VS, Jin Y, et al. D1 receptor alleles predict PET metabolic correlates of clinical response to clozapine. Mol Psychiatry 2003;8(1):109–13.
46. Potkin SG, Kennedy JL, Basile VS. Combining brain imaging and pharmacogenetics in understanding clinical response in Alzheimer's disease and schizophrenia. In: Lerer B, editor. Pharmacogenetics of psychotropic drugs. Cambridge, UK: Cambridge University Press; 2002.
47. Howes OD, Bose SK, Turkheimer F, et al. Dopamine synthesis capacity before onset of psychosis: a prospective [18F]-DOPA PET imaging study. Am J Psychiatry 2011;168(12):1311–7.
48. Jauhar S, Veronese M, Nour MM, et al. Determinants of treatment response in first-episode psychosis: an 18F-DOPA PET study. Mol Psychiatry 2019;24(10): 1502–12.
49. Koob GF, Volkow ND. Neurocircuitry of addiction. Neuropsychopharmacology 2010;35(1):217–38.
50. Everitt BJ, Robbins TW. Neural systems of reinforcement for drug addiction: from actions to habits to compulsion. Nat Neurosci 2005;8:1481–9.

51. Volkow ND, Fowler JS, Wang G-J. The addicted human brain viewed in the light of imaging studies: brain circuits and treatment strategies. Neuropharmacology 2004;47(Suppl 1):3–13.
52. Volkow ND, Kim SW, Wang G-J, et al. Acute alcohol intoxication decreases glucose metabolism but increases acetate uptake in the human brain. Neuroimage 2013;64:277–83.
53. Bjork JM, Gilman JM. The effects of acute alcohol administration on the human brain: insights from neuroimaging. Neuropharmacology 2014;84:101–10.
54. Volkow ND, Ma Y, Zhu W, et al. Moderate doses of alcohol disrupt the functional organization of the human brain. Psychiatry Res 2008;162(3):205–13.
55. Bralet M-C, Mitelman SA, Goodman CR, et al. Fluorodeoxyglucose positron emission tomography scans in patients with alcohol use disorder. Alcohol Clin Exp Res 2022;46:994–1010.
56. Kania A, Porco N, Caravaggio F. Measuring alcohol-induced striatal dopamine release in healthy humans with [11C]-Raclopride: a meta-analysis. Synapse 2025;79.
57. Mitchell JM, O'Neil JP, Janabi M, et al. Alcohol consumption induces endogenous opioid release in the human orbitofrontal cortex and nucleus accumbens. Sci Transl Med 2012;4:116ra6.
58. Ravan S, Martinez D, Slifstein M, et al. Molecular imaging in alcohol dependence. Handb Clin Neurol 2014;125:293–311.
59. Hirvonen J, Zanotti-Fregonara P, Umhau JC, et al. Reduced cannabinoid CB1 receptor binding in alcohol dependence measured with positron emission tomography. Mol Psychiatry 2013;18:916–21.
60. Akkus F, Mihov Y, Treyer V, et al. Metabotropic glutamate receptor 5 binding in male patients with alcohol use disorder. Transl Psychiatry 2018;8:17.
61. Clergue-Duval V, Questel F, Azuar J, et al. Brain 18FDG-PET pattern in patients with alcohol-related cognitive impairment. Eur J Nucl Med Mol Imaging 2020;47:281–91.
62. Walsh SL, Gilson SF, Jasinski DR, et al. Buprenorphine reduces cerebral glucose metabolism in polydrug abusers. Neuropsychopharmacology 1994;10: 157–70.
63. Jin L, Yuan M, Chen J, et al. Abnormal cerebral metabolism and metabolic connectivity in individuals with heroin dependence: an integrated resting-state PET/fMRI study in large-scale networks. J Psychiatry Neurosci 2023;48:E295–304.
64. Galynker II, Eisenberg D, Matochik JA, et al. Cerebral metabolism and mood in remitted opiate dependence. Drug Alcohol Depend 2007;90:166–74.
65. Prosser J, London ED, Galynker II. Sustained attention in patients receiving and abstinent following methadone maintenance treatment for opiate dependence: performance and neuroimaging results. Drug Alcohol Depend 2009;104(3):228–40.
66. Martinez D, Saccone PA, Liu F, et al. Deficits in dopamine D(2) receptors and presynaptic dopamine in heroin dependence: commonalities and differences with other types of addiction. Biol Psychiatry 2012;71(3):192–8.
67. Williams TM, Daglish MRC, Lingford-Hughes A, et al. Brain opioid receptor binding in early abstinence from opioid dependence: positron emission tomography study. Br J Psychiatry 2007;191:63–9.
68. Volkow ND, Mullani N, Gould KL, et al. Cerebral blood flow in chronic cocaine users: a study with positron emission tomography. Br J Psychiatry 1988;152:641–8.
69. London ED, Cascella NG, Wong DF, et al. Cocaine-induced reduction of glucose utilization in human brain. A study using positron emission tomography and [fluorine 18]-fluorodeoxyglucose. Arch Gen Psychiatry 1990;47:567–74.
70. Volkow ND, Hitzemann R, Wang GJ, et al. Long-term frontal brain metabolic changes in cocaine abusers. Synapse 1992;11:184–90.
71. Ferrando R, Barrachina A, Ferro A, et al. Alteraciones de la perfusión cerebral en consumidores activos de pasta base de cocaína. Rev Psiquiatr Urug 2009;73:51–62.
72. Proebstl L, Kamp F, Manz K, et al. Effects of stimulant drug use on the dopaminergic system: a systematic review and meta-analysis of in vivo neuroimaging studies. Eur Psychiatry 2019;59:15–24.
73. Volkow ND, Fowler JS, Wang GJ, et al. Dopamine in drug abuse and addiction: results of imaging studies and treatment implications. Arch Neurol 2007;64(11):1575–9.
74. Martinez D, Slifstein M, Nabulsi N, et al. Imaging glutamate homeostasis in cocaine addiction with the metabotropic glutamate receptor 5 positron emission tomography radiotracer [(11)C]ABP688 and magnetic resonance spectroscopy. Biol Psychiatry 2014;75:165–71.
75. Angarita GA, Worhunsky PD, Naganawa M, et al. Lower prefrontal cortical synaptic vesicle binding in cocaine use disorder: an exploratory 11 C-UCB-J positron emission tomography study in humans. Addict Biol 2022;27:e13123.
76. Volkow ND, Gillespie H, Mullani N, et al. Brain glucose metabolism in chronic marijuana users at baseline and during marijuana intoxication. Psychiatry Res Neuroimaging 1996;67:29–38.
77. Sevy S, Smith GS, Ma Y, et al. Cerebral glucose metabolism and D2/D3 receptor availability in young adults with cannabis dependence measured with positron emission tomography. Psychopharmacology (Berl) 2008;197:549–56.
78. Volkow ND, Wang G-J, Telang F, et al. Decreased dopamine brain reactivity in marijuana abusers is associated with negative emotionality and addiction severity. Proc Natl Acad Sci USA 2014;111: E3149–56.

79. D'Souza DC, Cortes-Briones JA, Ranganathan M, et al. Rapid changes in cannabinoid 1 receptor availability in cannabis-dependent male subjects after abstinence from cannabis. Biol Psychiatry Cogn Neurosci Neuroimaging 2016;1:60–7.
80. Dolan RJ, Bench CJ, Brown RG, et al. Regional cerebral blood flow abnormalities in depressed patients with cognitive impairment. J Neurol Neurosurg Psychiatry 1992;55:768–73.
81. Singh SB, Tiwari A, Katta MR, et al. The utility of PET imaging in depression. Front Psychiatry 2024;15: 1322118.
82. Kumar A, Newberg A, Alavi A, et al. Regional cerebral glucose metabolism in late-life depression and Alzheimer disease: a preliminary positron emission tomography study. Proc Natl Acad Sci USA 1993; 90:7019–23.
83. Smith GS, Workman CI, Protas H, et al. Positron emission tomography imaging of serotonin degeneration and beta-amyloid deposition in late-life depression evaluated with multi-modal partial least squares. Transl Psychiatry 2021;11:473.
84. Nummenmaa L, Karjalainen T, Isojärvi J, et al. Lowered endogenous mu-opioid receptor availability in subclinical depression and anxiety. Neuropsychopharmacology 2020;45:1953–9.
85. Schwartz JM, Baxter LR Jr, Mazziotta JC, et al. The differential diagnosis of depression. Relevance of positron emission tomography studies of cerebral glucose metabolism to the bipolar-unipolar dichotomy. JAMA 1987;258:1368–74.
86. Blumberg HP, Stern E, Martinez D, et al. Increased anterior cingulate and caudate activity in bipolar mania. Biol Psychiatry 2000;48:1045–52.
87. Brooks JO, Hoblyn JC, Woodard SA, et al. Corticolimbic metabolic dysregulation in euthymic older adults with bipolar disorder. J Psychiatr Res 2009;43(5): 497–502.
88. Schumer MC, Chase HW, Rozovsky R, et al. Prefrontal, parietal, and limbic condition-dependent differences in bipolar disorder: a large-scale meta-analysis of functional neuroimaging studies. Mol Psychiatry 2023;28(7):2826–38.
89. Brooks JO, Hoblyn JC, Ketter TA. Metabolic evidence of corticolimbic dysregulation in bipolar mania. Psychiatry Res 2010;181(2):136–40.
90. Cervenka S, Frick A, Bodén R, et al. Application of positron emission tomography in Psychiatry—methodological developments and future directions. Transl Psychiatry 2022;12(1):248.
91. Ducharme S, Dols A, Laforce R, et al. Recommendations to distinguish behavioural variant frontotemporal dementia from psychiatric disorders. Brain 2020; 143:1632–50.
92. Vijverberg EGB, Wattjes MP, Dols A, et al. Diagnostic accuracy of MRI and additional [18F]FDG-PET for behavioral variant frontotemporal dementia in patients with late onset behavioral changes. J Alzheimers Dis 2016;53:1287–97.
93. Bergeron D, Beauregard J-M, Guimond J, et al. Clinical impact of a second FDG-PET in atypical/unclear dementia syndromes. J Alzheimers Dis 2016;49: 695–705.
94. Thientunyakit T, Muangpaisan W, Minoshima S. 18F-FDG PET for dementia evaluation: co-pathologies, new diseases, and its roles in the era of antiamyloid treatment. Semin Nucl Med 2025;55(4):526–37.
95. Saleh N, Blaise C, Daoudi A, et al. Brain 18FDG-PET pattern in cognitively impaired elderly patients with bipolar disorder. Int J Bipolar Disord 2024;12(1):45.
96. Musat EM, Marlinge E, Leroy M, et al. Characteristics of bipolar patients with cognitive impairment of suspected neurodegenerative origin: a multicenter cohort. J Pers Med 2021;11:1183.
97. Kosek S, Kilsved E, Danfors T, et al. Regional metabolic abnormalities in autoimmune encephalitis: a meta-analysis of 498 cases with brain FDG PET. Clin Nucl Med 2025;50:208–13.
98. Berndorfler BD, Warwick JM, Doruyter AGG. Role of F-18 FDG PET-CT in neuropsychiatric systemic lupus erythematosus. Compr Psychiatry 2024;132:152480.
99. Guedj E, Campion JY, Dudouet P, et al. 18F-FDG brain PET hypometabolism in patients with long COVID. Eur J Nucl Med Mol Imaging 2021;48(9): 2823–33.

Brain [18F]FDG-PET in Subjective Cognitive Complaints

From Diagnostic Gap to Neurobiological Insight

Eric Guedj, MD, PhD[a,*], Antoine Verger, MD, PhD[b], Tatiana Horowitz, MD, MSc[a]

KEYWORDS

• FDG PET • Subjective cognitive complaints • Mild traumatic brain injury • Preclinical Alzheimer's disease • Long COVID • Hypometabolism • Diaschisis • Metacognition

KEY POINTS

- Subjective cognitive complaints are heterogeneous and do not correspond to a single operational definition across clinical populations.
- FDG PET provides a systems-level measure of cerebral metabolism that may help bridge subjective experience, objective cognitive performance, and brain dysfunction.
- In subjective cognitive decline, FDG PET can contribute to multimodal stratification within the Alzheimer's disease biomarker framework, although its clinical role is better established in mild cognitive impairment (MCI) and dementia.
- In persistent symptoms after mild traumatic brain injury, FDG PET findings suggest possible diffuse metabolic or network-level abnormalities.
- In long COVID and related postinfectious syndromes, FDG PET has identified hypometabolic patterns, while cognitive symptoms may be subjective or objectively measurable, particularly in attention and executive domains.

INTRODUCTION

Patients frequently report disabling cognitive difficulties despite normal, borderline, or only partially explanatory neuropsychological testing and structural imaging findings. This subjective-objective dissociation is evident in subjective cognitive decline (SCD), mild traumatic brain injury (mTBI), and postinfectious syndromes such as long COVID. These settings expose the limited sensitivity of conventional tools to early or distributed dysfunction.

These subjective cognitive complaints (SCC) encompasses perceived impairments in memory, attention, executive function, and cognitive fluency, including changes in effort, clarity, and subjective continuity. In SCD, complaints may represent the earliest symptomatic stage of

[a] Aix-Marseille University (AMU), Department of Nuclear Medicine, Timone Hospital, IMoTheP Team, Institut Fresnel, Marseille, France; [b] Department of Nuclear Medicine, Nancyclotep Imaging Platform, IADI Laboratory, INSERM U1254, Université de Lorraine, Nancy, France
* Corresponding author. Laboratoire de Médecine Nucléaire, Hôpital de la Timone, 264 rue Saint Pierre, 13005 Marseille, France.
E-mail address: eric.guedj@univ-amu.fr

PET Clin 21 (2026) 553–560
https://doi.org/10.1016/j.cpet.2026.05.004

Abbreviations	
AD	Alzheimer's disease
MTBI	mild traumatic brain injury
SCD	subjective cognitive decline

Alzheimer's disease (AD), preceding measurable impairment and sometimes correlating with amyloid burden and longitudinal decline.[1–6] Amyloid positivity reaches approximately 27% across SCD cohorts and increases with age.[7] SCD remains heterogeneous, as complaints may also reflect affective symptoms, sleep disorders, personality traits, or aging variability.[8,9] Persistent symptoms after mTBI and postinfectious syndromes, often reported as brain fog, similarly occur with limited or nonspecific structural correlates, although objective cognitive deficits may be present in subsets.[10–16]

These observations raise a fundamental question: do subjective complaints lack biological validity, or do they reveal the limitations of our current clinical metrics ? Increasing evidence supports the latter interpretation. FDG PET, by measuring cerebral glucose metabolism as an integrative proxy of synaptic activity, neurovascular coupling, and neuroglial energetic demand, provides a systems-level biomarker capable of interrogating precisely the functional layer at which SCC may arise.[9,17]

This narrative and conceptual review focuses on selected contexts in which FDG PET may help bridge SCC and objective network-level dysfunction. Evidence is strongest and most integrated within biomarker frameworks in SCD, and more heterogeneous in long COVID and persistent mTBI, where symptom definitions, objective cognitive status, mechanisms, comorbidity, timing, and methodology influence interpretation.

SCC AS A CROSS-DOMAIN CLINICAL PHENOTYPE

Across SCD, mTBI, and postinfectious syndromes, patients may report cognitive inefficiency, reduced endurance, attentional instability, and altered self-experience, often without proportional objective deficits. SCC is used here as a pragmatic cross-domain construct rather than a single nosologic entity, because definitions and populations vary substantially. Subjective complaints may sometimes reflect large-scale brain dysfunction, but this interpretation requires condition-specific caution.

In aging, SCD illustrates a temporal dissociation in which subjective complaints may precede objective impairment. Subjective symptoms have been associated with amyloid burden in cognitively normal individuals[1] and predict longitudinal cognitive decline in several cohorts,[2–6] suggesting that subjective awareness may capture early biological changes when conventional cognitive measures remain insensitive.

In mTBI, persistent symptoms are common and frequently disproportionate to findings on routine assessments.[10] Complaint severity correlates more strongly with fatigue, anxiety, depression, and posttraumatic stress than with injury severity markers, suggesting that SCC may reflect altered network efficiency and metacognitive monitoring rather than focal structural damage.[10,18] This emphasizes the need for biomarkers able to detect distributed physiologic consequences of injury while accounting for affective, sleep-related, and contextual modulators.

Postinfectious syndromes provide a third expression of this dissociation. In long COVID, patients frequently report cognitive slowing, attentional instability, fatigue, dysautonomia, reduced endurance, and brain fog; however, several cohorts also document measurable cognitive abnormalities, particularly in attentional and executive domains. FDG PET studies identify hypometabolic networks involving orbitofrontal/olfactory regions, limbic structures, brainstem, and cerebellum across independent cohorts.[11–16] These findings support a biological basis for symptoms that are often considered nonspecific, poorly explained, or difficult to objectify with conventional assessments.

Taken together, these settings suggest that SCC or related cognitive complaints may reflect distributed dysfunction involving systems subserving cognitive control, salience processing, interoception, and self-monitoring, with different levels of evidence across conditions.

WHY CONVENTIONAL ASSESSMENTS MISS THE SIGNAL

Structural MR imaging detects macroscopic lesions, atrophy, and vascular pathology, whereas neuropsychological testing quantifies performance under standardized conditions. Both are indispensable, but SCC often emerge at a level not optimally captured by either modality. Part of the challenge is semantic: SCC is heterogeneous and lacks a single operational definition. Clinically, complaints often reflect reduced efficiency, fluctuating vulnerability, or altered monitoring of effort rather than overt failure on conventional metrics.

On the other hand, many patients reporting SCC perform within normal limits in the structured environment of formal testing, yet struggle in everyday settings requiring multitasking, rapid adaptation, sustained effort, or resistance to distraction. The problem is not whether a cognitive operation can still be performed, but how much effort is required to maintain it, how stable performance remains over time, and how resilient the system is under real-life demands. These dimensions are only partially reflected in standard neuropsychological scores.

A second limitation concerns timing and imaging sensitivity. Molecular and functional alterations can precede MR imaging-visible structural changes and conventional cognitive decline,[9,17] especially in preclinical AD, where amyloid and tau pathology may already be present while structural imaging remains noncontributive.[1,2,9,19–21] In mTBI and postinfectious syndromes, however, the issue is not simply that structural abnormalities occur later. Conventional MR imaging is often nonexplanatory at the individual level, whereas quantitative group-level approaches may detect subtle structural effects. In this line, UK Biobank longitudinal MR imaging data after severe acute respiratory syndrome coronavirus 2 (SARS-CoV-2) infection showed gray matter and global brain volume changes at the population level.[22] Post-COVID brain involvement should therefore not be viewed as limited to metabolic or physiologic abnormalities, although such group-level structural signals differ from routine individual MR imaging interpretation.

Of note, clinicoradiological dissociations are not exceptional in neurology. Diaschisis illustrates how a focal insult can induce remote dysfunction across connected networks, producing symptoms disproportionate to visible lesion burden. By analogy, SCC may reflect impaired network integration, altered hub efficiency, or reduced large-scale coordination rather than localized tissue destruction. FDG PET is well positioned because it interrogates the metabolic expression of network function at the systems level.[9,17]

FDG PET AS A NETWORK-LEVEL BIOMARKER

FDG PET measures regional cerebral glucose utilization, tightly coupled to synaptic activity, neurovascular coupling, and neuroglial energetic demand.[17] Although it does not directly measure cognition, it captures one of its most relevant physiologic substrates: the metabolic support of distributed brain networks. This makes FDG PET particularly informative when symptoms are clinically salient but structural imaging remains normal or minimally informative. Importantly, FDG PET complements rather than duplicates MRI. Structural and metabolic alterations can dissociate spatially and temporally, reflecting distinct biological processes.[9,17] In some patients, MR imaging may remain normal while FDG PET shows functionally meaningful abnormalities; in others, structural damage may be visible with relatively modest metabolic cortical consequences at a given stage.

A key strength of FDG PET in SCC is that it operates at the level where complaints are most likely to arise. SCC may reflect altered network efficiency, reduced fluency of information processing, instability under load, or impaired integration across distributed systems—not purely focal phenomena. FDG PET therefore provides a biologically plausible bridge between subjective experience and objective dysfunction by revealing abnormalities in the metabolic organization of large-scale networks.[9,17]

In SCD, FDG PET occupies a nuanced position. Overt AD-like hypometabolism is less common than in MCI or dementia,[9] but subtle early changes may involve focal regions or vulnerable nodes before the full temporoparietal/posterior cingulate AD pattern.[9,23] The right middle temporal gyrus has been proposed as an early metabolic seed region for SCD, correlating with complaint severity and memory performance.[23] On the other hand, real-world memory-clinic data including subjective cognitive impairment and MCI suggest a high negative predictive value of normal FDG PET for dementia conversion and CSF biomarker evidence of neurodegeneration.[24] Normal FDG PET does not exclude biologically relevant SCC, particularly in very early, non-neurodegenerative, or biomarker-negative cases; abnormal FDG PET in context may strengthen the case for an evolving neurobiological process.

In chronic mTBI or persistent postconcussion cohorts, FDG PET studies have reported metabolic abnormalities despite normal or minimally informative computed tomography (CT)/MR imaging, including cerebrocerebellar hypometabolism, blast-versus blunt-force differences, and mixed patterns associated with symptoms, mood, or cognition.[25–30] These studies were not restricted to pure SCC populations. Recent PET/MR imaging work also suggests persistent abnormalities of glucose metabolism and cerebral blood flow, including possible neurovascular uncoupling.[31] Interpretation must account for heterogeneity in injury mechanism, timing, comorbidity, cognitive status, and methodology.[27,29]

Among postinfectious syndromes, long COVID provides the most developed FDG PET model, but available cohorts are again not limited to isolated subjective complaints. Across adult, pediatric, outpatient, multicenter, and longitudinal studies, recurrent hypometabolism has been reported in orbitofrontal/olfactory-related, limbic/paralimbic, brainstem, and cerebellar regions.[11–16] This is clinically relevant because long COVID combines patient-reported brain fog, fatigue, cognitive slowing, reduced endurance, anosmia-related symptoms, and dysautonomia with objectively measurable cognitive impairment in many patients, particularly in attentional and executive domains. FDG PET may therefore correlate not only with subjective complaints but also with neuropsychological deficits, symptom burden, and reduced cognitive endurance.[12–16] Of note, chronic fatigue syndrome/myalgic encephalomyelitis and fibromyalgia may be even more symptom-defined comparators for SCC than many long COVID cohorts, because fatigue, cognitive effort, brain fog, pain, and subjective functional limitation are central features only partly captured by conventional testing. This comparison should not be interpreted as implying that FDG PET abnormalities provide a signature of a *functional* condition. On the contrary, clinically relevant FDG PET abnormalities at the individual level are usually absent or nonspecific in primary psychiatric disorders, even though group-level metabolic differences may be reported in research settings. The presence of reproducible metabolic, neuroimmune, or interoceptive-network alterations in symptom-defined conditions should therefore be interpreted as evidence of measurable brain-system involvement rather than as a psychiatric or purely unexplained label.

These observations support a pattern-based and network-informed reading of FDG PET, with different certainty across conditions. In SCD, early signals may arise from focal hubs before canonical AD patterns. In mTBI and long COVID, distributed abnormalities may suggest altered network integrity, but interpretation should remain cautious because cohorts are heterogeneous, diagnostic certainty varies, and symptoms may be subjective, objective, systemic, or mixed.

A UNIFYING FRAMEWORK

In SCD, the upstream mechanism is plausibly early neurodegeneration propagating through network-dependent processes, with possible diaschisis-like remote hypometabolism before overt atrophy.[9,17] In mTBI, disconnection is plausible, although metabolic expression remains heterogeneous.[25–31] In postinfectious and related symptom-defined syndromes, PET evidence is compatible with neuroimmune, neuroglial, autonomic, and metabolic dysregulation affecting distributed systems.[32–37]

What unifies these conditions is not a single mechanism but the level at which dysfunction may be expressed. Salience, default mode, frontoparietal, limbic, and brainstem-cerebellar systems contribute to cognitive fluency, effort regulation, interoception, and self-monitoring. Partial disruption may produce major subjective consequences without frank collapse on standard tests, helping explain why symptom burden may diverge from visible lesion load.

This framework also helps move beyond a simplistic dichotomy between structurally visible lesions and unexplained symptoms. Network dysfunction may be biologically grounded without being anatomically obvious, and subjectively experienced symptoms may be real and clinically consequential even when conventional biomarkers are negative. FDG PET is valuable because it captures the downstream functional expression of these diverse processes in vivo.

Metacognitive mechanisms provide an additional interpretative layer. SCC can be conceptualized as arising not only from object-level cognitive dysfunction but also from altered monitoring of cognitive efficiency, effort, and predictability.[38] In early stages of neurodegenerative disease, preserved monitoring may increase awareness of subtle dysfunction, whereas progression may lead to reduced awareness or anosognosia.[18,38] In mTBI, postinfectious syndromes, and related symptom-defined conditions, altered monitoring may interact with fatigue, interoception, autonomic symptoms, pain, sleep disturbance, and affective load. FDG PET does not measure metacognition directly, but it may provide an objective correlate of the brain systems supporting cognitive efficiency, salience regulation, and self-monitoring, thereby improving interpretation and communication under diagnostic uncertainty.

INTEGRATION WITH MOLECULAR IMAGING

Amyloid PET demonstrates that a subset of SCD individuals harbor early AD pathology, although its relationship with complaints is influenced by affective and metacognitive factors.[1,8,39] Amyloid burden appears more strongly associated with worries about decline than with complaint severity.[39] Hippocampal encoding activity can predict subjective complaints independently of amyloid deposition and prior memory change.[3] Tau PET also supports the biological basis of SCC, with entorhinal tau pathology associated with complaints in cognitively normal individuals.

Within the amyloid tau neurodegeneration (ATN) research framework, FDG PET can be conceptualized as a downstream marker of neurodegeneration or neuronal dysfunction, helping distinguish amyloid-positive states without clear metabolic impact from those with established network-level dysfunction.[20,21] Real-world data support its negative predictive value in subjective cognitive impairment (SCI)/MCI populations.[24] Clinically, however, current FDG PET guidelines mainly concern objective cognitive impairment, particularly MCI and dementia, rather than isolated SCD.[40] This mismatch is a limitation and a possible target for future guideline evolution. In postinfectious and related syndromes, translocator protein (TSPO) PET studies suggest neuroinflammation in subsets of patients, complementing FDG PET assessment of network dysfunction.[32,33]

CLINICAL INTEGRATION

FDG PET should be interpreted as a contextual, pattern-based biomarker, not an isolated test. In SCD, it is best positioned as a stratification tool when downstream neurodegenerative impact must be assessed within a multimodal work-up. In mTBI, it may be useful in selected patients with persistent symptoms, functional impact, and nonexplanatory MR imaging. In long COVID, it may serve as a problem-solving biomarker in patients with disabling symptoms and limited or discordant objective findings.[11–16] Across settings, its relevance depends on coherence between pattern, phenotype, timing, and multimodal context.

Its contribution extends beyond diagnosis. When FDG PET reveals a coherent metabolic abnormality consistent with phenotype, it can reduce uncertainty, support rehabilitation, and improve communication. This is especially relevant in syndromes where patients encounter skepticism. Overinterpretation must be avoided: imaging is not a binary arbiter of whether symptoms are real but one tool for integrating subjective and biological dimensions.

METHODOLOGICAL CONSIDERATIONS AND FUTURE DIRECTIONS

The clinical utility of FDG PET in SCC depends on methodological rigor. Because expected abnormalities are often subtle, acquisition, reconstruction, interpretation, and reporting should follow brain FDG PET procedural standards.[40] Glycemia, uptake environment, recent stimulation, medication, sleep deprivation, motion, pain, and systemic illness may influence metabolism. Technical parameters are equally important, including uptake time, injected activity, acquisition duration, scanner performance, attenuation/scatter correction, reconstruction algorithm, resolution recovery, smoothing, partial-volume effects, and compatibility with the normative database. Standardized conditions, harmonized protocols, and documentation of confounders are essential, particularly in multicenter and longitudinal studies.

Analytical choices also play a major role. Normalization strategies and reference region selection can substantially alter the apparent extent and topography of hypometabolism. This is particularly important in long COVID and related postinfectious syndromes, and also mTBI, where commonly used reference regions such as the brainstem or cerebellum may themselves be involved.[11–16] Inappropriate normalization may attenuate, distort, or mask relevant abnormalities. Similar caution applies in aging populations, where partial volume effects and concomitant atrophy can complicate interpretation.

Whenever possible, semiquantitative or quantitative analyses anchored to age-adjusted normative databases should complement visual reading. Mild deviations may fall within physiologic variability, and similar patterns may arise from different processes, particularly in mTBI where affective symptoms, sleep disturbance, pain, medications, and injury heterogeneity shape the phenotype. FDG PET findings are therefore rarely specific in isolation; their value depends on coherence between pattern, symptoms, chronology, and multimodal context. SCC heterogeneity itself remains a limitation, encompassing distinct populations, symptom profiles, objective cognitive statuses, and mechanisms.

Future research should focus on homogeneous, operationally defined populations with careful characterization of symptom profile, objective cognitive status, affective and sleep comorbidities, disease stage, and time from insult. Harmonized FDG PET acquisition/analysis, longitudinal designs linking symptoms to objective performance, metabolic and molecular changes, and network-based approaches will be essential. In mTBI, larger prospective cohorts should stratify by injury mechanism, timing, comorbidity, cognitive status, and conventional/advanced MR imaging findings to determine whether FDG PET patterns are prognostic, treatment-responsive, or primarily explanatory. Multimodal integration including neuroinflammation imaging may enable more precise phenotyping.[9,17,31–33]

SUMMARY

Across preclinical AD, persistent symptoms after mTBI, and postinfectious syndromes, patients may report cognitive or cognitive-like complaints not fully explained by conventional structural imaging or standard neuropsychology. These settings should not be considered equivalent. SCD is most directly aligned with SCC and most integrated within AD biomarker frameworks. By contrast, mTBI and long COVID cohorts are more heterogeneous, often include mixed subjective and objective impairments, and are influenced by injury mechanism, timing, fatigue, affective and sleep comorbidities, systemic symptoms, and methodology.

FDG PET occupies a distinctive but context-dependent position. It does not replace MR imaging, neuropsychological testing, amyloid PET, tau PET, or fluid biomarkers but may complement them by interrogating the metabolic expression of distributed brain function. Its value is clearest in SCD when assessing downstream neurodegenerative impact within a multimodal framework, and more exploratory in mTBI and postinfectious syndromes, where studies suggest but do not definitively establish large-scale metabolic-network abnormalities.[9,11–17,25–37]

More broadly, FDG PET supports a cautious shift from dismissing subjective complaints as nonspecific noise toward considering them as potentially meaningful signals requiring structured investigation. Future work should rely on better-defined populations, standardized phenotyping, objective cognitive characterization, harmonized PET methodology, and longitudinal multimodal designs. Within such frameworks, FDG PET may improve stratification, interpretation, and communication in patients whose main difficulty is not always poor test performance but altered cognitive efficiency, endurance, or self-monitoring.

CLINICS CARE POINTS

- Subjective cognitive complaints are clinically meaningful but heterogeneous; clinicians should characterize the cognitive domain involved, objective cognitive status, functional impact, mood, sleep, fatigue, pain, medications, and systemic comorbidities.
- FDG PET should not be requested as a generic test for subjective cognitive complaints, but as a context-dependent biomarker aimed at answering a defined clinical question.
- In subjective cognitive decline, FDG PET is most useful when integrated into a multimodal Alzheimer's disease biomarker framework, particularly to assess downstream neurodegenerative impact.
- The clinical role of FDG PET is better established in mild cognitive impairment and dementia than in isolated subjective cognitive decline; isolated subjective complaints should not be overinterpreted as neurodegeneration without supportive clinical or biomarker evidence.
- A normal FDG PET may help lower the probability of near-term neurodegenerative progression in selected memory-clinic populations, but it does not exclude very early Alzheimer's disease, non-neurodegenerative causes, or biologically relevant subjective symptoms.
- In persistent symptoms after mild traumatic brain injury, FDG PET may reveal diffuse or network-level abnormalities despite nonexplanatory structural imaging, but findings are heterogeneous and should be interpreted cautiously.
- In post-concussion presentations, fatigue, sleep disturbance, anxiety, depression, posttraumatic stress, pain, medications, and injury mechanism are major interpretive confounders and should be documented in the report.
- In long COVID and related post-infectious syndromes, FDG PET may support objective evidence of brain-system involvement in selected patients, particularly when symptoms are disabling and conventional investigations are unrevealing or discordant.
- Recurrent hypometabolic patterns in long COVID should not be used as a binary diagnostic criterion, because cohorts are heterogeneous and cognitive symptoms may be subjective, objective, systemic, or mixed.
- FDG PET reports should emphasize pattern-based interpretation rather than isolated regional findings, and should explicitly address clinical coherence, differential diagnosis, and limits of specificity.
- Semi-quantitative analysis may improve reproducibility, but normalization strategy, reference-region selection, age-adjusted normative database, and scanner/protocol harmonization are critical, especially when abnormalities are subtle.
- Reference regions such as the cerebellum or brainstem should be used cautiously in post-infectious syndromes, because these regions may themselves be involved in the metabolic pattern.
- FDG PET findings should support clinical reasoning, rehabilitation planning, and patient communication, but should not be presented as a stand-alone arbiter of whether symptoms are "real" or disease-specific.

DISCLOSURE

No competitive interests.

REFERENCES

1. Amariglio RE, Becker JA, Carmasin J, et al. Subjective cognitive complaints and amyloid burden in cognitively normal older individuals. Neuropsychologia 2012;50(12):2880–6.
2. Amariglio RE, Buckley RF, Mormino EC, et al. Amyloid-associated increases in longitudinal report of subjective cognitive complaints. Alzheimer's Dement 2018;4:444–9.
3. Chen X, Farrell ME, Rundle MM, et al. The relationship of functional hippocampal activity, amyloid deposition, and longitudinal memory decline to memory complaints in cognitively healthy older adults. Neurobiol Aging 2021;105:245–53.
4. Hohman TJ, Beason-Held LL, Lamar M, et al. Subjective cognitive complaints and longitudinal changes in memory and brain function. Neuropsychology 2011;25(1):125–30.
5. Timmers T, Ossenkoppele R, Verfaillie SCJ, et al. Amyloid PET and cognitive decline in cognitively normal individuals: the SCIENCe project. Neurobiol Aging 2019;79:50–8.
6. Vogel JW, Varga Dolezalova M, La Joie R, et al. Subjective cognitive decline and β-amyloid burden predict cognitive change in healthy elderly. Neurology 2017;89(19):2002–9.
7. Jansen WJ, Janssen O, Tijms BM, et al. Prevalence estimates of amyloid abnormality across the Alzheimer disease clinical spectrum. JAMA Neurol 2022;79(3):228–43.
8. Perrotin A, La Joie R, de La Sayette V, et al. Subjective cognitive decline in cognitively normal elders from the community or from a memory clinic: differential affective and imaging correlates. Alzheimer's Dement 2017;13(1):64–72.
9. Wang X, Huang W, Su L, et al. Neuroimaging advances regarding subjective cognitive decline in preclinical Alzheimer's disease. Mol Neurodegener 2020;15:55.
10. Hoge CW, McGurk D, Thomas JL, et al. Mild traumatic brain injury in U.S. soldiers returning from Iraq. N Engl J Med 2008;358(5):453–63.
11. Guedj E, Million M, Dudouet P, et al. ^{18}F-FDG brain PET hypometabolism in post-SARS-CoV-2 infection: substrate for persistent/delayed disorders? Eur J Nucl Med Mol Imag 2021;48(2):592–5.
12. Guedj E, Campion JY, Dudouet P, et al. ^{18}F-FDG brain PET hypometabolism in patients with long COVID. Eur J Nucl Med Mol Imag 2021;48(9):2823–33.
13. Verger A, Kas A, Dudouet P, et al. Visual interpretation of brain hypometabolism related to neurological long COVID: a French multicentric experience. Eur J Nucl Med Mol Imag 2022;49(9):3197–202.
14. Goehringer F, Bruyere A, Doyen M, et al. Brain ^{18}F-FDG PET imaging in outpatients with post-COVID-19 conditions: findings and associations with clinical characteristics. Eur J Nucl Med Mol Imag 2023; 50(4):1084–9.
15. Horowitz T, Dudouet P, Campion JY, et al. Persistent brain metabolic impairment in long COVID patients with persistent clinical symptoms: a nine-month follow-up [^{18}F]FDG-PET study. Eur J Nucl Med Mol Imag 2024;51(11):3215–22.
16. Morand A, Campion JY, Lepine A, et al. Similar patterns of [^{18}F]FDG brain PET hypometabolism in paediatric and adult patients with long COVID: a paediatric case series. Eur J Nucl Med Mol Imag 2022;49(3):913–20.
17. Chételat G. Multimodal neuroimaging in Alzheimer's disease: early diagnosis, physiopathological mechanisms, and impact of lifestyle. J Alzheimers Dis 2018;64(s1):S199–211.
18. Prigatano GP. Disturbances of self-awareness and rehabilitation of patients with traumatic brain injury. J Head Trauma Rehabil 2005;20(1):19–29.
19. Buckley RF, Hanseeuw B, Schultz AP, et al. Region-specific association of subjective cognitive decline with tauopathy independent of global β-amyloid burden. JAMA Neurol 2017;74(12):1455–63.
20. Ebenau JL, Timmers T, Wesselman LMP, et al. ATN classification and clinical progression in subjective cognitive decline. Neurology 2020;95(1):e46–58.
21. Eliassen CF, Reinvang I, Selnes P, et al. Biomarkers in subtypes of mild cognitive impairment and subjective cognitive decline. Brain Behav 2017;7: e00685.
22. Douaud G, Lee S, Alfaro-Almagro F, et al. SARS-CoV-2 is associated with changes in brain structure in UK Biobank. Nature 2022;604(7907):697–707.
23. Dong QY, Li TR, Jiang XY, et al. Glucose metabolism in the right middle temporal gyrus could be a potential biomarker for subjective cognitive decline. Alzheimers Res Ther 2021;13:134.
24. Heyer S, Simon M, Doyen M, et al. ^{18}F-FDG PET can effectively rule out conversion to dementia and the presence of CSF biomarker of neurodegeneration: a real-world data analysis. Alzheimers Res Ther 2024;16(1):182.
25. Peskind ER, Petrie EC, Cross DJ, et al. Cerebrocerebellar hypometabolism associated with repetitive blast exposure mild traumatic brain injury in 12 Iraq war veterans with persistent post-concussive symptoms. Neuroimage 2011;54(Suppl 1):S76–82.
26. Mendez MF, Owens EM, Reza Berenji G, et al. Mild traumatic brain injury from primary blast vs. blunt forces: post-concussion consequences and functional neuroimaging. NeuroRehabilitation 2013; 32(2):397–407.
27. Byrnes KR, Wilson CM, Brabazon F, et al. FDG-PET imaging in mild traumatic brain injury: a critical review. Front Neuroenerg 2014;5:13.
28. Komura A, Kawasaki T, Yamada Y, et al. Cerebral glucose metabolism in patients with chronic mental

and cognitive sequelae after a single blunt mild traumatic brain injury without visible brain lesions. J Neurotrauma 2019;36(5):641–9.
29. Teichner EM, You JC, Hriso C, et al. Alterations in cerebral glucose metabolism as measured by 18F-fluorodeoxyglucose-PET in patients with persistent postconcussion syndrome. Nucl Med Commun 2021;42(7):772–81.
30. Bischof GN, Cross DJ. Brain trauma imaging. J Nucl Med 2023;64(1):20–9.
31. Heholt J, Patel R, Vedaei F, et al. Simultaneous arterial spin labeling functional MRI and fluorodeoxyglucose PET in mild chronic traumatic brain injury. J Neuroradiol 2024;51(5):101211.
32. Nakatomi Y, Mizuno K, Ishii A, et al. Neuroinflammation in patients with chronic fatigue syndrome/myalgic encephalomyelitis: an ^{11}C-(R)-PK11195 PET study. J Nucl Med 2014;55(6):945–50.
33. Mueller C, Fang YH, Jones C, et al. Evidence of neuroinflammation in fibromyalgia syndrome: a [^{18}F] DPA-714 positron emission tomography study. Pain 2023;164(10):2285–95.
34. Tirelli U, Chierichetti F, Tavio M, et al. Brain positron emission tomography (PET) in chronic fatigue syndrome: preliminary data. Am J Med 1998;105(3A): 54S–8S.
35. Siessmeier T, Nix WA, Hardt J, et al. Observer independent analysis of cerebral glucose metabolism in patients with chronic fatigue syndrome. J Neurol Neurosurg Psychiatry 2003;74(7):922–8.
36. Yunus MB, Young CS, Saeed SA, et al. Positron emission tomography in patients with fibromyalgia syndrome and healthy controls. Arthritis Rheum 2004;51(4):513–8.
37. Usui C, Soma T, Hatta K, et al. A study of brain metabolism in fibromyalgia by positron emission tomography. Prog Neuropsychopharmacol Biol Psychiatry 2017;75:120–7.
38. Nelson TO, Narens L. Metamemory: a theoretical framework and new findings. In: Bower GH, editor. The psychology of learning and motivation, 26. Academic Press; 1990. p. 125–73.
39. Verfaillie SCJ, Timmers T, Slot RER, et al. Amyloid-β load is related to worries, but not to severity of cognitive complaints in individuals with subjective cognitive decline: the SCIENCe project. Front Aging Neurosci 2019;11:7.
40. Guedj E, Varrone A, Boellaard R, et al. EANM procedure guidelines for brain PET imaging using [^{18}F]FDG, version 3. Eur J Nucl Med Mol Imag 2022;49(2):632–51.

Fluorodeoxyglucose PET and Consciousness

Cyrus Ayubcha, MD, PhD[a], Thomas J. Werner, MSE[b], Abass Alavi, MD[c], Andrew B. Newberg, MD[d,e,*]

KEYWORDS

• Consciousness • Awareness • Wakefulness • Meditation • Brain injury • Cognition • Emotion

KEY POINTS

- Fluorodeoxyglucose (FDG) PET neuroimaging has been widely used to investigate the neural basis of consciousness across a broad range of states.
- Neuroimaging research has also examined intentionally altered states of consciousness, including those induced by meditation and psychedelic substances, to better understand variations in conscious experience.
- Studying consciousness with FDG PET presents methodological and conceptual challenges that limit interpretation of neuroimaging findings related to subjective experience.

INTRODUCTION

Consciousness remains among the most intricate and elusive dimensions of human existence to investigate. A central challenge lies in that although every individual possesses consciousness, we are inherently confined within our own subjective awareness, making fully objective examination extraordinarily difficult. Because consciousness is fundamentally experiential, the primary way to access another person's mental state is through self-report. Yet the very act of asking someone to describe their present experience inevitably modifies that experience. This introduces methodological complications, particularly when attempting to correlate neurophysiological measures, such as functional brain imaging, with lived subjective states.

Even defining consciousness presents conceptual difficulty.[1] In the medical clinical context, consciousness is often equated with wakefulness. For example, when evaluating a patient following a head injury or cerebrovascular event, clinicians may describe the patient as conscious if the individual is awake and responsive to external stimuli. However, beyond this pragmatic medical usage, scholars in philosophy, neuroscience, theology, and consciousness studies generally interpret consciousness as awareness. In humans, this frequently entails self-awareness. A video camera may register the same visual field perceived by the human eye, but unlike a person, it lacks awareness that it is perceiving. Human consciousness thus includes reflexive awareness—the awareness of being aware.

[a] Department of Neurosurgery, Harvard Medical School, Boston, MA, USA; [b] Department of Radiology, Hospital of the University of Pennsylvania, University of Pennsylvania Perelman School of Medicine, Philadelphia, PA, USA; [c] Division of Nuclear Medicine, Department of Radiology, Hospital of the University of Pennsylvania, University of Pennsylvania Perelman School of Medicine, Philadelphia, PA, USA; [d] Department of Radiology, Sidney Kimmel Medical College, Thomas Jefferson University, Philadelphia, PA, USA; [e] Department of Integrative Medicine and Nutritional Sciences, Sidney Kimmel Medical College, Thomas Jefferson University, Philadelphia, PA, USA

* Corresponding author. Department of Integrative Medicine and Nutritional Sciences, 789 East Lancaster Avenue, Suite 110, Villanova, PA 19085.

E-mail address: Andrew.newberg@jefferson.edu

PET Clin 21 (2026) 561–571
https://doi.org/10.1016/j.cpet.2026.04.001

Abbreviations

BOLD	blood-oxygenation-level-dependent
DMN	default mode network
EEG	electroencephalography
fMRI	functional MR imaging
MCS	minimally conscious state
MRS	magnetic resonance spectroscopy
NIR	near-infrared imaging
SPECT	single photon emission computed tomography
UWS	unresponsive wakefulness syndrome

Awareness appears to operate across multiple levels, spanning biological, psychological, and potentially spiritual dimensions, each grounded in varying degrees in neurobiology. Prior conceptual models have proposed several categories or tiers of awareness.[2] The most basic level is instinctual awareness, typically operating at an organismic level. Even simple life forms demonstrate rudimentary responsiveness to environmental stimuli that supports survival, integrating sensory input with adaptive response. In organisms possessing a nervous system, such awareness likely involves structures including the thalamus, nucleus accumbens, periaqueductal gray, and limbic circuitry, reflecting fundamental approach–avoidance and emotionally mediated processes.

A subsequent level involves habitual responsiveness, characterized by learning and memory formation. Through repeated experience, organisms develop patterned behaviors related to feeding, social interaction, and reproduction. Neural substrates associated with such learned behaviors likely include midbrain structures, the cerebellum, and posterior neocortical regions. More complex still is intentional decision-making, which prominently characterizes human cognition. This level incorporates language, affective evaluation, and goal-directed planning. Neural correlates commonly implicated include the dorsolateral prefrontal cortex and temporoparietal association cortices. Executive processes—such as organizing daily activities, preparing a grocery list, or planning travel—require integration of present conditions with anticipated future outcomes. Intentional awareness, therefore, entails temporal integration within a consciously guided decision framework.

Another dimension of awareness is creative imagination. Processes such as spontaneous mind-wandering, daydreaming, and associative ideation fall within this domain. Creative cognition has been associated with activity in the default mode network (DMN), as well as coordinated interactions between hemispheres. Sensory, emotional, and higher order cognitive processes converge in generative and novel configurations. In research conducted by our group, highly creative individuals demonstrated distinctive activation patterns within both default mode and executive control networks compared to individuals reporting average creativity levels[3] (**Fig. 1**).

At still more complex levels are self-reflective awareness and what may be termed transformational awareness. These forms frequently overlap with spiritual or existential dimensions of experience, involving symbolic and intuitive processing of the self and its relationship to others. Transformational awareness encompasses profound states such as mystical or enlightenment experiences. Neuroimaging investigations have implicated distributed networks in these states, including the anterior cingulate cortex, insula, thalamus, brainstem structures, limbic regions, and frontoparietal circuits. Notably, such higher order states appear to rely on coordinated activity across multiple neural systems rather than a single localized structure.

Given these gradations of awareness, neuroimaging offers a compelling—though methodologically and philosophically complex—approach to examining the neural substrates of consciousness. Numerous brain regions have been proposed as potential "centers" of consciousness, yet no study has definitively identified a singular anatomic source or mechanism that generates conscious experience. A particularly challenging question concerns how consciousness might arise from neuronal firing patterns, electrical oscillations, neurotransmitter dynamics, and the vast network of neural interconnections within the brain. No empirical investigation has successfully isolated the fundamental origin of conscious experience, a dilemma often described as the "hard problem" of consciousness.[4]

This unresolved question has led some scholars to propose that consciousness may be an emergent property arising from complex neurobiological interactions, speculated to be related to quantum interactions within the microtubules of neurons.[5] Importantly, others suggest it may not be reducible to biological mechanisms alone. Across diverse philosophic and spiritual traditions, consciousness has even been regarded as "primary"—constituting the foundational substance of reality from which material phenomena emerge.[6] Both Buddhist and Hindu philosophic systems emphasize the notion of consciousness as fundamental to existence. Nevertheless, even if consciousness is ontologically primary, it clearly interacts intimately with brain function. Accordingly, neuroimaging remains a valuable methodological tool

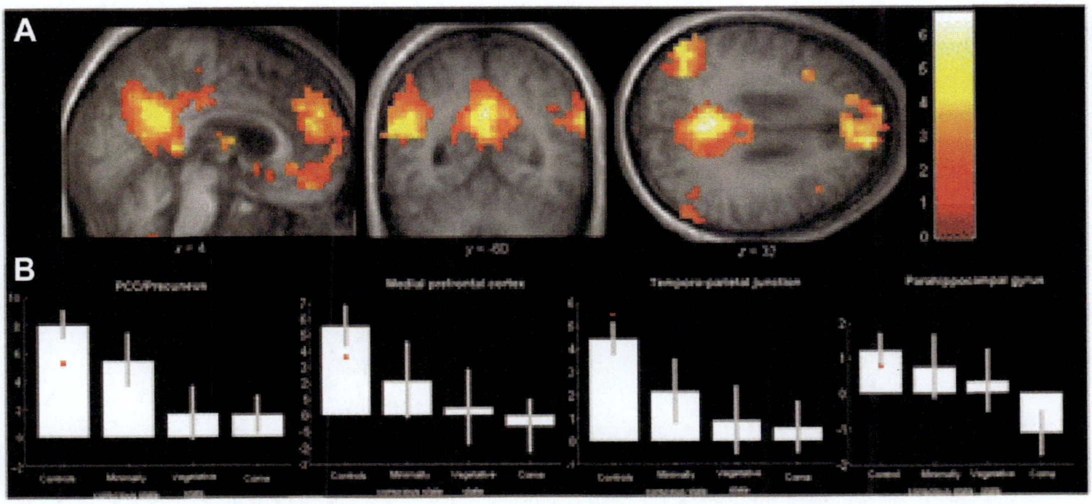

Fig. 1. Default network connectivity correlates with the level of consciousness, ranging from healthy controls, to minimally conscious, vegetative then comatose patients. (*A*) Areas showing a linear correlation between default network connectivity and consciousness. Results are thresholded for display at uncorrected $P < .05$ and rendered on the mean T1 structural image of the patients. (*B*) Mean Z-scores and 90% confidence interval for default network connectivity in posterior cingulate cortex (PCC)/precuneus, temporo-parietal junction, medial prefrontal cortex, and parahippocampal gyrus across patient populations. Locked-in syndrome patient Z-scores are displayed for illustrative purposes as an additional red circles overlaid on control population data. (*From* Reproduced with permission from Vanhaudenhuyse A, et al.[53] Vanhaudenhuyse A, Noirhomme Q, Tshibanda LJ, et al. Default network connectivity reflects the level of consciousness in non-communicative brain-damaged patients. Brain 2010;133(Pt 1):161–71. https://doi.org/10.1093/brain/awp313; Reproduced with permission.[53])

for investigating how conscious states, and consciousness itself, correlate with neural processes.

These questions have also contributed to the development of a field referred to as neurotheology, an interdisciplinary approach examining the relationship between brain function and religious or spiritual phenomena.[7] Many deeply meaningful religious experiences, including mystical or enlightenment states, are understood as altered states of consciousness.[8] Thus, neurotheological research may serve as a useful bridge in the broader effort to investigate consciousness through neuroimaging methodologies.

NEUROIMAGING OF CONSCIOUSNESS

Neuroimaging offers multiple avenues for investigating consciousness, largely because conscious experience can fluctuate across a spectrum—from diminished states such as coma or anesthesia to heightened or altered states induced by meditation, pharmacologic agents, or spiritual practices. These variations provide experimental entry points for examining how brain structure and function relate to subjective awareness.

Among the principal imaging modalities used in consciousness research are PET, single photon emission computed tomography (SPECT), and MR imaging (**Fig. 2**).

PET and SPECT imaging, both grounded in nuclear medicine techniques, contribute meaningfully to consciousness research. Both provide robust quantitative assessments of physiologic parameters that might be associated with various states of consciousness. Although these modalities require administration of radioactive tracers, they are generally considered safe in research and clinical contexts. Importantly, they can be applied in situations less compatible with MR imaging environments. For example, PET and SPECT might be used during spiritual practices involving movement or postural variation that might induce altered states of consciousness since injection of the tracer can be performed outside of the scanner environment. Several studies of this type have been performed during various mind–body practices that alter consciousness (see later discussion).

One particularly compelling application of PET and SPECT involves the investigation of neurotransmitter systems during different conscious states. Radioligands are available for numerous neurotransmitter pathways, including serotonin, dopamine, gamma-aminobutyric acid, and endogenous opioid systems—each of which may plausibly contribute to variations in awareness.[9] Beyond measuring overall neurotransmitter activity, these tracers can target presynaptic and

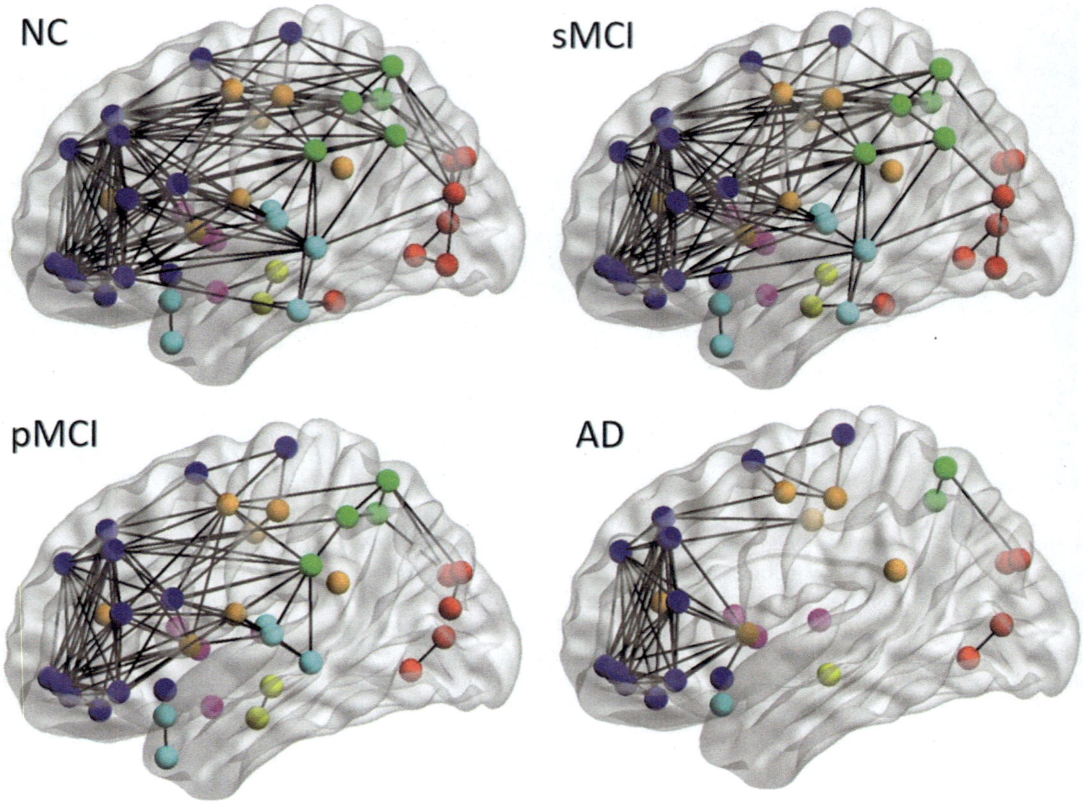

Fig. 2. The lateral view of mean individual intrahemispheric connectivity graphs of NC, sMCI, pMCI, and AD. The intrahemispheric connectivity graphs were visualized for 4 groups and obtained by thresholding the correlation coefficient matrix using the threshold of 0.4354. The intrahemispheric connections are indicated by black lines and nodes are represented by different colors (*deep blue* for frontal; *light blue* for temporal; *green* for parietal; *red* for occipital; *pink* for thalamus, pallidum, caudate, putamen, amygdala; *yellow* for hippocampus; and *deep yellow* for other regions). (*From* Image reprinted without changes from Huang SY, et al.[54] under the Creative Commons Attribution 4.0 International License (CC BY). https://creativecommons.org/licenses/by/4.0/). Huang S-Y, Hsu J-L, Lin K-J, et al. A Novel Individual Metabolic Brain Network for 18F-FDG PET Imaging. Front Neurosci 2020;14:344. https://doi.org/10.3389/fnins.2020.00344.[54])

postsynaptic receptors, transporters, and even glial-associated binding sites. Such capabilities allow researchers to explore neurochemical correlates of altered states of consciousness with considerable specificity.

Functional MR imaging (fMRI) has been especially valuable for assessing physiologic parameters such as functional connectivity and regional cerebral blood flow, and, through magnetic resonance spectroscopy (MRS), certain neurotransmitter concentrations.[9] Because many fMRI paradigms include a resting-state scan as a baseline condition, researchers can compare network activity across individuals, including those experiencing altered states of consciousness. Differences in connectivity patterns or perfusion can thus be identified between typical wakefulness and other states such as sleep or anesthesia.[10,11]

However, interpretation of fMRI signals requires caution. The blood-oxygenation-level-dependent (BOLD) signal reflects changes in blood oxygenation mediated by neurovascular coupling rather than direct neuronal activity, and emerging evidence suggests that this relationship is not uniform across brain regions. Some areas, especially within the default mode, may exhibit discordant relationships between BOLD signal changes and underlying oxygen metabolism, indicating that changes in cerebral blood flow do not always reliably index neuronal activity. These findings challenge the canonical interpretation of BOLD fMRI and suggest that quantitative approaches integrating measures of oxygen metabolism may provide a more accurate characterization of neural function.[10] MRS adds another dimension by estimating concentrations of specific neurochemicals; however, it does not directly measure receptor density, receptor binding, or affinity—parameters more commonly evaluated using PET or SPECT methodologies.

These techniques face conceptual and methodological challenges when applied to consciousness research. One central difficulty concerns defining the "resting" conscious state. It is not self-evident that resting-state cerebral metabolism or perfusion accurately captures a stable or uniform conscious condition. Some investigators have proposed, based on fMRI findings, that consciousness is better conceptualized as an inherently dynamic process in which shifting interactions among core neural networks underpin transitions from one state to another.[11] Structural or morphometric imaging avoids the need to define a resting mental state, but introduces other limitations, including accurate anatomic segmentation, susceptibility to motion artifact, and the inherent difficulty of delineating fine-grained structures. Moreover, structural imaging is relatively insensitive to rapid, state-dependent neural changes that likely characterize fluctuations in consciousness.

A common assumption in neuroscience is that specific aspects of consciousness correspond to activity within particular brain regions, for instance, emotional experience with limbic activation. Yet, it is equally plausible that conscious experience reflects dynamic transitions in neural activity rather than static regional activation. In this view, the process of changes such as increasing synchronization or shifting connectivity—may be more closely linked to conscious phenomena than any single steady-state pattern.[12] Future research will need to clarify how evolving neural dynamics correspond to subjective awareness, and fMRI, with its capacity to assess network-level interactions, is likely to remain central to this effort.

Additional methodologies have also been employed in the study of altered states, including electroencephalography (EEG), near-infrared imaging (NIR), and magnetoencephalography. EEG, among the earliest tools used to examine meditative states, remains particularly valuable due to its excellent temporal resolution.[13] The relatively unobtrusive placement of an electrode cap allows individuals to engage in many contemplative practices with minimal interference. However, EEG provides limited spatial precision, making it difficult to localize the exact anatomic sources of recorded electrical activity.

Across all modalities, a major challenge lies in capturing conscious states as they occur. Some meditative practices or psychedelic-induced states can be studied within an MR imaging scanner, provided participants can remain sufficiently still. Other states, however, may not be compatible with the constraints of MR imaging acquisition and instead require alternative approaches such as PET, SPECT, EEG, or NIR. Selecting the appropriate neuroimaging method thus depends not only on the physiologic variable of interest but also on the practical feasibility of studying a given state of consciousness during its natural expression.

STUDYING SPECIFIC ASPECTS OF CONSCIOUSNESS

Consciousness can be disrupted in numerous clinical conditions. Traumatic brain injury, neoplasms, cerebrovascular accidents, and inflammatory disorders may all impair awareness to varying degrees. Neuroimaging plays a crucial role in identifying the regions affected by such insults and clarifying how those areas contribute to conscious experience.[14] In a similar vein, neurodegenerative disorders—including Alzheimer's disease and Parkinson's disease—can alter cognition and awareness over time. Epilepsy also has important implications for consciousness, particularly temporal lobe epilepsy, which has been associated in some cases with atypical spiritual or mystical-type experiences.[15] Psychiatric illnesses provide additional windows into altered consciousness. Schizophrenia, for example, may profoundly distort perception, self-experience, and reality testing. Dissociative identity disorder (formerly termed multiple personality disorder) is especially intriguing in this regard, as individuals appear to shift between distinct identity states, each with differing patterns of memory, affect, and behavior. Functional neuroimaging during such shifts may offer insight into how conscious states transition within the same individual.[16]

Another rapidly expanding area of investigation involves studying the effects of psychedelic compounds. Contemporary clinical research is evaluating psychedelics as potential treatments for depression, anxiety disorders, and posttraumatic stress disorder. These agents induce marked alterations in perception, cognition, affect, and sense of self, often including changes in ego boundaries and self-referential processing.[17] One methodological advantage of studying psychedelics is that their primary neurochemical mechanisms are relatively well characterized. Classic agents such as psilocybin and lysergic acid diethylamide exert strong effects on the serotonergic system, particularly at 5-hydroxytryptamine receptor 2A (5-HT2A) receptors. Neuroimaging studies have begun to characterize how these compounds modify functional connectivity, cerebral blood flow, and network organization.[18,19] Some investigations have also compared psychedelic-induced states with other altered states, such as those achieved through hypnosis, to explore shared or divergent neural mechanisms.[20]

Among nonpharmacologic approaches, spiritual and contemplative practices, especially meditation and prayer, have been extensively examined. These approaches can induce altered states of consciousness during the practice itself, but they may also produce enduring trait-level changes in brain structure and function. Thus, the concept of enlightenment or spiritual maturation can refer both to a transient experiential state and to a persistent transformation in the individual. Neuroimaging research has explored both immediate state effects during practice and long-term adaptations associated with sustained engagement in contemplative disciplines.

Multiple imaging studies have identified structural and functional brain differences in experienced meditators who frequently report altered states of awareness.[21] Regions implicated include portions of the frontal and parietal lobes, limbic structures, and large-scale networks such as the salience network and the DMN. Longitudinal and cross-sectional studies suggest that specific meditation programs may influence cognition, emotional regulation, and attentional processes over extended periods. These effects are related to, but distinct from, acute neural changes observed during meditation itself.[22] For instance, meditation training has been associated with altered neural responses during emotional and cognitive tasks, as reflected in functional imaging findings.[23–27] Morphometric MR imaging studies have also reported increased cortical thickness or gray matter volume—particularly within frontal regions and prefrontal cortex—in long-term practitioners compared to nonmeditators.[28] Such findings have been observed both within specific traditions and when practitioners from diverse contemplative backgrounds are analyzed collectively. Earlier research from our group demonstrated differences in cerebral blood flow in regions including the midbrain, thalamus, putamen, caudate, prefrontal cortex, and parietal cortex in long-term meditators relative to controls.[29] Nevertheless, many of these investigations have emphasized neural correlates of meditation without directly measuring how subjective consciousness itself is altered (**Fig. 3**).

Some research has grouped individuals practicing varied techniques—such as Zen Buddhism, Kriya yoga, Vipassana, Kundalini yoga, and other unspecified methods—into a single meditator cohort for comparison with nonmeditators.[29] This

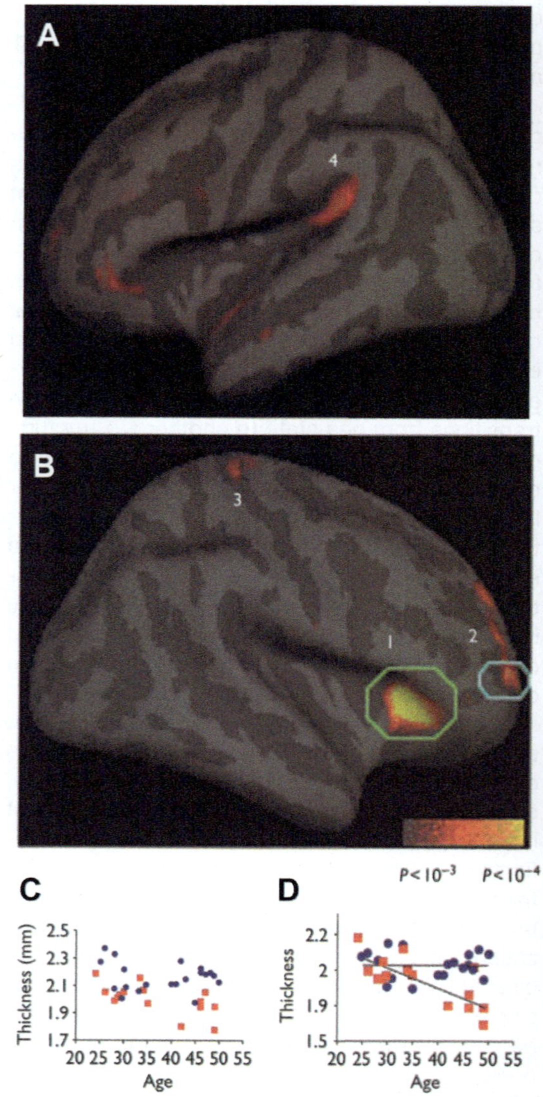

Fig. 3. Cortical regions thicker in meditators than in controls. (*A* and *B*) Statistical map depicting between-group differences in thickness at each point on the cortical surface overlaid on the inflated average brain. All points meeting a $P < .01$ threshold (uncorrected) are displayed to better illustrate the anatomic extent of the areas and the relative specificity of the findings. Numbered regions: (1) insula, (2) Brodmann area (BA) 9/10, (3) somatosensory cortex, (4) auditory cortex. (*C* and *D*) Scatter plot of mean cortical thickness of each participant in the subregion above threshold within each circled region of (*C*) insula and (*D*) BA 9/10, plotted versus age. Meditation participants: blue circles; control participants: red squares. (*From* Reproduced with permission from Lazar SW et al.[55] Lazar SW, Kerr CE, Wasserman RH, et al. Meditation experience is associated with increased cortical thickness. Neuroreport 2005;16(17):1893–7.[55])

heterogeneous approach may reveal shared or potentially universal neural adaptations associated with contemplative practice. However, studying specific meditation forms individually allows for greater precision in identifying distinct neural signatures linked to particular techniques.

Despite this heterogeneity, important findings have emerged. For example, there is increased cortical gyrification, quantified as mean curvature across the cortical surface, in meditators, particularly within the left precentral gyrus, right fusiform gyrus, right cuneus, and bilateral anterior dorsal insula. Moreover, the degree of gyrification correlated positively with years of meditation practice. Other analyses have identified larger gray matter volumes in meditators within the right orbitofrontal cortex, right thalamus, left inferior temporal gyrus, and right hippocampus.[30] Differences in hippocampal volume and microstructural characteristics have likewise been observed in long-term practitioners compared to nonmeditators.[31]

Diffusion tensor imaging studies have further demonstrated increased white matter connectivity in experienced meditators, both globally and particularly between hemispheres.[32,33] Significant group differences have been reported in tracts such as the corticospinal tract, superior longitudinal fasciculus, and uncinate fasciculus. These findings suggest that sustained contemplative practice may enhance structural integration across distributed neural systems, potentially reflecting repeated engagement of attention, cognitive control, and emotional regulation networks.

Mindfulness meditation, derived from ancient contemplative traditions, has received substantial attention in modern neuroscience. Because mindfulness explicitly cultivates awareness of present-moment experience, it is directly relevant to the study of consciousness. Practices commonly include focused attention on the breath, systematic body scanning, and loving-kindness meditation.[34] Morphometric MR imaging investigations have shown that long-term mindfulness practitioners exhibit increased gray matter density or volume in regions associated with introspection, emotional regulation, and self-referential processing.[35] Structural adaptations have been observed in the hippocampus, a region central to learning and memory.[36] Increased cortical thickness has also been reported in frontal regions, the hippocampus, and the right insula among long-term practitioners.[37]

Functional neuroimaging studies indicate that mindfulness practice is associated with modifications in DMN connectivity, a network implicated in self-referential thinking and mind-wandering.[38] Enhanced functional connectivity within or modulation of this network in experienced practitioners may correspond to a shift toward greater present-centered awareness and less self-referential mental states.[35] Additionally, mindfulness training appears to influence neural responses to emotional stimuli, with altered activation patterns in the amygdala and prefrontal cortex consistent with improved emotional regulation and decreased reactivity.[39]

Overall, contemplative neuroscience increasingly supports the notion that meditation can produce enduring alterations in both brain structure and functional organization. Long-term practitioners demonstrate neural changes suggestive of enhanced attentional control, emotional balance, and self-awareness. Continued research into these sustained adaptations offers valuable insight into the brain's capacity for neuroplasticity and into how disciplined mental training may shape consciousness itself over time.

Studying Disorders of Consciousness

In clinical neurology, "consciousness" is operationally understood as having 2 separable components[40]: (1) arousal/wakefulness and (2) content/awareness (ie, the capacity for conscious experience and purposeful interaction). Importantly, patients may be conscious but poorly responsive (eg, severe motor impairment), meaning that responsiveness is an imperfect proxy for awareness.[41] This clinical framing is foundational for interpreting neuroimaging findings in disorders of consciousness and for avoiding diagnostic circularity (defining consciousness only by behavior).

Neuroanatomically, a sustained reduction in the level of consciousness typically reflects either (1) widespread bilateral hemispheric dysfunction (eg, diffuse hypoxic–ischemic injury or toxic–metabolic encephalopathy) or (2) disruption of key subcortical arousal pathways in the upper brainstem/diencephalon and their thalamocortical projections. Clinically, this underlies the classic emergency distinction between structural causes of coma (mass lesions, brainstem injury, and hemorrhage) versus diffuse/metabolic causes (systemic derangements, intoxication, and global hypoxia), a distinction that remains crucial even in the modern neuroimaging era.[40,42]

Standardized behavioral assessment remains the diagnostic cornerstone (eg, Coma Recovery Scale–Revised), yet misclassification is common when diagnosis relies on nonstandardized bedside impressions. Studies comparing clinical consensus to standardized instruments have reported that a substantial fraction of patients labeled vegetative/unresponsive may actually demonstrate reproducible signs consistent with minimally conscious state (MCS) when formally tested. These realities motivate an evidence-based, multimodal approach in which FDG PET, fMRI, and EEG are used as adjuncts—not replacements—to structured bedside examination.[43,44]

Early PET investigations demonstrated that patients in a vegetative state exhibit global cerebral metabolism reduction to approximately 40% to 50% of normal values.[45] Importantly, this hypometabolism is not uniformly distributed, but rather the association cortices, especially in the precuneus and posterior cingulate cortex, show disproportionate decreases.[46] These midline regions are also central components of the DMN, which has been implicated in self-referential processing and conscious awareness as described earlier (**Fig. 4**).

Laureys and colleagues[2] reported that recovery of consciousness was associated with restoration of metabolic activity within a frontoparietal network, rather than simple normalization of global metabolism. This finding shifted theoretic models from a purely arousal-based framework to one emphasizing large-scale network integration as a substrate for conscious experience.

FDG PET has proven particularly valuable in distinguishing unresponsive wakefulness syndrome (UWS, formerly vegetative state), and the MCS. In a landmark study, Stender and colleagues[47] demonstrated that FDG PET classified patients with disorders of consciousness more accurately than bedside behavioral assessment alone. Using quantitative metabolic thresholds within the frontoparietal networks, PET achieved diagnostic accuracy exceeding 80% in differentiating UWS from MCS. Patients in MCS typically exhibit partial preservation of metabolism in the lateral frontoparietal cortices, whereas patients with UWS show

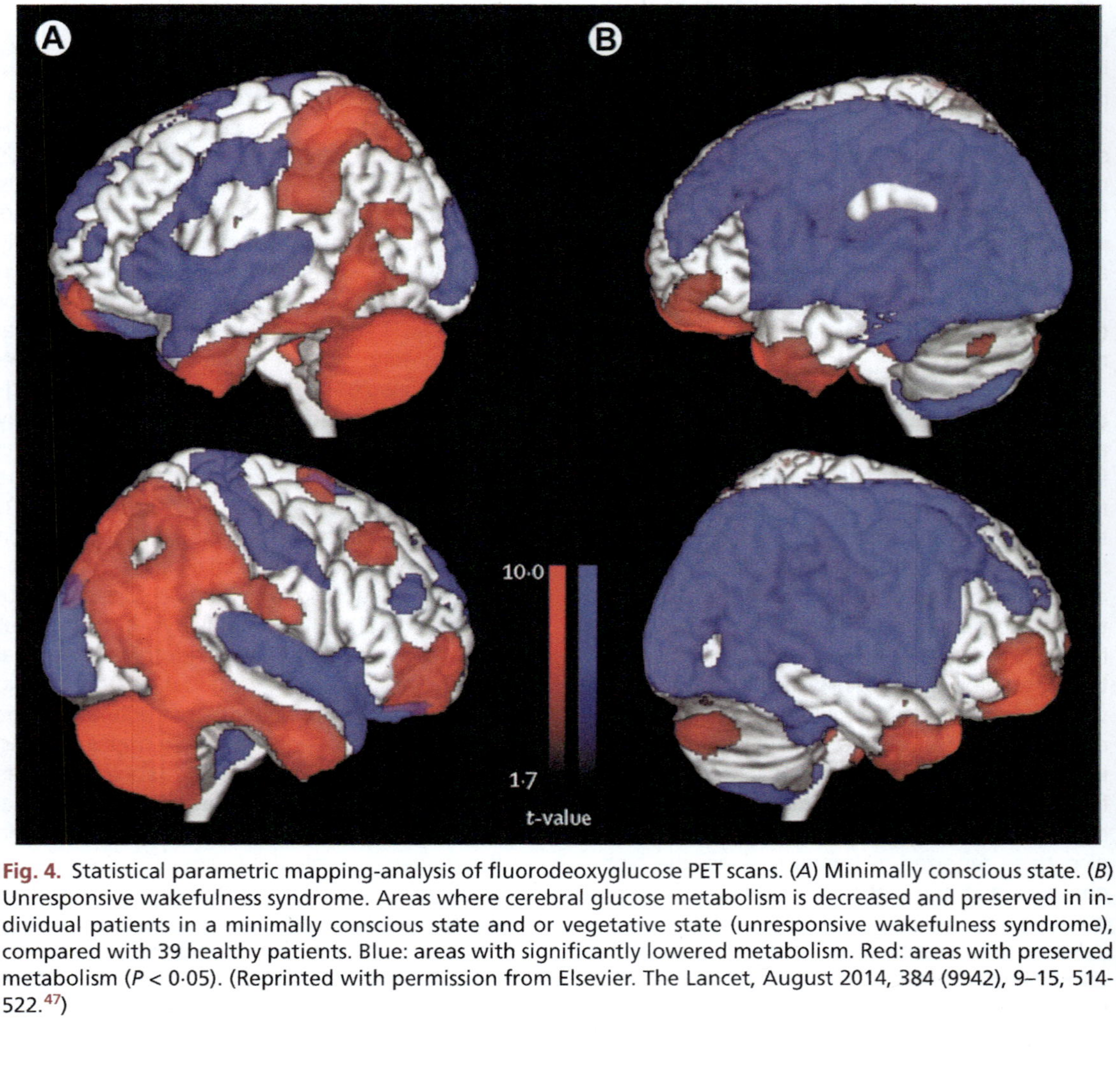

Fig. 4. Statistical parametric mapping-analysis of fluorodeoxyglucose PET scans. (*A*) Minimally conscious state. (*B*) Unresponsive wakefulness syndrome. Areas where cerebral glucose metabolism is decreased and preserved in individual patients in a minimally conscious state and or vegetative state (unresponsive wakefulness syndrome), compared with 39 healthy patients. Blue: areas with significantly lowered metabolism. Red: areas with preserved metabolism ($P < 0{\cdot}05$). (Reprinted with permission from Elsevier. The Lancet, August 2014, 384 (9942), 9–15, 514-522.[47])

more profound and widespread metabolic depression.[11] Furthermore, preservation of metabolism in the precuneus and posterior cingulate cortex appears particularly discriminative. These findings underscore the importance of associative cortical regions in supporting minimal but reproducible signs of awareness.

Beyond diagnosis, FDG PET may offer prognostic insight as well. Preservation of cortical metabolism, particularly in frontoparietal and thalamic regions, has been associated with a higher likelihood of clinical recovery.[48] Conversely, diffuse and severe metabolic suppression predicts a poor neurologic outcome. A separate prospective cohort study found that metabolic activity within the posteromedial cortex was strongly associated with long-term functional recovery in patients with severe head injury.[49] This region is highly interconnected with thalamic and prefrontal structures, forming a hub of the “mesocircuit” model of consciousness.[50] According to this framework, impaired thalamocortical connectivity leads to widespread cortical downregulation, whereas restoration of thalamic output may reactivate distributed cortical networks. FDG PET provides an in vivo method to assess this mesocircuit integrity.

There is also a clinical entity called “covert consciousness” or cognitive motor dissociation, in which patients lacking overt behavioral responsiveness demonstrate preserved brain network activity. While task-based fMRI has revealed command-following in some behaviorally unresponsive patients, FDG PET offers a complementary resting-state metabolic perspective. Patients demonstrating higher metabolic activity in the association cortices, even in the absence of behavioral responsiveness, are more likely to show evidence of covert awareness on advanced neuroimaging paradigms.[51] Thus, FDG PET may serve as a screening modality to identify candidates for more sophisticated cognitive testing or neuromodulatory interventions.

FDG PET findings correlate with other measures of network integrity, including resting-state fMRI connectivity and EEG complexity metrics.[52] Multimodal approaches enhance diagnostic precision by combining metabolic, structural, and electrophysiologic data. For example, preserved metabolism in the posterior cingulate cortex often parallels preserved functional connectivity within the DMN. Hybrid PET/MR imaging systems are likely to further enable simultaneous assessment of metabolism and structural integrity, facilitating comprehensive evaluation of both focal injury and distributed network dysfunction.

It should also be emphasized that beyond physiologic evaluation, the accurate classification of disordered consciousness has profound ethical and clinical consequences, influencing decisions regarding prognosis, rehabilitation, and life-sustaining therapies. Given the substantial risk of misdiagnosis using behavioral assessment alone,[43] incorporation of FDG PET into diagnostic algorithms may reduce diagnostic error and improve individualized care. However, barriers remain, including cost, limited availability, reading expertise, and the need for standardized quantitative thresholds. Ongoing multicenter efforts aim to harmonize analytical approaches and validate metabolic biomarkers across institutions. Emerging PET tracers targeting neuroinflammation, synaptic density, and tau pathology may further refine the understanding of states of persistent unconsciousness. Additionally, FDG PET may serve as an outcome biomarker in trials evaluating pharmacologic agents (eg, amantadine), neuromodulation (eg, deep brain stimulation and transcranial stimulation), or sensory stimulation protocols. As conceptual models of consciousness increasingly emphasize distributed cortical integration and thalamocortical interactions, FDG PET remains uniquely positioned to quantify the metabolic substrate of these networks in vivo.

SUMMARY

FDG PET has assumed a central role in investigations of consciousness from both a clinical and philosophic perspective. By measuring regional cerebral glucose metabolism, PET scanning enables the systematic evaluation of brain activity across normal waking states, physiologic alterations such as sleep, atypical states including meditation, and pathologic conditions encompassed within disorders of consciousness. Through these applications, PET imaging has substantially advanced the understanding of the neurophysiological substrates that support awareness and cognition. Ongoing research will continue to refine models of the relationship between brain function and conscious experience, and PET is likely to remain a prominent tool in elucidating these complex interactions.

CLINICS CARE POINTS

- FDG PET may be used to study various normal states of consciousness.
- FDG PET may be used to study various abnormal states of consciousness.
- FDG PET can be considered in consciousness studies to help better understand the nature of consciousness.

DISCLOSURE

Nothing to disclose.

REFERENCES

1. Cardeña E, Berkovich-Ohana A, Valli K, et al. A consensus taxonomy of altered (nonordinary) states of consciousness: Bringing order to disarray. Psychology of Consciousness: theory, Research, and Practice. Advance Online Publication 2025. https://doi.org/10.1037/cns0000431.
2. Newberg AB, Waldman MR. How enlightenment changes your brain: the new science of transformation. New York, NY: Penguin Random House; 2016.
3. Chrysikou EG, Jacial C, Yaden DB, et al. Differences in brain activity patterns during creative idea generation between eminent and non-eminent thinkers. NeuroImage 2020;220:117011.
4. Brogaard B, Gatzia DE. What can neuroscience tell us about the hard problem of consciousness? Frontiers in neuroscience 2016;10:395.
5. Hameroff S. Consciousness, cognition and the neuronal cytoskeleton–A new paradigm needed in neuroscience. Frontiers in molecular neuroscience 2022;15:869935.
6. D'Aquili EG, Newberg AB. The mystical mind. Minneapolis (MN): Augsburg Press; 1999.
7. Newberg AB. Neurotheology: how science can enlighten us about spirituality. New York, NY: Columbia University Press; 2018.
8. Yaden DB, Newberg AB. The varieties of spiritual experience: 21st century research and perspectives. New York, NY: Oxford; 2022.
9. Newberg AB, Iversen J. The neural basis of the complex mental task of meditation: neurotransmitter and neurochemical considerations. Medical Hypothesis 2003;61(2):282–91.
10. Epp SM, Castrillón G, Yuan B, et al. BOLD signal changes can oppose oxygen metabolism across the human cortex. Nat Neurosci 2026;29(5):1225–36.
11. Cavanna F, Vilas MG, Palmucci M, et al. Dynamic functional connectivity and brain metastability during altered states of consciousness. NeuroImage 2018;180(Pt B):383–95.
12. Edelman GM, Gally JA, Baars BJ. Biology of consciousness. Front Psychol 2011;2:4.
13. Deolindo CS, Ribeiro MW, Aratanha MA, et al. A critical analysis on characterizing the meditation experience through the electroencephalogram. Front Syst Neurosci 2020;14:53.
14. Boly M. Measuring the fading consciousness in the human brain. Current opinion in neurology 2011;24(4):394–400.
15. Lin K, Marx C, Caboclo LO, et al. Sign of the Cross (Signum Crucis): observation of an uncommon ictal manifestation of mesial temporal lobe epilepsy. Epilepsy & behavior : E&B 2009;14(2):400–3.
16. Lebois LAM, Kumar P, Palermo CA, et al. Deconstructing dissociation: a triple network model of trauma-related dissociation and its subtypes. Neuropsychopharmacology : official publication of the American College of Neuropsychopharmacology 2022;47(13):2261–70.
17. Griffiths RR, Johnson MW, Richards WA, et al. Psilocybin-occasioned mystical-type experience in combination with meditation and other spiritual practices produces enduring positive changes in psychological functioning and in trait measures of prosocial attitudes and behaviors. Journal of psychopharmacology (Oxford, England) 2018;32(1):49–69.
18. Carhart-Harris RL, Erritzoe D, Williams T, et al. Neural correlates of the psychedelic state as determined by fMRI studies with psilocybin. Proc Natl Acad Sci USA 2012;109(6):2138–43.
19. Mortaheb S, Fort LD, Mason NL, et al. Dynamic functional hyperconnectivity after psilocybin intake is primarily associated with oceanic boundlessness. Biol Psychiatry Cogn Neurosci Neuroimaging 2024;9(7):681–92.
20. Moujaes F, Rieser NM, Phillips C, et al. Comparing neural correlates of consciousness: from psychedelics to hypnosis and meditation. Biological psychiatry. Cognitive neuroscience and neuroimaging 2024;9(5):533–43.
21. Luders E, Kurth F. The neuroanatomy of long-term meditators. Curr Opin Psychol 2019;28:172–8.
22. Afonso RF, Kraft I, Aratanha MA, et al. Neural correlates of meditation: a review of structural and functional MRI studies. Front Biosci (Schol Ed) 2020;12:92–115. PMID: 32114450.
23. Manna A, Raffone A, Perrucci MG, et al. Neural correlates of focused attention and cognitive monitoring in meditation. Brain Res Bull 2010;82(1–2):46–56. PMID: 20223285.
24. Travis F. Transcendental experiences during meditation practice. Ann N Y Acad Sci 2014;1307:1–8. PMID: 24673148.
25. Lin Y, Tang R, Braver TS. Investigating mindfulness influences on cognitive function: on the promise and potential of converging research strategies. Psychon Bull Rev 2021;29(4):1198–222.
26. Zhang Q, Wang Z, Wang X, et al. The effects of different stages of mindfulness meditation training on emotion regulation. Front Hum Neurosci 2019;13:208.
27. Whitfield T, Barnhofer T, Acabchuk R, et al. The effect of mindfulness-based programs on cognitive function in adults: a systematic review and meta-analysis. Neuropsychol Rev 2022;32(3):677–702.
28. Luders E, Kurth F, Mayer EA, et al. The unique brain anatomy of meditation practitioners: alterations in cortical gyrification. Front Hum Neurosci 2012;6:34.

29. Newberg AB, Wintering N, Waldman MR, et al. Cerebral blood flow differences between long-term meditators and non-meditators. Conscious Cogn 2010; 19(4):899–905. PMID: 20570534.
30. Luders E, Toga AW, Lepore N, et al. The underlying anatomical correlates of long-term meditation: larger hippocampal and frontal volumes of gray matter. Neuroimage 2009;45(3):672–8.
31. Luders E, Kurth F, Toga AW, et al. Meditation effects within the hippocampal complex revealed by voxel-based morphometry and cytoarchitectonic probabilistic mapping. Front Psychol 2013;4:398.
32. Luders E, Phillips OR, Clark K, et al. Bridging the hemispheres in meditation: thicker callosal regions and enhanced fractional anisotropy (FA) in long-term practitioners. Neuroimage 2012;61(1):181–7.
33. Luders E, Clark K, Narr KL, et al. Enhanced brain connectivity in long-term meditation practitioners. Neuroimage 2011;57(4):1308–16.
34. Lizama-Lefno A, Mojica K, Serrat M, et al. Mindfulness components and their clinical efficacy: a critical review of an ongoing debate. Healthcare (Basel) 2026;14(2):196. Published 2026 Jan 13.
35. Brewer JA, Worhunsky PD, Gray JR, et al. Meditation experience is associated with differences in default mode network activity and connectivity. Proc Natl Acad Sci U S A 2011;108(50):20254–9.
36. Hölzel BK, Carmody J, Vangel M, et al. Mindfulness practice leads to increases in regional brain gray matter density. Psychiatry Res 2011;191(1):36–43.
37. Lazar SW, Bush G, Gollub RL, et al. Functional brain mapping of the relaxation response and meditation. Neuroreport 2000;11(7):1581–5.
38. Garrison KA, Zeffiro TA, Scheinost D, et al. Meditation leads to reduced default mode network activity beyond an active task. Cogn Affect Behav Neurosci 2015;15(3):712–20.
39. Desbordes G, Negi LT, Pace TW, et al. Effects of mindful-attention and compassion meditation training on amygdala response to emotional stimuli in an ordinary, non-meditative state. Front Hum Neurosci 2012;6:292.
40. Posner JB, Saper CB, Schiff ND, et al. Plum and Posner's diagnosis and treatment of Stupor and coma. 5th edition. Oxford University Press; 2019. https://doi.org/10.1093/med/9780190208875.001.0001.
41. Giacino JT, Ashwal S, Childs N, et al. The minimally conscious state: definition and diagnostic criteria. Neurology 2002;58(3):349–53.
42. Saper CB, Scammell TE, Lu J. Hypothalamic regulation of sleep and circadian rhythms. Nature 2005; 437(7063):1257–63.
43. Schnakers C, Vanhaudenhuyse A, Giacino J, et al. Diagnostic accuracy of the vegetative and minimally conscious state: clinical consensus versus standardized neurobehavioral assessment. BMC Neurology 2009;9:35.
44. Bender A, Jox RJ, Grill E, et al. Persistent vegetative state and minimally conscious state: a systematic review and meta-analysis of diagnostic procedures. Deutsches Ärzteblatt International 2015;112(14): 235–42.
45. Levy DE, Sidtis JJ, Rottenberg DA, et al. Differences in cerebral blood flow and glucose utilization in vegetative versus locked-in patients. Ann Neurol 1987;22(6):673–82.
46. Laureys S, Goldman S, Phillips C, et al. Impaired effective cortical connectivity in vegetative state: preliminary investigation using PET. Neuroimage 1999;9(4):377–82.
47. Stender J, Gosseries O, Bruno MA, et al. Diagnostic precision of PET imaging and functional MRI in disorders of consciousness: a clinical validation study. Lancet 2014;384(9942):514–22.
48. Thibaut A, Bruno MA, Ledoux D, et al. Metabolic activity in external and internal awareness networks in severely brain-damaged patients. J Neurotrauma 2012;29(5):778–89.
49. Fridman EA, Beattie BJ, Broft A, et al. Regional cerebral metabolic patterns demonstrate the role of anterior forebrain mesocircuit dysfunction in the severely injured brain. Proc Natl Acad Sci U S A 2014;111-(17):6473–8.
50. Schiff ND. Disorders of consciousness. Lancet 2009;374(9704):2059–70.
51. Monti MM, Vanhaudenhuyse A, Coleman MR, et al. Willful modulation of brain activity in disorders of consciousness. N Engl J Med 2010;362(7):579–89.
52. Demertzi A, Soddu A, Faymonville ME, et al. Hypnotic modulation of resting state fMRI default mode and extrinsic network connectivity. Prog Brain Res 2011;193:309–22.
53. Vanhaudenhuyse A, Noirhomme Q, Tshibanda LJ, et al. Default network connectivity reflects the level of consciousness in non-communicative brain-damaged patients. Brain 2010;133(Pt 1):161–71.
54. Huang S-Y, Hsu J-L, Lin K-J, et al. A novel individual metabolic brain network for 18F-FDG PET imaging. Front. Neurosci 2020;14:344. https://doi.org/10.3389/fnins.2020.00344.
55. Lazar SW, Kerr CE, Wasserman RH, et al. Meditation experience is associated with increased cortical thickness. Neuroreport 2005;16(17):1893–7.

Fluorodeoxyglucose PET Scans in the Integrative Medicine Setting

Andrew B. Newberg, MD[a,b,*], Yining Hua, MSc, PhD[c],
Cyrus Ayubcha, MD, PhD[d], Daniel A. Monti, MD[e]

KEYWORDS

• FDG PET • Neuroimaging • Oncology imaging • Screening • Integrative medicine • Chronic disease

KEY POINTS

- In integrative medicine, FDG PET assesses regional brain glucose metabolism to evaluate mental function, neuropsychiatric disorders, aging, and early neurodegenerative disease.
- Whole-body FDG PET assesses systemic metabolic activity, helping detect occult malignancies, inflammatory conditions, and other metabolically active diseases.
- FDG PET complements clinical evaluation and other imaging modalities, including SPECT, CT, and MRI, in selected integrative medicine applications.

INTRODUCTION

Functional imaging has dramatically expanded our understanding of the biological mechanisms underlying a variety of neurologic and medical disorders. Fluorodeoxyglucose (FDG) PET imaging of the brain provides the ability to observe changes associated with various mental states and neuropsychiatric disorders. FDG PET of the brain also has the ability to determine the current status of a person's brain providing some indication of age-related effects and the potential development of neurodegenerative disorders such as Alzheimer's disease (AD). The challenge is determining how best to use information from FDG PET scans of the brain in the clinical setting.

In addition, FDG PET of the body can be used for the general assessment of body physiology with the specific goal of screening for occult cancers. Areas of inflammation may also be discovered and evaluated in the context of the patient's health status.

Thus, FDG PET imaging can be a useful adjunct in selected integrative medicine contexts for evaluating disease processes in the brain and body. This article reviews the potential indications for FDG PET scanning in the integrative medicine setting. It also considers FDG PET within the broader application of functional imaging studies that may also include SPECT and MR imaging.

FLUORODEOXYGLUCOSE PET SCANS FOR PATIENTS IN THE INTEGRATIVE MEDICINE SETTING

Many patients who present to integrative medicine practices have the primary goal of staying healthy including both the brain and body. They want to

[a] Department of Integrative Medicine and Nutritional Sciences; [b] Department of Radiology, Research at the Marcus Institute of Integrative Health, Thomas Jefferson University, Philadelphia, PA, USA; [c] Department of Epidemiology, Harvard T.H. Chan School of Public Health, Boston, MA, USA; [d] Department of Neurosurgery, Harvard Medical School, Boston, MA, USA; [e] Department of Integrative Medicine and Nutritional Sciences, Marcus Institute of Integrative Health, Thomas Jefferson University, Philadelphia, PA, USA
* Corresponding author. Department of Integrative Medicine and Nutritional Sciences, Thomas Jefferson University, 789 East Lancaster Avenue, Suite 110, Villanova, PA 19085.
E-mail address: Andrew.newberg@jefferson.edu

PET Clin 21 (2026) 573–585
https://doi.org/10.1016/j.cpet.2026.06.001

Abbreviations	
ACC	anterior cingulate cortex
AD	Alzheimer's disease
COVID-19	coronavirus disease 2019
CT	computed tomography
DLPFC	dorsolateral prefrontal cortex
DMN	default mode network
DMPFC	dorsomedial prefrontal cortex
FDG	fluorodeoxyglucose
fMRI	functional magnetic resonance imaging
FUO/IUO	fever or inflammation of unknown origin
MBSR	mindfulness-based stress reduction
OCD	obsessive-compulsive disorder
OFC	orbitofrontal cortex
PTSD	posttraumatic stress disorder
rCBF	regional cerebral blood flow
SPECT	single photon emission computed tomography
SPECT	single photon emission computed tomography
TMS	transcranial magnetic stimulation

understand their starting point—that is, their physiologic age rather than just their chronologic age. They want to understand if there are underlying, occult issues in their body, such as inflammation or cancer, that might be corrected through various lifestyle modifications.

For such patients, a screening FDG PET scan of the brain and/or body might provide some unique clinical opportunities. Scan findings can be correlated with clinical history of past illnesses, current symptoms, or even other testing such as genetic, gut health, or other laboratory tests. For example, a patient who has the apolipoprotein E (APOE) ε3/ε4 genetic profile might be particularly interested to know whether their brain has early findings of cognitive impairment or AD. And if such findings exist, they might be interested in aggressively modifying their lifestyle including diet and nutrition, weight, diabetes risk, and smoking and alcohol behaviors. They might also be interested in doing things to enhance brain function such as increasing physical activity, engaging brain training techniques, and ensuring good sleep habits.

FDG PET imaging can provide important information about inflammation in the body.[1] Studies have found that FDG uptake can arise in inflamed joints or other soft tissues. FDG uptake in blood vessels may be particularly important for identifying inflammation or possibly atherosclerosis.

What many patients presenting to ingrative medicine (IM) clinics want to know about is the potential presence of occult cancers. A whole body PET scan can help detect cancers in many organs including breast, colon, lung, and pancreas among others. While not fully recognized as a screening tool, even incidental findings such as a focus in the thyroid can have up to a 60% chance of representing malignancy.[2] It is important to be clear with patients that some cancers are not particularly hypermetabolic. Some breast cancers will not be detected, and prostate cancer is one of the most common cancers that often is not hypermetabolic.[3] Thus, an FDG PET scan can be helpful but must be interpreted with caution. One of the major criticisms of using screening tools such as FDG PET is the potential for detecting incidental findings that can lead to significant distress and costly workup. Thus, it is important for the reader to be aware of the underlying likelihood of cancer in a given patient and evaluate the scan appropriately. As research proceeds, it might be found that patients with an increased risk for cancer such as a first-degree relative or history of smoking should have scans read more aggressively, whereas those who are unlikely to have cancer based on history should have scans read more conservatively.

Beyond generally healthy patients presenting for overall screening, FDG PET scans can be particularly helpful in patients with known disorders of the brain or body. Some of the more common health issues are considered later.

WHOLE-BODY FLUORODEOXYGLUCOSE PET IMAGING FOR OCCULT MALIGNANCY AND INFLAMMATION

Evaluation of Occult Malignancy in High-risk Patients

Whole-body FDG PET has emerged as a pivotal imaging modality in clinical oncology and inflammatory disease evaluation. The technique exploits the increased glucose metabolism characteristic of many cancer cells and activated inflammatory cells, providing functional information that complements anatomic imaging. Whole-body FDG-PET (often combined with computed tomography [CT] or MR imaging) allows a comprehensive assessment of the entire body in a single imaging session, making it particularly valuable in patients with occult malignancies or unexplained systemic inflammation.

Occult malignancy refers to clinically suspected or biologically inferred cancer that remains undetected by routine imaging and clinical assessment. Whole-body FDG PET has been widely studied in this context, both in patients with suspected cancers such as in paraneoplastic syndromes, and idiopathic inflammatory conditions associated with cancer. A systematic review and meta-analysis covering 1293 patients with suspected paraneoplastic syndromes found that whole-body FDG PET or FDG PET/CT had a pooled sensitivity of approximately 81% and specificity of approximately 88% for detecting underlying malignancy, with the diagnostic odds ratio indicating high overall accuracy.[4]

Fluorodeoxyglucose PET for Cancer Screening

In the integrative medicine setting, many patients have no specific history of cancer, but may have a family history or other reasons to be concerned about cancer and are eager to undergo screening in order to detect any cancer as early as possible. There are several studies evaluating the use of whole-body FDG PET or PET/CT scans to screen *otherwise healthy, asymptomatic* individuals for cancer. The results indicate that while FDG PET may be capable of screening for cancers, the overall evidence does not support it as a routine population-wide screening tool.

A large Japanese cohort study (Nishidai clinic) involving nearly 4900 asymptomatic volunteers found that FDG PET screening identified cancers in about 0.7% of participants.[5] In a study linked to the *Osaka Cancer Registry*, screening of 1762 asymptomatic adults, FDG PET (often combined with other modalities) yielded a sensitivity of approximately 85%, specificity of approximately 86%, and positive predictive value of approximately 10% for detecting cancers within 1 year of screening.[6]

The potential problem with using FDG PET as a screening tool is that across several studies, the prevalence of occult cancers detected by FDG PET in healthy people has been typically around 1% to 2% of screened individuals. These detection rates are much lower than for targeted screening programs such as colonoscopy or mammography.[7] Thus, more than half of PET-positive findings did not correspond to confirmed cancer on follow-up. The authors concluded that such a low detection rate does not justify routine screening in otherwise healthy adults.

FLUORODEOXYGLUCOSE PET FOR THE EVALUATION OF INFLAMMATION

Because FDG accumulates in activated inflammatory cells, whole-body FDG PET has been utilized in patients with fever or inflammation of unknown origin (FUO/IUO). In a large retrospective study of 300 patients, FDG PET/CT demonstrated overall sensitivity of 80.2% and specificity of 89.8% for identifying the cause of FUO/IUO, with a very high specificity (100%) specifically for malignancy in this cohort.[8] A meta-analysis indicated that FDG PET has demonstrated excellent performance detecting infectious and inflammatory processes with reported sensitivities of approximately 80% and specificities of approximately 85% in suspected infections.[9] These results are superior compared to other nuclear medicine imaging techniques such as Gallium-67 scintigraphy, and support the use of FDG PET when conventional workup fails to localize a source of systemic inflammation.

In the integrative medicine setting, the potential value of FDG PET for evaluating patients for inflammatory processes is less clear since inflammation is often detected with sensitive laboratory tests making it less likely to be detected with imaging. Symptoms such as chronic pain or chronic fatigue might have an inflammatory source which can be small, indolent, and take up undetectable amounts of FDG. Ideally, the use of FDG PET in the integrative medicine setting would be used judiciously with carefully selected patients. For example, patients with more localized signs or symptoms (eg, sinus pain and gastrointestinal disturbances) might be more likely to yield a positive finding on FDG PET.[10,11] FDG PET is particularly useful when considering a variety of inflammatory disorders such as sarcoidosis, large vessel vasculitis, musculoskeletal infections, joint prosthesis or implant-related complications, human immunodeficiency virus-related infections, and miscellaneous indications, such as immunoglobulin G4-related systemic disease.[12]

PET IMAGING OF THE BRAIN

By examining parameters such as regional cerebral glucose metabolism, cerebral blood flow, and neurotransmitter system activity, imaging modalities including PET, single photon emission computed tomography (SPECT), and functional magnetic resonance imaging (fMRI) have contributed substantially to improved diagnosis, characterization of pathophysiology, and monitoring of treatment effects. Beyond conventional clinical applications, these techniques may be particularly valuable in evaluating therapeutic strategies within integrative medicine.

One of the major strengths of functional neuroimaging lies in its ability to reveal the individualized neural patterns associated with specific disorders. Rather than viewing psychiatric and neurologic illnesses as uniform entities, imaging allows clinicians and researchers to identify which brain structures and functional networks are most affected in a given patient. Such individualized mapping holds promise for more personalized treatment approaches. Moreover, neuroimaging offers a powerful method for investigating the mechanisms of action underlying integrative interventions. Techniques such as acupuncture, meditation, and other mind–body therapies can be studied directly in terms of their effects on neural activity. Elucidating these mechanisms is essential for enabling these integrative approaches to be used in standard medical practice.

In clinical PET imaging, FDG is the most commonly used tracer since measuring cerebral glucose metabolism and its patterns can be very useful in helping with the diagnosis of various neuropsychiatric conditions (**Fig. 1**). Several amyloid and tau protein binding tracers are now available for evaluating AD pathology. In SPECT imaging, tracers such as technetium labeled agents (eg, ^{99m}Tc hexamethylpropylene-amine oxime and ethyl cysteinate dimer) assess regional cerebral blood flow (rCBF), and ^{123}I ioflupane (DaTscan) is employed to measure dopamine transporter binding in the evaluation of Parkinson's disease. In addition to these clinically approved agents, numerous investigational tracers have been developed to assess a wide range of neurotransmitter systems and disease-related targets, providing highly specific molecular information.

FLUORODEOXYGLUCOSE PET IN PSYCHIATRIC CONDITIONS FREQUENTLY ENCOUNTERED IN THE INTEGRATIVE MEDICINE SETTING

In the integrative medicine setting, patients often present with one of a number of psychiatric symptoms or disorders. In this setting, additional imaging of the brain can be helpful not only for confirmation but also to help understand the underlying neurophysiology of the patient, and even potentially guide therapy.

Neuroimaging in Depression

Functional neuroimaging has played a central role in advancing our understanding of depressive disorders. Early investigations primarily examined the biological mechanisms underlying depression, whereas more recent research has emphasized the clinical utility of imaging for identifying subtypes, estimating prognosis, and guiding individualized treatment strategies. A key consideration is that depression, like many psychiatric illnesses, is highly heterogeneous. Distinct patients may exhibit dysfunction in different neural circuits, which may account for variations in symptom presentation and therapeutic response.

Across studies using PET and SPECT (**Fig. 2**), one of the most consistent observations in depression is a generalized reduction in cerebral blood flow and glucose metabolism. Early FDG PET research demonstrated that individuals with late-onset depression showed widespread cortical and subcortical hypometabolism, with relative sparing of the basal ganglia. A meta-analysis reported decreased metabolism in the bilateral insula, left putamen, right caudate, and cingulate gyrus, alongside increased metabolism in the right thalamus and vermis.[13] The degree of hypometabolism has also been correlated with depression severity as measured by both self-report and clinician

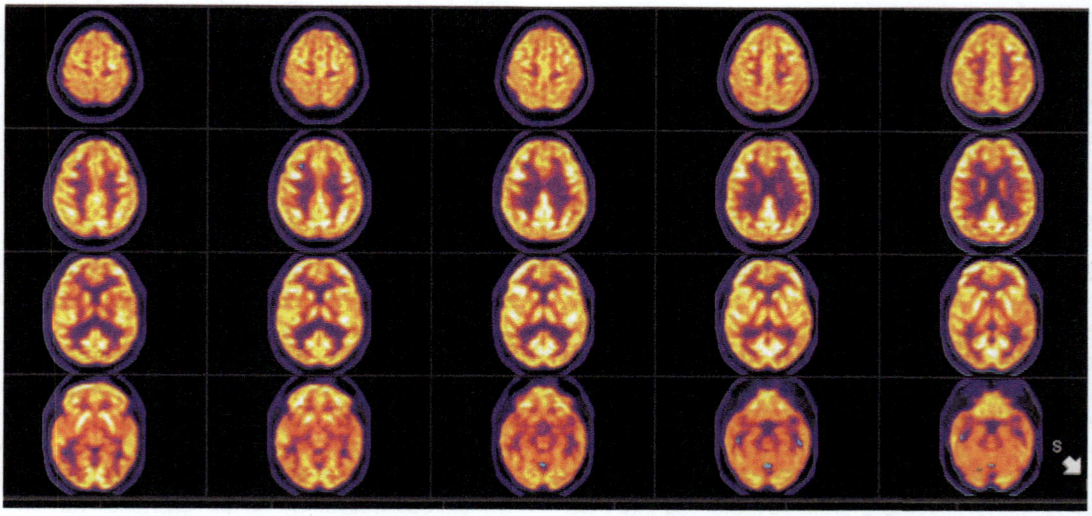

Fig. 1. Normal FDG PET scan from a healthy individual without any neuropsychiatric disorder. The scan demonstrates uniform metabolism throughout the cortical and subcortical structures.

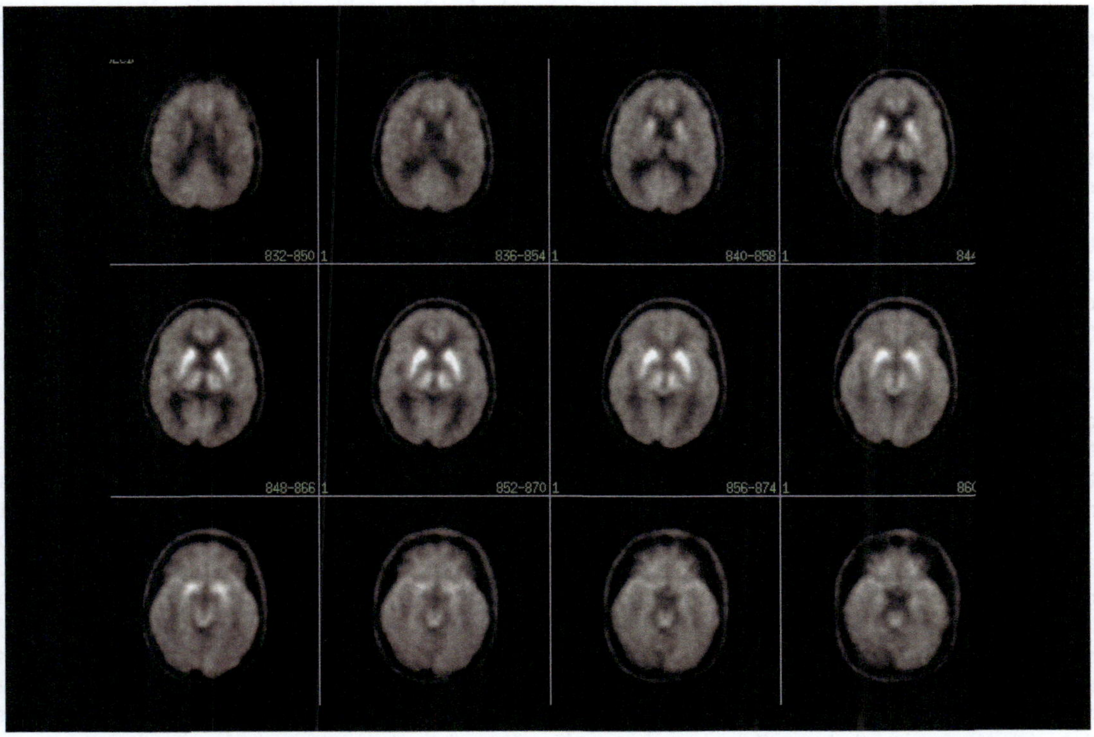

Fig. 2. An FDG-PET scan of a patient with major depression shows a global cortical decrease in metabolism relative to the subcortical structures.

ratings.[14] Depressive severity has been positively associated with metabolism in the cingulate gyrus, thalamus, and basal ganglia, whereas sleep disturbance correlates with increased limbic and basal ganglia metabolism.[15] Decreased metabolism in the midbrain, in particular, may be associated with poor outcome and higher remittance rate in patients with depression.[16]

Comorbid anxiety appears to influence metabolic patterns. Patients with depressive and anxiety symptoms have demonstrated hypermetabolism in the right parahippocampal region and left anterior cingulate cortex (ACC), along with hypometabolism in the cerebellum, left fusiform gyrus, superior temporal cortex, angular gyrus, and insula.[17] FDG PET scans in young patients with cancer showed that hypometabolism in the ventral prefrontal cortex, hippocampus, and amygdala after treatment predicted future depression.[18]

FDG PET studies examining treatment effects generally demonstrate a trend toward metabolic normalization with clinical improvement. For example, successful treatment with paroxetine has been associated with increased metabolism toward normative levels in the inferior frontal gyrus and prefrontal cortex,[19] as well as decreased hypermetabolism in insular and limbic regions.[20]

Neuroimaging has also been applied to integrative therapies such as transcranial magnetic stimulation (TMS). PET data demonstrated that hypermetabolism in the left dorsolateral prefrontal cortex (DLPFC) predicted antidepressant response to 1 Hz repetitive TMS, whereas hypometabolism predicted response to 20 Hz stimulation.[21] Supportive data comes from fMRI and SPECT studies that have linked pretreatment activation or perfusion patterns, particularly in the anterior cingulate and ventromedial prefrontal cortex, to TMS responsiveness.[22,23]

From an integrative medicine perspective, imaging studies have begun to evaluate complementary therapies. In drug-naïve patients with major depressive disorder (MDD), electroacupuncture at the GV20 point altered functional connectivity within the default mode network (DMN), including increased connectivity between posterior and anterior cingulate regions.[24] Laser acupuncture has also been shown to modulate inferior parietal and cerebellar activity.[25] Although these physiologic changes are promising, further research is required to clarify their relationship to clinical improvement and underlying mechanisms.

Neuroimaging in Anxiety

Anxiety, and its relationship to stress, is a common problem in patients presenting to integrative medicine practitioners. The anxiety may be primary in that they have an anxiety disorder or anxiety associated with depression. Commonly patients seeking integrative medicine have chronic health problems including pain and fatigue, which causes significant anxiety and stress. Patients have stress about the discomfort of the symptoms, their unpredictability, and the lack of certainty about their prognosis. Patients also have anxiety about the implications of these disorders for their general life and well-being. Such disorders can interfere with many important life activities such as a patient's job, relationships, and hobbies. Helping patients navigate anxiety and stress is an important role for integrative medicine practitioners and sometimes functional imaging can provide important information regarding diagnosis or management.

The neural substrate underlying anxiety differs in important ways from those implicated in depression. PET imaging has been instrumental in clarifying the neurophysiological mechanisms of stress and anxiety. Key structures include the hippocampus, amygdala, and prefrontal cortex, components of the limbic system that regulate the hypothalamic–pituitary–adrenal axis and modulate the stress response. Early H_2O PET studies demonstrated that patients with anxiety disorders exhibit increased rCBF in the right parahippocampal gyrus at rest compared with healthy controls.[26]

Integrative approaches to anxiety have likewise been examined with neuroimaging. Studies of mindfulness-based stress reduction (MBSR) in social anxiety disorder have demonstrated increased dorsomedial prefrontal cortex (DMPFC) activity during negative self-referential tasks, along with altered temporal dynamics of neural responses in the DMPFC and posterior cingulate cortex.[27,28] When compared with aerobic exercise, both MBSR and exercise significantly reduced anxiety symptoms, though each intervention was associated with distinct neural changes. FDG PET imaging has also shown changes in frontal and thalamic activity during meditation practices (**Fig. 3**), potentially underlying their anxiolytic benefits. These findings raise important questions regarding the differing mechanisms through which integrative therapies exert clinical effects.

Neuroimaging in Obsessive–compulsive Disorder

PET and SPECT imaging have been widely applied to the study of obsessive–compulsive disorder (OCD). Converging evidence implicates dysfunction within the cortico-striato-thalamo-cortical (CSTC) circuitry,[29] particularly involving the orbitofrontal cortex (OFC). Many studies have demonstrated increased cerebral metabolism in the OFC and caudate nuclei in patients with OCD (**Fig. 4**).[30] Hypermetabolism in the cingulate gyrus has also been reported.[31] Conversely, several investigations have identified hypometabolism in bilateral parietal regions, with some noting a negative correlation between obsessive–compulsive symptom severity and right parietal rCBF. Dysfunction in parietal areas, particularly the angular and supramarginal gyri, may contribute to the cognitive and attentional abnormalities observed in OCD.

Functional imaging has also been used to assess therapeutic response. Higher baseline glucose metabolism in the OFC has been associated with greater improvement following behavioral therapy but poorer outcomes with fluoxetine.[32] Behavioral therapy responders have shown significant bilateral reductions in caudate metabolism after treatment.[33] Additionally, lower pretreatment OFC metabolism predicted greater symptom improvement with paroxetine.[34] These findings suggest that distinct metabolic patterns may help predict differential response to behavioral versus pharmacologic interventions.

Although neuroimaging studies specifically evaluating integrative therapies in OCD are lacking, imaging has been used to predict response to conventional treatments. One study[35] found that improvement with fluoxetine correlated with smaller pretreatment gray matter volume in the right middle lateral OFC, whereas cognitive behavioral therapy (CBT) response was associated with larger pretreatment gray matter volume in the right medial prefrontal cortex. Given the increasing number of clinical trials examining acupuncture, meditation, and related integrative approaches in OCD,[36] future neuroimaging studies could provide critical mechanistic insights.

Neuroimaging in Posttraumatic Stress Disorder

Posttraumatic stress disorder (PTSD) is characterized by dysregulation within fronto-limbic circuitry, particularly involving prefrontal cortical regions, the amygdala, hippocampus, and related paralimbic structures. Functional neuroimaging studies consistently demonstrate altered rCBF and glucose metabolism within these networks following traumatic exposure.

An FDG PET study of 15 patients with PTSD demonstrated decreased metabolic activity in the cingulate gyri, precuneus, insula, hippocampus,

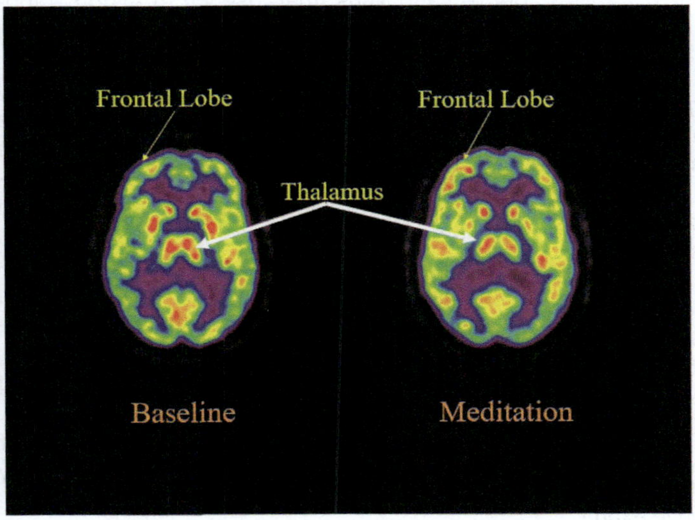

Fig. 3. FDG PET scans of a subject at rest and while performing a meditation task. During meditation, there is increased metabolism in the frontal lobes (*arrow*) and decreased metabolism in the thalami (*thick arrow*). These structures are involved in stress and anxiety pathways and the observed effects in these scans may provide physiologic support for the antianxiety effects of such practices.

prefrontal cortex, occipital lobe, and language-related areas.[37] In contrast, relatively increased activity was observed in the fusiform gyrus, superior temporal lobe, and cerebellum. These findings reinforce the model of impaired top–down cortical regulation with relative hyperactivity in sensory and limbic regions.

Additional rCBF studies comparing trauma-exposed individuals with and without PTSD have provided further insight. During recollection of traumatic memories, patients with PTSD exhibited increased activation in the OFC and anterior temporal poles, accompanied by decreased blood flow in anterior frontal and left inferior frontal regions.[38] A follow-up study from the same group reported reduced medial frontal gyrus activity during trauma recall.[39] Symptom severity correlated positively with right amygdala blood flow and negatively with medial frontal gyrus activity, supporting a model of exaggerated amygdala responsivity coupled with diminished medial prefrontal inhibitory control.

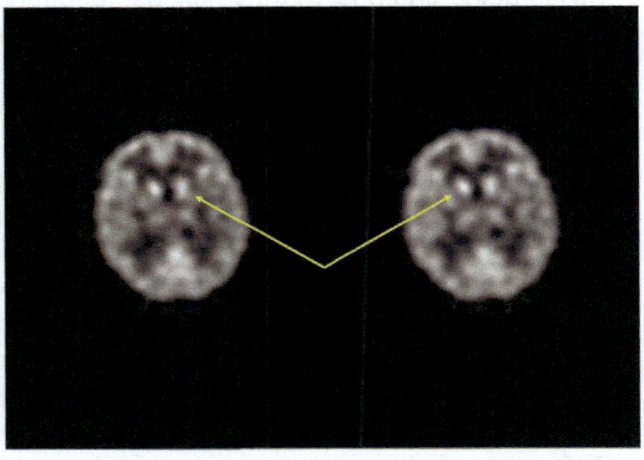

Fig. 4. FDG-PET of a patient with OCD showing increased glucose metabolism in the caudate nuclei bilaterally (*arrows*).

Functional MR imaging studies have examined neural changes associated with psychotherapeutic interventions. A study by Monti and colleagues[40] reported that the NeuroEmotional technique significantly reduced traumatic stress symptoms in patients with cancer and was associated with decreased reactivity in the parahippocampal region and brainstem.

Another study[41] demonstrated that mindfulness-based exposure therapy increased DMN functional connectivity between the posterior cingulate cortex, DLPFC, and ACC. Enhanced connectivity correlated with reductions in avoidance and hyperarousal symptoms, indicating improved integration between self-referential and regulatory networks.

FLUORODEOXYGLUCOSE PET IN NEUROLOGIC CONDITIONS FREQUENTLY ENCOUNTERED IN THE INTEGRATIVE MEDICINE SETTING

In the integrative medicine setting, patients often present with one of a number of neurologic symptoms or disorders. Some of the more common issues relate to cognitive impairment and possible dementia as well as patients with a history of head injury. Symptoms such as chronic pain or fatigue are also common and FDG PET of the brain or body may help elucidate the nature of such symptoms. In this setting, PET imaging can be helpful not only for confirmation of a clinical diagnosis but also to help understand the underlying neurophysiology of the patient, and even potentially guide therapy.

Fluorodeoxyglucose PET in Alzheimer's Disease

Numerous studies have evaluated the diagnostic performance of FDG PET in identifying AD in patients with cognitive symptoms. Early large studies reported that FDG PET can distinguish AD subjects from healthy controls with high sensitivity. For example, Silverman and colleagues[42] demonstrated sensitivities around 94% with specificities near 73% when comparing clinically diagnosed AD against controls using metabolic patterns consistent with AD hypometabolism. Similar findings across the literature place sensitivity generally in the range of 90% to 96% and specificity between 63% and 89% for detecting AD in symptomatic patients.

Because metabolic alterations can precede overt cognitive decline, many studies have examined FDG PET's ability to predict which individuals with MCI will progress to AD dementia. Systematic reviews and meta-analyses focusing on MCI cohorts report a wide range of diagnostic accuracies. In 1 meta-analysis of FDG PET in patients with MCI, pooled sensitivity was approximately 79% and pooled specificity was approximately 74% for predicting conversion to AD dementia, with substantial between-study variability.[43] Other systematic reviews show similarly broad ranges of reported test performance: sensitivities from approximately 56% to 100% and specificities from approximately 24% to 100%, depending on analytical metric and study methodology.[44]

Although FDG PET has been primarily studied in symptomatic populations, there is growing interest in identifying metabolic changes in cognitively normal individuals at elevated dementia risk (eg, APOE ε4 carriers or those with subjective cognitive decline). In a study of over 200 patients with amnestic MCI, 3 subtypes emerged regarding FDG PET findings.[45] Hippocampal sparing-cortical hypometabolism was associated with younger age and the highest level of AD CSF pathology. Hippocampal/cortical hypometabolism was associated with a high percentage of APOE ε3/ε4 or ε4/ε4 carriers, and medial-temporal hypometabolism was associated with older age, a low AD-CSF pathology, and a benign course. Within the whole cohort, the severity of temporo-parietal hypometabolism was correlated with AD-CSF pathology and correlated with the rate of progression of cognitive decline.

Negative FDG PET findings in at-risk individuals have shown high negative predictive values of approximately 85% for AD in some "real-world" cohorts for ruling out imminent conversion to dementia.[46] Thus, the absence of hypometabolism is associated with lower short-term risk of progression.

The strengths of FDG PET also include its ability to help diagnose other disease entities that are part of the differential diagnosis of cognitive impairment including other neurodegenerative disorders such as frontotemporal dementia, or even late life depression.[47]

However, FDG PET also has limitations. Sensitivity and specificity vary with disease stage, analytical methods (visual vs quantitative), and comparison standards. Specific patterns of hypometabolism overlap with other dementias, necessitating careful interpretation in conjunction with clinical, neuropsychological, structural imaging, and other biomarker data. High costs and limited availability further constrain widespread routine use.

Thus, FDG PET can be useful in the integrative medicine setting when working with patients presenting with cognitive impairment. It can help clarify the diagnosis as well as provide some prognostic information. Given that the present treatment is largely related to lifestyle modifications related to diet and nutrition, adequate sleep, and appropriate nutritional supplementation.

NEUROIMAGING IN CHRONIC CONCUSSION

Chronic concussion, often categorized within mild traumatic brain injury, is primarily a neurologic condition but frequently manifests with psychiatric and cognitive symptoms, including depression, anxiety, fatigue, irritability, and executive dysfunction. In the United States, more than 1.5 million individuals sustain traumatic brain injuries annually, with approximately 80,000 to 90,000 experiencing long-term disability. While structural imaging in the acute phase is essential to exclude fractures or intracranial hemorrhage, patients with persistent postconcussion symptoms often have normal CT or MR imaging findings. In these cases, functional and metabolic neuroimaging can provide critical diagnostic and prognostic information.[48]

One of the central goals of neuroimaging in chronic concussion is to identify objective physiologic abnormalities that correlate with clinical symptoms. Demonstrating measurable metabolic or perfusion deficits can validate patients' experiences, particularly when symptoms are otherwise attributed to psychological factors or malingering. Thus, functional imaging offers both clinical and psychosocial value by substantiating the biological basis of persistent symptoms.

FDG PET studies demonstrate that focal lesions—such as cortical contusions, intracranial hematomas, and encephalomalacia—typically exhibit localized hypometabolism corresponding to structural damage (**Fig. 5**). However, subdural and epidural hematomas may produce more diffuse cortical hypometabolism, sometimes affecting the contralateral hemisphere[49] or contralateral cerebellum—crossed cerebellar diaschisis.[50]

Diffuse axonal injury, a hallmark of concussion-related pathology, is associated with widespread and focal cortical hypometabolism.[51] These effects may reflect disruption of interhemispheric callosal fibers projecting to visual association regions. In patients with multiple injuries, metabolic patterns may be heterogeneous, and no single characteristic PET signature is universally observed.

Functional neuroimaging in chronic concussion provides an opportunity to identify region-specific dysfunction that may inform targeted treatment strategies. For example, hypometabolism in frontal regions may support interventions aimed at enhancing executive function, including cognitive rehabilitation, neurofeedback, or noninvasive neuromodulation.

Integrative approaches such as meditation practices may augment frontal lobe regulation and network connectivity, while neurofeedback may help normalize aberrant oscillatory or connectivity patterns. As quantitative biomarkers evolve, neuroimaging may facilitate personalized therapeutic planning and objective monitoring of treatment response.

LONG CORONAVIRUS DISEASE 2019

Long coronavirus disease 2019 (COVID-19) refers to the clinical condition in which symptoms continue for at least 2 months and persist beyond 3 months after an acute, symptomatic, probable, or confirmed severe acute respiratory syndrome coronavirus 2 infection.[52] These ongoing symptoms have no other identifiable cause and frequently include symptoms such as cognitive difficulties, headaches, anxiety, depression, and other neuropsychiatric features.[53] In recent years, FDG PET has been applied to investigate the neural substrates of long COVID-19. Group-level analyses have identified a characteristic pattern of reduced glucose metabolism involving the orbitofrontal and olfactory cortices, (para)limbic regions, brainstem, and cerebellum.[54] This constellation of findings on FDG PET has been described as a "hypometabolic signature" of neuro-COVID-19 and has subsequently been replicated in larger cohorts.[55]

Importantly, in long COVID-19, brain areas with hypometabolism have been associated with clinical measures. In outpatients with post-COVID-19 conditions, the extent of hypometabolic clusters correlated with the number of symptoms reported during the initial infection, the time elapsed since symptom onset, ongoing fatigue, and language impairment. In a cross-sectional study of patients with postacute sequelae of COVID-19 evaluated using FDG PET, reduced metabolism in the frontal regions was linked to impaired concentration and mood disturbances.[56] Medial temporal hypometabolism was associated with memory complaints, and pontine hypometabolism correlated with paresthesia.

These findings have generated interest in FDG PET as a potential biomarker for persistent neurologic symptoms, and could be useful in the integrative medicine community in which practitioners encounter patients seeking care

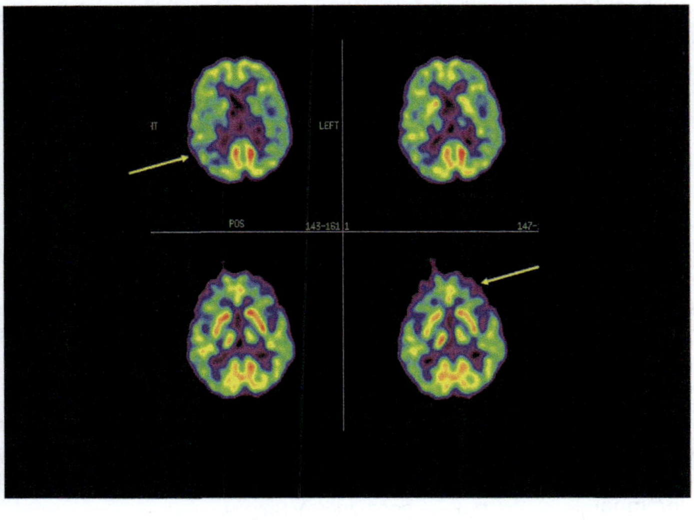

Fig. 5. FDG-PET of a patient with prior head injury and persistent symptoms showing areas of decreased glucose metabolism primarily in the frontal and temporal regions (*arrows*).

for long COVID-19. However, longitudinal voxel-based analyses have shown that, in patients with prolonged complaints, hypometabolic regions often remain largely stable over time, with only modest improvement in the pons and cerebellum under less stringent statistical thresholds.[57] Furthermore, at the individual patient level, applying the typical neuro-COVID-19 hypometabolic pattern through visual interpretation in a large multicenter cohort of patients yielded negative results in up to half of cases.[58] This variability suggests that individual-level interpretation can be challenging, requiring experienced readers and careful methodological approaches. Subtle metabolic changes and technical considerations, such as the selection of an appropriate reference region for normalization, particularly given possible white matter involvement, may complicate accurate assessment. Additional research is needed to determine the diagnostic value of FDG PET in long COVID-19 and whether it can be used to predict or follow response to therapeutic interventions.

SUMMARY

Functional neuroimaging, particularly with FDG PET, has substantially advanced our understanding of disorders affecting affective, cognitive, and behavioral regulation. These are conditions and symptoms that patients have who present for integrative medicine approaches for treatment. Looking forward, there is considerable opportunity to integrate functional neuroimaging into the evaluation of both conventional and integrative therapeutic interventions. PET, SPECT, and fMRI may serve as tools to characterize mechanisms of action, identify predictive biomarkers, and monitor physiologic response to treatment. Such research will be essential for delineating optimal therapeutic strategies, clarifying potential risks, and supporting evidence-based expansion of integrative modalities within neuropsychiatric and neurologic care.

CLINICS CARE POINTS

- Functional brain imaging can provide objective information about regional brain function, helping clinicians better characterize neurological and psychiatric disorders and supporting a more individualized approach to diagnosis and treatment planning.
- PET, SPECT, and functional MRI offer complementary information about cerebral metabolism, blood flow, neurotransmitter function, and structural and functional connectivity, allowing clinicians to select the imaging modality best suited to the patient's clinical question.
- In integrative medicine, functional neuroimaging can be used not only to evaluate disease processes but also to investigate the mechanisms and therapeutic effects of interventions such as meditation, acupuncture, neurofeedback, and other complementary therapies, facilitating evidence-based integration into clinical practice.
- Whole-body FDG PET is highly sensitive for detecting metabolically active malignancies and inflammatory processes, but abnormal FDG uptake is not specific for cancer and must always be interpreted within the clinical context.
- Routine whole-body FDG PET screening is not typically recommended for asymptomatic individuals because of false-positive findings, radiation exposure, cost, and the absence of evidence demonstrating improved mortality.
- Whole-body FDG PET may provide clinical value in carefully selected high-risk patients, such as those with hereditary cancer syndromes, suspected recurrent malignancy, or unexplained paraneoplastic syndromes, when used as part of an individualized diagnostic strategy.

DISCLOSURE

None of the authors have any conflicts to disclose.

REFERENCES

1. Kung BT, Seraj SM, Zadeh MZ, et al. An update on the role of ^{18}F-FDG-PET/CT in major infectious and inflammatory diseases. Am J Nucl Med Mol Imaging 2019;9(6):255–73.
2. Chen W, Parsons M, Torigian DA, et al. Evaluation of thyroid FDG uptake incidentally identified on FDG-PET/CT imaging. Nucl Med Commun 2009;30(3):240–4.
3. Jadvar H. FDG PET in prostate cancer. PET Clin 2009;4(2):155–61.
4. Sheikhbahaei S, Marcus CV, Fragomeni RS, et al. Whole-body ^{18}F-FDG PET and ^{18}F-FDG PET/CT in Patients with Suspecped Paraneoplastic Syndrpme: A Systematsc Review ans Meta-Analrsis of Diameta-ac Accuracy. J Nucl Med 2017;58(7):1031–6.
5. Kojima S, Zhou B, Teramukai S, et al. Cancer screening of healthy volunteers using whole-body 18F-FDG-PET scans: the nishidai clinic study. Eur J Cancer 2007;43(12):1842–8.

6. Sengoku T, Matsumura K, Usami M, et al. Diagnostic accuracy of FDG-PET cancer screening in asymptomatic individuals: use of record linkage from the Osaka Cancer Registry. Int J Clin Oncol 2014; 19(6):989–97.
7. Chan HP, Liu WS, Liou WS, et al. Comparison of FDG-PET/CT for cancer detection in populations with different risks of underlying malignancy. In Vivo 2020;34(1):469–78.
8. Weitzer F, Nazerani Hooshmand T, Pernthaler B, et al. Diagnostic value of F-18 FDG PET/CT in fever or inflammation of unknown origin in a large single-center retrospective study. Sci Rep 2022;12(1): 1883.
9. Treglia G. Diagnostic performance of ^{18}F-FDG PET/CT in Infectiousiand Inflammatoiy Diseases adcording to Published peta-Analymeta-a. ontrast Media Mol Imaging 2019;2019:3018349.
10. Pijl JP, Nienhuis PH, Kwee TC, et al. Limitations and pitfalls of FDG-PET/CT in infection and inflammation. Semin Nucl Med 2021;51(6):633–45.
11. Glaudemans AW, de Vries EF, Galli F, et al. The use of (18)F-FDG-PET/CT for diagnosis and treatment monitoring of inflammatory and infectious diseases. Clin Dev Immunol 2013;2013:623036.
12. Vaidyanathan S, Patel CN, Scarsbrook AF, et al. FDG PET/CT in infection and inflammation–current and emerging clinical applications. Clin Radiol 2015; 70(7):787–800.
13. Su L, Cai Y, Xu Y, et al. Cerebral metabolism in major depressive disorder: a voxel-based meta-analysis of positron emission tomography studies. BMC Psychiatry 2014;14(1):321.
14. Milak MS, Keilp J, Parsey RV, et al. Regional brain metabolic correlates of self-reported depression severity contrasted with clinician ratings. J Affect Disord 2010;126(1):113–24.
15. Milak MS, Parsey RV, Keilp J, et al. Neuroanatomic correlates of psychopathologic components of major depressive disorder. Arch Gen Psychiatry 2005; 62(4):397–408.
16. Milak MS, Parsey RV, Lee L, et al. Pretreatment regional brain glucose uptake in the midbrain on PET may predict remission from a major depressive episode after three months of treatment. Psychiatry Res 2009;173(1):63–70.
17. Reiman EM, Raichle ME, Robins E, et al. Neuroanatomical correlates of a lactate-induced anxiety attack. Arch Gen Psychiatry 1989;46(6): 493–500.
18. Liu N, Sun J, Jiang Y, et al. Brain metabolic vulnerability in 18-F FDG PET/CT predict future depression risk in young cancer survivors. Transl Psychiatry 2025;15(1):459.
19. Brody AL, Saxena S, Silverman DHS, et al. Brain metabolic changes in major depressive disorder from pre- to post-treatment with paroxetine. Psychiatry Research: Neuroimaging 1999;91(3):127–39.
20. Kennedy SH, Evans KR, Krüger S, et al. Changes in regional brain glucose metabolism measured with positron emission tomography after paroxetine treatment of major depression. Am J Psychiatr 2001; 158(6):899–905.
21. Kimbrell TA, Little JT, Dunn RT, et al. Frequency dependence of antidepressant response to left prefrontal repetitive transcranial magnetic stimulation (rTMS) as a function of baseline cerebral glucose metabolism. Biol Psychiatry 1999;46(12):1603–13.
22. Langguth B, Wiegand R, Kharraz A, et al. Pre-treatment anterior cingulate activity as a predictor of antidepressant response to repetitive transcranial magnetic stimulation (rTMS). Neuroendocrinol Lett 2007;28(5):633–8.
23. Kito S, Hasegawa T, Koga Y. Cerebral blood flow ratio of the dorsolateral prefrontal cortex to the ventromedial prefrontal cortex as a potential predictor of treatment response to transcranial magnetic stimulation in depression. Brain Stimul 2012; 5(4):547–53.
24. Deng D, Liao H, Duan G, et al. Modulation of the default mode network in first-episode, Drug-naïve major depressive disorder via acupuncture at baihui (GV20) acupoint. Front Hum Neurosci 2016;10:230.
25. Quah-Smith I, Suo C, Williams MA, et al. The antidepressant effect of laser acupuncture: a comparison of the resting brain's default mode network in healthy and depressed subjects during functional magnetic resonance imaging. Med Acupunct 2013;25(2): 124–33.
26. Reiman EM, Butler FK, Raichle ME, et al. A focal brain abnormality in panic disorder, a severe form of anxiety. Nature 1984;310(5979):683–5.
27. Goldin P, Ziv M, Jazaieri H, et al. MBSR vs aerobic exercise in social anxiety: FMRI of emotion regulation of negative self-beliefs. Soc Cognit Affect Neurosci 2013;8(1):65–72.
28. Goldin P, Ziv M, Jazaieri H, et al. Randomized controlled trial of mindfulness-based stress reduction versus aerobic exercise: effects on the self-referential brain network in social anxiety disorder. Front Hum Neurosci 2012;6:295.
29. Menzies L, Chamberlain SR, Laird AR, et al. Integrating evidence from neuroimaging and neuropsychological studies of obsessive-compulsive disorder: the orbitofronto-striatal model revisited. Neurosci Biobehav Rev 2008;32(3):525–49.
30. Insel TR, Winslow JT. Neurobiology of obsessive compulsive disorder. Psychiatr Clin 1992;15(4):813–24.
31. Swedo SE, Schapiro MB, Grady CL, et al. Cerebral glucose metabolism in childhood-onset obsessive-compulsive disorder. Arch Gen Psychiatry 1989; 46(6):518–23.

32. Brody AL, Saxena S, Schwartz JM, et al. FDG-PET predictors of response to behavioral therapy and pharmacotherapy in obsessive compulsive disorder. Psychiatry Research: Neuroimaging 1998; 84(1):1–6.
33. Schwartz JM, Stoessel PW, Baxter LR, et al. Systematic changes in cerebral glucose metabolic rate after successful behavior modification treatment of obsessive-compulsive disorder. Arch Gen Psychiatry 1996;53(2):109–13.
34. Saxena S, Brody AL, Maidment KM, et al. Localized orbitofrontal and subcortical metabolic changes and predictors of response to paroxetine treatment in obsessive-compulsive disorder. Neuropsychopharmacology 1999;21(6):683–93.
35. Hoexter MQ, Dougherty DD, Shavitt RG, et al. Differential prefrontal gray matter correlates of treatment response to fluoxetine or cognitive-behavioral therapy in obsessive-compulsive disorder. Eur Neuropsychopharmacol 2013;23(7):569–80.
36. Zhang Z, Wang X, Tan Q, et al. Electroacupuncture for refractory obsessive-compulsive disorder: a pilot waitlist-controlled trial. J Nerv Ment Dis 2009;197(8): 619–22.
37. Molina ME, Isoardi R, Prado MN, et al. Basal cerebral glucose distribution in long-term post-traumatic stress disorder. World J Biol Psychiatr 2010;11(2 Pt 2):493–501.
38. Shin LM, McNally RJ, Kosslyn SM, et al. Regional cerebral blood flow during script-driven imagery in childhood sexual abuse-related PTSD: a PET investigation. Am J Psychiatry 1999;156(4):575–84.
39. Shin LM, Orr SP, Carson MA, et al. Regional cerebral blood flow in the amygdala and medial prefrontal cortex during traumatic imagery in male and female Vietnam veterans with PTSD. Arch Gen Psychiatry 2004;61(2):168–76.
40. Monti DA, Tobia A, Stoner M, et al. Neuro emotional technique effects on brain physiology in cancer patients with traumatic stress symptoms: preliminary findings. J Cancer Surviv 2017;11(4):438–46.
41. King AP, Block SR, Sripada RK, et al. Altered default mode network (DMN) resting state functional connectivity following a mindfulness-based exposure therapy for posttraumatic stress disorder (PTSD) in combat veterans of Afghanistan and Iraq. Depress Anxiety 2016;33(4):289–99.
42. Silverman DH, Small GW, Chang CY, et al. Positron emission tomography in evaluation of dementia: regional brain metabolism and long-term outcome. JAMA 2001;286(17):2120–7.
43. Zhang S, Han D, Tan X, et al. Diagnostic accuracy of 18 F-FDG and 11 C-PIB-PET for prediction of short-term conversion to Alzheimer's disease in subjects with mild cognitive impairment. 2012. In: Database of abstracts of reviews of effects (DARE): quality-assessed reviews [Internet]. York (UK): Centre for Reviews and Dissemination (UK); 1995. Available at: https://www.ncbi.nlm.nih.gov/books/NBK91536/.
44. Smailagic N, Lafortune L, Kelly S, et al. 18F-FDG PET for prediction of conversion to Alzheimer's disease dementia in people with mild cognitive impairment: an updated systematic review of test accuracy. J Alzheimers Dis 2018;64(4):1175–94.
45. Caminiti SP, De Francesco S, Tondo G, et al. FDG-PET markers of heterogeneity and different risk of progression in amnestic MCI. Alzheimer's Dement 2024;20(1):159–72.
46. Heyer S, Simon M, Doyen M, et al. ^{18}F-FDG PET can effectively rule out conversion to dementia and the presence of CSF biomarker of neurodegeneration: a real-world data analysis. Alzheimers Res Ther 2024;16(1):182.
47. Kumar A, Newberg A, Alavi A, et al. Regional cerebral glucose metabolism in late-life depression and Alzheimer disease: a preliminary positron emission tomography study. Proc Natl Acad Sci U S A 1993; 90(15):7019–23.
48. Teichner EM, You JC, Hriso C, et al. Alterations in cerebral glucose metabolism as measured by 18F-fluorodeoxyglucose-PET in patients with persistent postconcussion syndrome. Nucl Med Commun 2021;42(7):772–81.
49. George JK, Alavi A, Zimmerman RA, et al. Metabolic (PET) correlates of anatomic lesions (CT/MRI) produced by head trauma (abstract). J Nucl Med 1989; 30:802.
50. Alavi A, Mirot A, Newberg A, et al. Fluorine-18-FDG evaluation of crossed cerebellar diaschisis in head injury. J Nucl Med 1997;38(11):1717–20.
51. Nakashima T, Nakayama N, Miwa K, et al. Focal brain glucose hypometabolism in patients with neuropsychologic deficits after diffuse axonal injury. AJNR Am J Neuroradiol 2007;28(2):236–42.
52. Soriano JB, Murthy S, Marshall JC, et al, WHO Clinical Case Definition Working Group on Post-COVID-19 Condition. WHO Clinical Case Definition Working Group on Post-COVID-19 Condition. A clinical case definition of post-COVID-19 condition by a Delphi consensus. Lancet Infect Dis 2022;22(4):e102–7.
53. van Kessel SAM, Olde Hartman TC, Lucassen PLBJ, et al. Post-acute and long-COVID-19 symptoms in patients with mild diseases: a systematic review. Fam Pract 2022;39(1):159–67.
54. Guedj E, Campion JY, Dudouet P, et al. ^{18}F-FDG brain PET hypometabolism in patients with long COVID. Eur J Nucl Med Mol Imaging 2021;48(9): 2823–33.
55. Martini AL, Carli G, Kiferle L, et al. Time-dependent recovery of brain hypometabolism in neuro-COVID-19 patients. Eur J Nucl Med Mol Imaging 2022; 50(1):90–102.
56. Rozenblum L, Debroucker T, Habert MO, et al. Cognitive impairment and brain metabolic changes

in post-acute sequelae of COVID-19: insights from an [18 F]FDG PET/CT cohort study. Clin Nucl Med 2025;50(3):e146–53.

57. Horowitz T, Dudouet P, Campion JY, et al. Persistent brain metabolic impairment in long COVID patients with persistent clinical symptoms: a nine-month follow-up [18F]FDG-PET study. Eur J Nucl Med Mol Imaging 2024;51(11):3215–22.

58. Verger A, Kas A, Dudouet P, et al. Visual interpretation of brain hypometabolism related to neurological long COVID: a French multicentric experience. Eur J Nucl Med Mol Imaging 2022;49(9):3197–202.

How Fluorine-18-labeled Fluorodeoxyglucose PET Changed Clinical Practice in Central Nervous System Disorders

Eric Guedj, MD, PhD[a,*], Andrew B. Newberg, MD[b,c], Abass Alavi, MD[d]

KEYWORDS

• [18F]FDG PET • Brain metabolism • Neuroimaging • Biomarkers • Central nervous system • Neurodegenerative disorders • Epilepsy • Autoimmune encephalitis

KEY POINTS

- Fluorine-18-labeled fluorodeoxyglucose ([18F]FDG) PET provides an integrated, physiologically grounded measure of neuronal and synaptic dysfunction, often detecting abnormalities before structural imaging becomes informative.
- Pattern-based interpretation of regional brain metabolism has established [18F]FDG PET as a robust diagnostic tool in dementia, epilepsy, and selected neuroinflammatory conditions, while focal hypermetabolism is clinically informative in lymphoma.
- Standardization of acquisition, quantification, and interpretation has enabled reproducible, multicenter clinical use and facilitated guideline integration.
- In the biomarker era, [18F]FDG PET complements pathology-specific markers by characterizing downstream functional expression and network-level impairment.
- Emerging network-based and artificial intelligence-driven analyses further extend its role in prognosis, patient stratification, and precision neurology.

Fifty years is a long time in clinical neuroscience, long enough for a method to evolve from conceptual breakthrough to routine clinical infrastructure, and for its clinical meaning to be repeatedly reshaped by new diseases, therapeutic advances, and evolving evidentiary frameworks. When the autoradiographic deoxyglucose method developed by Sokoloff and colleagues was translated in vivo to humans with fluorine-18-labeled fluorodeoxyglucose ([18F]FDG) in 1976, metabolic imaging moved from experimental neurophysiology to a clinically interpretable map of brain function.[1–4] This brain-first trajectory remains important, because the later success of [18F]FDG PET in oncology should not obscure its foundational role in clinical neuroscience. What followed was not merely a technical success. [18F]FDG PET established a new diagnostic language: spatially organized brain patterns of hypometabolism and, in selected neoplastic,

[a] Aix Marseille University, APHM, CNRS, Centrale Marseille, Institut Fresnel, Timone Hospital, CERIMED, Nuclear Medicine Department, Marseille, France; [b] Department of Integrative Medicine and Nutritional Sciences; [c] Department of Radiology, Research at the Marcus Institute of Integrative Health, Thomas Jefferson University, Philadelphia, PA, USA; [d] Division of Nuclear Medicine, Department of Radiology, Hospital of the University of Pennsylvania, Philadelphia, PA, USA
* Corresponding author. Laboratoire de Médecine Nucléaire, Hôpital de la Timone, 264 rue Saint Pierre, 13005 Marseille, France.
E-mail address: eric.guedj@univ-amu.fr

PET Clin 21 (2026) 587–592
https://doi.org/10.1016/j.cpet.2026.06.002

Abbreviations	
[18F]FDG	fluorine-18-labeled fluorodeoxyglucose
CNS	central nervous system
COVID-19	coronavirus disease 2019
EEG	electroencephalogram

inflammatory, and infectious settings, hypermetabolism, that clinicians could recognize, discuss, and act upon.

In today's biomarker landscape, with the increasing clinical use of amyloid and tau PET, more innovative synaptic and neuroinflammatory tracers, and rapidly expanding blood-based assays, [18F]FDG PET may appear insufficiently specific. Yet this apparent limitation is also the source of its enduring value. Rather than indexing a single upstream molecular signature, [18F]FDG PET captures an integrated downstream phenotype of neuronal and synaptic dysfunction, often before MR imaging becomes clearly informative, and reflects, to varying degrees, neurovascular coupling, circuit integrity, and systemic physiology. This integrative signal gained stronger mechanistic grounding through work on neuron-glia metabolic coupling, particularly the astrocyte-centered framework developed by Pellerin and Magistretti,[5] which moved interpretation beyond a simplistic neuron-only model. At the same time, renewed interest in cerebral energetics across neurologic disease—including insulin-resistance hypotheses in Alzheimer's disease and the possible central nervous system (CNS) relevance of metabolic modulators such as glucagon-like peptide-1 (GLP-1) receptor agonists and metformin—has brought metabolic imaging back into pathophysiological discussions.[6] In that sense, [18F]FDG PET did more than accompany the biomarker era: it helped define some of its core clinical principles—quantification, pattern-based inference, standardization, and multicenter comparability—and remains well positioned as a durable functional biomarker within precision neurology.[7,8]

FROM TRACER CHEMISTRY TO CLINICALLY INTERPRETABLE PHYSIOLOGY

The early history of [18F]FDG PET is inseparable from the deoxyglucose method itself: the idea that a glucose analog could quantify local cerebral metabolism as a proxy for functional activity.[2–4] The autoradiographic research of Sokoloff and colleagues[3] provided the conceptual and operational foundation. The first human [18F]FDG studies, led by teams including Alavi and Reivich, represented far more than a technical milestone: they showed that metabolic imaging could depict brain function with clinically meaningful contrast.[1,4] Kinetic modeling enabled quantitative estimation of local cerebral glucose utilization in humans, transforming [18F]FDG PET from an elegant image into a quantitatively interpretable physiologic signal.[4]

In parallel, radiochemistry matured from experimental synthesis to reproducible production suitable for clinical use.[2] PET instrumentation, attenuation correction strategies, and quantitative workflows also improved, strengthening reproducibility and enabling more robust interindividual and longitudinal comparisons. Regional metabolic abnormalities associated with neurodegeneration and epilepsy could be detected even when structural imaging was normal, equivocal, or nonspecific. [18F]FDG PET, therefore, introduced a new diagnostic logic: disease could be approached as a spatially structured metabolic signature, not only as a clinical syndrome or an anatomic lesion.

FROM NETWORK SIGNATURES TO FOCAL LESION ASSESSMENT: DEMENTIA, EPILEPSY, AND NEURO-ONCOLOGY

As scanners became more widely available and analytical workflows matured, [18F]FDG PET shifted from physiologic demonstration to clinically actionable interpretation. In dementia and epilepsy, this evolution largely took the form of reproducible network-level signatures. In neuro-oncology, by contrast, [18F]FDG PET was more often used as a focal lesion tool, exploiting hypermetabolic contrast in selected clinical scenarios rather than disease-defining topographies. This transition was enabled not only by broader access to PET, but also by the emergence of structured reading approaches and semiquantitative support tools, including normalization strategies, region-of-interest methods, and voxel-based comparisons with reference datasets.[7,8] [18F]FDG PET was no longer simply "showing metabolism"; it was generating interpretable evidence that could be communicated, taught, and defended in multidisciplinary care.

In cognitive disorders, [18F]FDG PET became a practical tool for differential diagnosis when clinical phenotypes overlapped and MR imaging remained inconclusive. Distinctive hypometabolic distributions such as temporoparietal and posterior cingulate involvement in typical Alzheimer's disease, frontotemporal abnormalities in frontotemporal lobar degeneration, and later more specific supportive signatures such as the cingulate island sign in dementia with Lewy bodies proved particularly useful in real-world uncertainty.[9,10] What converted compelling images into clinical decisions was not pattern recognition alone, but the convergence of structured visual interpretation, semiquantitative support, and evidence that [18F]FDG PET improves diagnostic accuracy and confidence beyond expert clinical assessment.[9]

In movement disorders, [18F]FDG PET similarly extended clinical reasoning beyond the confirmation of nigrostriatal degeneration. By capturing extranigral cortical, subcortical, brainstem, and cerebellar involvement, it helped differentiate Parkinson's disease from atypical parkinsonian syndromes within a broader pattern-based diagnostic framework.[7,8]

In epilepsy, [18F]FDG PET became a cornerstone of presurgical evaluation, especially in MR imaging-negative cases, extratemporal epilepsies, and complex electroclinical presentations.[11] By demonstrating interictal hypometabolism consistent with the epileptogenic network, or with its dominant hub, it helped formulate hypotheses that could then be tested against electroencephalogram (EEG), MR imaging, and, when needed, invasive recordings. Over time, its role evolved from a putative localizing test to an integrated component of surgical decision-making, influencing candidacy, electrode implantation strategies, and operative planning.[11]

In neuro-oncology, the trajectory was more circumscribed. High physiologic cortical uptake limited sensitivity for many low-grade tumors and reduced lesion-to-background contrast in several settings. Even so, [18F]FDG PET retained value in selected questions, particularly for suspected recurrence versus treatment-related change, high-grade lesions, but above all for primary CNS lymphoma.[12,13] Its limitations, however, also accelerated the adoption of alternative tracers, most notably amino acid PET, where available. This more selective role should not be seen as failure, but as evidence of an important principle: [18F]FDG PET changed practice not by being universally optimal, but by being clinically useful where glucose metabolism mattered most.

Early experience also suggested that [18F]FDG PET could reveal functionally abnormal patterns in autoimmune encephalitis,[14] especially when structural imaging was unrevealing.

STANDARDIZATION AND COVERAGE: WHEN [18F]FDG PET BECAME "PRACTICE"

A decisive transition in the clinical life cycle of [18F]FDG PET was the shift from an available technology to a system-supported standard of care. This inflection point depended on more than scanner performance. It required procedural standards, harmonized acquisition and reconstruction, quality assurance, reader training, and, crucially, coverage and policy decisions that formalized indications and made clinical utility operational.[7,8,15]

The widespread deployment of PET/CT streamlined workflows, improved attenuation correction, facilitated anatomic coregistration, and helped standardize real-world practice. In many health systems, the expansion of whole-body oncologic PET also increased scanner infrastructure, radiopharmacy capacity, and trained personnel, indirectly improving access to brain PET. Multicenter harmonization, including cross-calibration, phantom validation, and progressively aligned reconstruction and normalization practices, made results more portable across sites, readers, and time, which was essential for both guideline development and payer acceptance.[7,8] This reproducibility also contributed to the educational diffusion of metabolic pattern recognition, allowing nuclear medicine physicians, neurologists, psychiatrists, and multidisciplinary teams to share a common interpretive framework.

In the United States, a pivotal policy milestone occurred in 2004, when the Centers for Medicare & Medicaid Services established national coverage for [18F]FDG PET in the differential diagnosis of Alzheimer's disease versus frontotemporal dementia under specific clinical conditions.[15] The criteria were restrictive, but the signal was unmistakable: [18F]FDG PET had crossed a threshold of evidence and utility sufficient to shape national policy. In Europe, harmonization efforts and procedural guidance similarly accelerated maturation, culminating in increasingly detailed recommendations on acquisition, interpretation, and reporting.[7,8] During this period, semiquantitative tools—normative databases, z-score mapping, three dimensional stereotactic surface projection, and voxel-based approaches—became increasingly embedded in practice. Interpretation shifted from "what the eye sees" to "what the reader can justify", a cultural change that remains central to contemporary biomarker imaging.[7–9]

THE BIOMARKER REVOLUTION AND THE REPOSITIONING OF FLUORINE-18-LABELED FLUORODEOXYGLUCOSE PET

From the mid-2010s onward, CNS diagnostics increasingly embraced pathology-specific biomarkers, including amyloid and tau PET, dopamine transporter and synaptic density imaging, neuroinflammatory tracers in research, and, more recently, blood-based biomarker panels. In this new ecosystem, [18F]FDG PET did not disappear; it was repositioned. Its main value became less the inference of upstream pathology and more the measurement of downstream functional consequence. It remained particularly relevant for differential diagnosis in atypical and mixed presentations, for phenotypic adjudication when biomarkers were discordant, and for assessing the severity and spatial distribution of functional impairment.[7,8]

At the same time, [18F]FDG PET analytics moved beyond regional uptake into network-oriented models. Approaches described as metabolic connectivity or covariance analysis use interregional relationships in glucose metabolism to derive graph-like representations of brain organization, complementing conventional topographic reads.[16] Although still primarily research-facing, these methods are conceptually aligned with the broader move toward multidimensional and AI-assisted biomarker interpretation, and they may prove especially valuable for prognosis, treatment stratification, and monitoring.

In dementia, professional guidance continues to support [18F]FDG PET as a clinically useful adjunct for differentiating Alzheimer's disease, frontotemporal degeneration, dementia with Lewy bodies, and related syndromes.[7–10] In the era of disease-modifying therapies and increasingly accessible blood biomarkers, this role may become more, not less, important, because upstream biomarker positivity does not by itself resolve phenotypic heterogeneity, stage, or clinical relevance. [18F]FDG PET helps answer a different question: what is the functional expression of the disease in this patient.

In movement disorders, metabolic pattern analysis has shown strong performance in distinguishing Parkinson's disease from atypical parkinsonian syndromes, particularly when early clinical assessment is uncertain or confounded by comorbidities.[17] The contribution of [18F]FDG PET here is not best framed as "PET versus clinician", but as a network-level constraint that stabilizes classification, shortens time to a more reliable diagnosis, and thereby affects prognosis, counseling, and trial eligibility.

In epilepsy, hybrid imaging—including PET-MR imaging instrumentation—and advanced postprocessing have further consolidated clinical impact. Integrated PET/MR workflows, improved reconstruction, and refined postprocessing have together enhanced lesion detection and presurgical localization in selected settings.[11] These developments do not replace multidisciplinary reasoning; they make [18F]FDG PET a more robust contributor to it.

Immune-mediated CNS disease has provided another important arena for renewed relevance. In autoimmune encephalitis, where MR imaging may be normal early and antibody results may be delayed, negative, or difficult to interpret, [18F]FDG PET has shown high sensitivity in several series and is associated with characteristic, although heterogeneous, patterns of cortical and subcortical metabolic abnormality.[14] The coronavirus disease 2019 (COVID-19) pandemic further catalyzed the use of brain [18F]FDG PET in postinfectious conditions, generating a large observational literature on post-COVID-19 condition and related neurocognitive symptoms.[18] This body of research highlighted a major strength of the technique: the ability to detect systems-level dysfunction before overt structural injury becomes apparent and to do so in a clinically interpretable manner.

WHY FLUORINE-18-LABELED FLUORODEOXYGLUCOSE PET CHANGED PRACTICE

Across indications, [18F]FDG PET has repeatedly changed management through a small number of durable mechanisms. First, it improves differential diagnosis when symptoms and MR imaging are nonspecific. Second, it constrains diagnostic reasoning at the network level, whether by localizing dysfunction in epilepsy or by identifying syndrome-relevant metabolic signatures in neurodegenerative and movement disorders.[9–11,17] Third, by quantifying the burden and distribution of functional impairment, it supports prognostic stratification. Fourth, as therapies become more targeted and heterogeneous, it helps refine treatment pathways by characterizing downstream functional phenotype. Fifth, its impact has been magnified by standardization, which allows results to be compared across readers, centers, and time.[7,8]

Importantly, these mechanisms translated into practical decisions rather than only diagnostic refinement. In cognitive disorders, [18F]FDG PET helped move patients from broad syndromic labels toward more pathophysiologically and topographically consistent diagnoses, thereby informing counseling, prognosis, prioritization of complementary biomarker testing, and selection for disease-specific pathways.[7–10] In epilepsy, its value was often expressed at the level of multidisciplinary strategy: refining the hypothesis of the epileptogenic network, guiding invasive EEG implantation, and increasing confidence in surgical planning when MR imaging and electroclinical data were incomplete or discordant.[11] In inflammatory and postinfectious conditions, it provided objective evidence of cerebral dysfunction in situations where conventional investigations could remain unrevealing, helping to structure follow-up and avoid premature nonspecific or purely psychogenic attribution.[14,18] Across these settings, the clinical contribution of [18F]FDG PET was, therefore, not limited to detecting an abnormal scan. It changed the evidentiary status of functional brain dysfunction and made it actionable within multidisciplinary care.

Taken together, these contributions are not tied to a single disease category or therapeutic era. They reflect a broader structural advantage of [18F]FDG PET: it is a physiologically grounded tool that maps clinically meaningful dysfunction at the level at which patients actually present, through symptoms, syndromes, and network failure.

THE NEXT REFRAMING

As the field marks the 50 year milestone of human [18F]FDG imaging, the next reframing is already underway. [18F]FDG PET is increasingly being integrated into multimodal diagnostic pathways that combine plasma biomarkers, MR imaging signatures, pathology-specific PET tracers, and, more broadly, systemic and brain-body perspectives on disease. In such an ecosystem, its comparative advantage is likely to remain phenotypic resolution: a robust and clinically legible map of downstream functional vulnerability that can contextualize upstream markers, arbitrate discordant results, and support individualized clinical reasoning.[7,8] This may be particularly relevant when pathology-specific biomarkers identify disease biology but do not fully explain symptom severity, clinical phenotype, or the spatial organization of impairment.

At 50 years, the case for [18F]FDG PET is, therefore, not nostalgic. It changed clinical practice because it taught neuroscience and medicine how to operationalize function: to quantify it, standardize it, compare it, and act on it. As CNS care becomes more precise, the need for reproducible measures of downstream functional integrity is likely to grow. In that future, [18F]FDG PET may be less a standalone test than one of the central functional backbones of integrated precision neurology.

CLINICS CARE POINTS

- [18F]FDG PET should be used to answer a defined clinical question, particularly when clinical assessment, MRI, or pathology-specific biomarkers are inconclusive or discordant.
- Interpretation should be pattern-based and clinically contextualized. Regional hypometabolism or hypermetabolism should be integrated with the patient's phenotype, disease stage, structural imaging, biological markers, and longitudinal course.
- In cognitive disorders, epilepsy, movement disorders, autoimmune encephalitis, and selected neuro-oncology settings, [18F]FDG PET contributes most by clarifying functional network involvement, supporting differential diagnosis, presurgical reasoning, prognostic assessment, or treatment-pathway decisions.
- [18F]FDG PET is not a direct marker of a single disease pathology. It reflects downstream neuronal, synaptic, glial, vascular, and network-level dysfunction, and should therefore be considered complementary to amyloid, tau, dopaminergic, inflammatory, or tumor-specific imaging biomarkers.
- Standardized acquisition, semiquantitative support, and structured reporting are essential to ensure reproducibility, communicate diagnostic confidence, and explicitly state limitations or discordance with other clinical data.

DISCLOSURE

Nothing to disclose.

REFERENCES

1. Hess S, Blomberg BA, Zhu HJ, et al. Historic images in nuclear medicine: 1976: the first issue of Clinical Nuclear Medicine and the first human FDG study. Clin Nucl Med 2014;39(8):701–3.
2. Fowler JS, Ido T. Initial and subsequent approach for the synthesis of 18FDG. Semin Nucl Med 2002;32(1):6–12.
3. Sokoloff L, Reivich M, Kennedy C, et al. The [14C]deoxyglucose method for the measurement of local cerebral glucose utilization: theory, procedure, and normal values in the conscious and anesthetized albino rat. J Neurochem 1977;28(5):897–916.
4. Reivich M, Kuhl D, Wolf A, et al. The [18F]fluorodeoxyglucose method for the measurement of local cerebral glucose utilization in man. Circ Res 1979;44(1):127–37.
5. Magistretti PJ, Pellerin L. Cellular mechanisms of brain energy metabolism. Relevance to functional brain imaging and to neurodegenerative disorders. Ann N Y Acad Sci 1996;777:380–7.
6. Ong LT, Sia CH. Interactions between antidiabetes medications and heart-brain axis. Curr Opin Endocrinol Diabetes Obes 2025;32(1):34–43.
7. Guedj E, Varrone A, Boellaard R, et al. EANM procedure guidelines for brain PET imaging using [18F]FDG, version 3. Eur J Nucl Med Mol Imag 2022;49(2):632–51.

8. Arbizu J, Morbelli S, Minoshima S, et al. SNMMI Procedure Standard/EANM Practice Guideline for Brain [18F]FDG PET imaging, version 2.0. J Nucl Med 2025;66(Suppl 2):S45–60.
9. Foster NL, Heidebrink JL, Clark CM, et al. FDG-PET improves accuracy in distinguishing frontotemporal dementia and Alzheimer's disease. Brain 2007; 130(Pt 10):2616–35.
10. Lim SM, Katsifis A, Villemagne VL, et al. The 18F-FDG PET cingulate island sign and comparison to 123I-beta-CIT SPECT for diagnosis of dementia with lewy bodies. J Nucl Med 2009;50(10):1638–45.
11. Traub-Weidinger T, Arbizu J, Garibotto V, et al. EANM practice guidelines for an appropriate use of PET and SPECT for patients with epilepsy. Eur J Nucl Med Mol Imag 2024;51(7):1891–908.
12. Parent EE, Johnson DR, Gleason T, et al. Neuro-Oncology Practice Clinical Debate: FDG PET to differentiate glioblastoma recurrence from treatment-related changes. Neurooncol Pract 2021;8(5):518–25.
13. Rozenblum L, Houillier C, Soussain C, et al. Role of positron emission tomography in primary central nervous system lymphoma. Cancers (Basel) 2022; 14(17):4071.
14. Jha S, Nagaraj C, Mundlamuri R, et al. FDG-PET in autoimmune encephalitis: utility, pattern of abnormalities, and correlation with autoantibodies. Ann Indian Acad Neurol 2022;25(6):1122–9.
15. Centers for Medicare & Medicaid Services. FDG PET for Dementia and Neurodegenerative Diseases. National Coverage Determination (NCD) 220.6.13. Issued September 15, 2004. Available at: https://www.cms.gov/medicare/coverage/evidence/dementia.
16. Cavaliere C, Galli A, Meneghini C, et al. Molecular connectivity studies of cerebral glucose metabolism and blood flow: a scoping review. Neurosci Biobehav Rev 2026;185:106623.
17. Meyer PT, Frings L, Rücker G, et al. 18F-FDG PET in parkinsonism: differential diagnosis and evaluation of cognitive impairment. J Nucl Med 2017;58(12): 1888–98.
18. Guedj E, Campion JY, Dudouet P, et al. 18F-FDG brain PET hypometabolism in patients with long COVID. Eur J Nucl Med Mol Imag 2021;48(9): 2823–33.

Future Directions for [18F]FDG PET in Central Nervous System Diseases

Eric Guedj, MD, PhD[a,*], Andrew B. Newberg, MD[b,c], Abass Alavi, MD[d]

KEYWORDS

• [18F]FDG PET • Brain metabolism • Metabolic connectivity • Artificial intelligence • Functional PET • Total-body PET • Standardization • Precision neurology

KEY POINTS

- [18F]FDG PET is evolving from a regional imaging modality into a computational and network-aware biomarker of distributed brain dysfunction.
- Its broader clinical impact will depend on standardized, reproducible, and scalable frameworks that enable robust deployment across centers.
- Artificial intelligence and advanced analytics may enhance individual-level interpretation, prognostication, and multimodal integration, provided they achieve clinical-grade validation.
- Emerging approaches, including dynamic [18F]FDG PET and total-body PET, extend the field toward temporal physiology and brain–body interactions.
- Within precision neurology, [18F]FDG PET is well positioned as a functional anchor that complements molecular and fluid biomarkers by reflecting the downstream expression of disease.

For five decades, brain [18F]FDG PET has provided a clinically valuable readout of neuronal and synaptic dysfunction across a broad spectrum of central nervous system (CNS) disorders. Its enduring relevance lies in its ability to capture an integrated functional phenotype that often reflects the downstream expression of network dysfunction more directly than structural imaging alone.[1,2] As molecular PET tracers continue to diversify, [18F]FDG PET may retain an important role in neurology, and an emerging one in psychiatry, by building on what it uniquely provides: a scalable representation of the functional expression of disease.

Against this background, three developments appear particularly important. First, [18F]FDG PET is evolving from a visually interpreted regional image into a more computational, network-aware, and potentially systems-level biomarker of brain dysfunction. Second, the broader scientific and clinical impact of this evolution will depend on standardized, multicenter, and clinically deployable frameworks that make [18F]FDG PET outputs portable, reproducible, and trustworthy across sites and populations.[3–5] Third, [18F]FDG PET is likely to retain a major role not in isolation, but as part of a multimodal precision-neurology ecosystem in which functional imaging complements molecular, structural, and fluid biomarkers. Together, these shifts suggest that the next phase of [18F]FDG PET in CNS disorders may be defined

[a] Aix Marseille University, APHM, CNRS, Centrale Marseille, Institut Fresnel, Timone Hospital, CERIMED, Nuclear Medicine Department, Marseille, France; [b] Department of Integrative Medicine and Nutritional Sciences, Research at the Marcus Institute of Integrative Health, Thomas Jefferson University, Philadelphia, PA, USA; [c] Department of Radiology, Research at the Marcus Institute of Integrative Health, Thomas Jefferson University, Philadelphia, PA, USA; [d] Division of Nuclear Medicine, Department of Radiology, Hospital of the University of Pennsylvania, Philadelphia, PA, USA
* Corresponding author. Laboratoire de Médecine Nucléaire, Hôpital de la Timone, 264 rue Saint Pierre, 13005 Marseille, France.
E-mail address: eric.guedj@univ-amu.fr

PET Clin 21 (2026) 593–597
https://doi.org/10.1016/j.cpet.2026.06.003
1556-8598/26/

Abbreviation	
CNS	central nervous system

less by a change in tracer identity than by a modernization of how its signal is represented, validated, and integrated into decision-making.

FROM IMAGES TO COMPUTATIONAL, NETWORK-LEVEL, AND SYSTEMS REPRESENTATIONS

A first transformation concerns the nature of the biomarker itself. In routine practice, [18F]FDG PET already combines expert visual assessment with semiquantitative support,[1,2] but the field is increasingly moving beyond the detection of regional uptake abnormalities toward structured, reproducible, and individually quantifiable representations of distributed network-level brain dysfunction.[6] In that sense, the future of [18F]FDG PET may depend not only on what it detects, but also on how its signal is modeled and expressed. Metabolic connectivity and graph-based approaches seek to capture distributed disease effects that may remain visually subtle yet clinically meaningful, including prodromal neurodegeneration, compensatory reorganization, and syndrome-relevant connectomic signatures.[6]

This network perspective is particularly relevant because many CNS disorders are clinically expressed through distributed dysfunction rather than isolated lesions. In Alzheimer's disease, frontotemporal degeneration, dementia with Lewy bodies and parkinsonian syndromes, the diagnostic value of [18F]FDG PET often resides in the spatial organization of hypometabolism.[1,2,7,8] In epilepsy, the clinically relevant signal may extend beyond the seizure onset zone to involve connected cortical and subcortical structures that shape surgical hypotheses and outcome prediction.[9] In immune-mediated or post-infectious conditions, metabolic abnormalities may similarly reflect systems-level disruption that is not captured by conventional structural imaging.[1,2,10] Future computational approaches should therefore preserve this clinical logic: they should not merely generate abstract network metrics, but translate distributed metabolic information into interpretable patterns that help clinicians understand why a patient presents with a given syndrome, why symptoms may exceed structural findings, and how disease expression may evolve over time.[1,2,6] However, their translational value will depend on moving beyond retrospective group-level contrasts toward individual-level inference that can improve patient phenotyping and clinical decision-making. In the near term, network-level [18F]FDG PET metrics are most likely to gain clinical traction in settings where [18F]FDG PET already contributes to care and where distributed dysfunction is central to interpretation, such as atypical dementias, parkinsonian syndromes, and epilepsy surgery pathways. Their usefulness will ultimately depend on demonstrating incremental value beyond conventional regional analyses, for example, through improved prognostication, subtype stratification, or monitoring of treatment-related network reconfiguration.[6]

A further extension of this trajectory concerns time-resolved physiology. Static [18F]FDG PET remains a powerful technique, but it provides only a temporally coarse representation of glucose utilization. The maturation of infusion protocols and high-sensitivity systems has renewed interest in dynamic [18F]FDG PET approaches, including functional PET (fPET), which may enable higher temporal resolution assessments of uptake during tasks or at rest.[11,12] Methodological resources comparing [18F]FDG-fPET with fMRI are especially valuable because they allow benchmarking of signal dynamics and spatial correspondence across modalities.[11,12] At present, these approaches remain largely confined to specialized research settings, and their clinical role is still emerging. Nonetheless, in selected contexts such as pharmacodynamic studies, assessment of network responsiveness, or mechanistic phenotyping, they may eventually broaden the scope of metabolic imaging. Beyond fPET itself, this logic may be particularly relevant for psychiatric and neuropsychiatric conditions, where metabolic abnormalities may be better interpreted as state-sensitive and context-sensitive network phenotypes than as fixed disease-specific signatures. For these applications, standardized uptake conditions and careful documentation of medication exposure, substance use, sleep, affective state, and task context will be essential to separate clinically meaningful signal from avoidable variability.[1,2]

Long axial field-of-view and total-body PET systems may extend this logic even further toward systems physiology. By markedly increasing sensitivity and anatomic coverage, these platforms make it increasingly feasible to examine brain metabolism in relation to whole-body dynamics within a single acquisition.[13,14] In disorders in which cerebral dysfunction is closely intertwined with systemic processes—including paraneoplastic syndromes, immune-mediated disease, infection-associated brain dysfunction, and treatment-related neurotoxicity—[18F]FDG PET may progressively contribute to a more integrated brain–body physiology framework.[13,14] This remains an emerging horizon rather than an established clinical standard, but it is conceptually consistent with the broader evolution of [18F]FDG PET from regional imaging toward networked and systemic representations of disease.

FROM EXPERT-CENTER PRACTICE TO STANDARDIZED, SCALABLE, AND CLINICALLY DEPLOYABLE [18F]FDG PET

The next challenge is therefore translational. If computationally enriched [18F]FDG PET is to move beyond expert centers, its outputs must remain robust, reproducible, and clinically interpretable across scanners, institutions, and patient populations.

A first requirement is technical robustness. Image enhancement, harmonization, and artificial intelligence-assisted analytical pipelines, ranging from denoising and resolution recovery to reconstruction-adjacent strategies, may improve effective sensitivity and reduce unwanted variability, particularly in low-dose protocols, shortened acquisitions, pediatric imaging, and high-throughput dementia workflows.[15] Automated quality control may add further value by systematizing tasks that expert teams often perform implicitly, such as detecting motion, injection-to-acquisition anomalies, off-target uptake patterns, or preprocessing failures before they influence interpretation. Computational pipelines may also support more robust spatial normalization, more consistent reference-region strategies, and more auditable feature extraction.[5,15] More broadly, the field must ensure that [18F]FDG PET processing is sufficiently stable, transparent, and reproducible to support downstream inference.[1,2,5] Within this framework, the clinical promise of artificial intelligence should be framed as an extension of structured reading.[15] In brain [18F]FDG PET, AI-assisted tools may help by highlighting subtle abnormalities, comparing individual patients with age-appropriate reference populations, and quantifying deviations from expected metabolic patterns. Such tools could be particularly valuable for supporting more consistent interpretation across centers with variable neuro-PET expertise, or for helping high-volume workflows prioritize cases requiring more detailed expert review. However, their outputs must remain actionable for clinicians. A probability score without anatomic localization, pathophysiological plausibility, or prognostic interpretation is unlikely to change practice. For this reason, AI-assisted interpretation should remain traceable, anatomically explicit, and designed to support expert-led review rather than produce opaque standalone outputs.[15]

A second requirement is data discipline. In this context, PET-BIDS provides a practical framework for structuring PET data and metadata in ways that facilitate aggregation, sharing, and reproducible analysis.[3] Likewise, consensus recommendations on the content and format of PET brain data in publications and archives clarify what should be reported to support interpretability and comparability across studies.[4] These standards are especially important because they shift reproducibility from an implicit expectation to an explicit methodological commitment. Yet the implementation gap remains substantial, and reproducibility audits continue to identify limitations in metadata completeness, preprocessing provenance, and analytical transparency.[5]

A third requirement is multicenter infrastructure. Because centralized pooling of clinical imaging data is increasingly constrained by privacy regulation, governance complexity, and institutional reluctance to export patient-level data, privacy-preserving approaches such as federated learning may offer a pragmatic route for multicenter [18F]FDG PET research.[16] Their value lies in enabling model development across more diverse scanner ecosystems and patient populations while limiting data movement. However, such frameworks will only be useful if combined with harmonized acquisition protocols, locked preprocessing pipelines, clearly defined outcomes, and transparent reporting of performance, including subgroup analyses and failure modes.[16]

Ultimately, deployability will require more than technical performance. [18F]FDG PET-derived tools will need to demonstrate external validity across centers, vendors, protocols, and demographic strata, while generating outputs that are interpretable, calibrated, and prospectively useful. In practice, the decisive benchmark will be whether these tools inform patient management, whether through additional testing, intensified follow-up, referral, or treatment selection.[15,17,18] In Europe, the AI Act further reinforces the need for risk management, data quality, transparency, documentation, and human oversight for high-risk systems.[19] Standardization, validation, and regulation should therefore be viewed as successive steps in the same translational pathway.

POSITIONING [18F]FDG PET WITHIN MULTIMODAL PRECISION NEUROLOGY

The final issue is strategic where [18F]FDG PET fits within the biomarker ecosystem of modern neurology and psychiatry. In many CNS pathways, it is now interpreted alongside plasma biomarkers, pathology-specific PET tracers, and MRI. Its future relevance is therefore unlikely to rest on competing with more disease-specific markers at the molecular level. Rather, [18F]FDG PET may retain a distinctive role as a functional anchor, capturing the downstream expression of disease burden, resilience, and network vulnerability in a way that often aligns closely with symptoms and disability.[1,2]

This positioning matters because multimodal precision neurology does not simply require more biomarkers; it requires biomarkers that answer different questions. Pathology-specific tracers and fluid markers may identify molecular processes, but they do not necessarily reflect how those processes are functionally expressed at the level of cerebral networks or clinical impairment. Interestingly, [18F]FDG PET occupies an important intermediate space between biology and phenotype. This intermediate position may become increasingly important as disease-modifying strategies expand. In Alzheimer's disease, for example, amyloid or tau biomarkers may establish biological eligibility for targeted interventions, but they do not fully determine the clinical phenotype, the degree of network failure, or the coexistence of non-Alzheimer contributors to cognitive impairment. Similarly, in movement disorders, autoimmune encephalitis, epilepsy, and psychiatric presentations, molecular or structural markers may be necessary but insufficient to explain the patient-level burden of disease. [18F]FDG PET can help bridge this gap by documenting whether, where, and how cerebral function is already compromised. Its role in precision neurology should therefore be understood not as competing with molecular biomarkers, but as contextualizing them within the functional architecture of the living brain.[1,2,6] It may be especially useful when upstream markers are discordant, when symptoms are disproportionate to structural damage, or when clinicians need a more integrated assessment to constrain differential diagnosis or estimate trajectory. Operationally, this argues for reports and decision-support outputs that explicitly connect metabolic patterns with the clinical question, the degree of diagnostic confidence, and the recommended next step in the biomarker pathway. Such clinically oriented reporting would help ensure that increasingly complex analytical outputs remain understandable, comparable, and actionable for multidisciplinary teams across centers.[1,2]

Parkinsonian syndromes provide a practical example of this question-driven logic: presynaptic dopaminergic imaging may help establish whether nigrostriatal degeneration is present, whereas [18F]FDG PET can be more informative for identifying which distributed degenerative syndrome best explains the clinical phenotype. Similar reasoning should guide future multimodal pathways, in which each biomarker is selected according to the clinical question rather than according to a generic hierarchy of technological specificity.[1,2,8]

Recent work using deep learning to predict progression trajectories, metabolic change, or cognitive decline from [18F]FDG PET illustrates one possible direction, particularly when models are coupled with explainability strategies that identify the imaging features driving prognostic output.[17,18] However, the decisive benchmark will remain prospective clinical utility. [18F]FDG PET will be most relevant in precision neurology not when it produces the most sophisticated models, but when it improves the timing, confidence, or appropriateness of clinical decisions within multimodal pathways.

SUMMARY

Taken together, these developments suggest a realistic roadmap for the coming years. [18F]FDG PET may be reframed as a computational and network-aware biomarker, embedded in standardized and clinically deployable infrastructures, and positioned more explicitly within multimodal precision-neurology pathways. These are not independent agendas, but interdependent ones. Computational sophistication without standardization will not scale; standardization without clinical integration will not matter; and multimodal relevance without robust functional phenotyping will remain incomplete. The future of brain [18F]FDG PET in CNS disorders is therefore unlikely to depend on a single breakthrough. Rather, it may emerge from the convergence of better representations, better infrastructures, and better clinical integration. The key challenge will be to ensure that these advances remain clinically meaningful. A future in which [18F]FDG PET produces increasingly sophisticated metrics but fails to influence diagnosis, prognosis, treatment selection, or patient communication would represent a missed opportunity. Conversely, if computational modeling, harmonized infrastructures, and multimodal integration are developed around clinically relevant questions, [18F]FDG PET could gain renewed clinical importance. Its future strength may lie precisely in its ability to connect scales: molecular biology, network dysfunction, systemic physiology, clinical phenotype, and therapeutic decision-making. Under those conditions, [18F]FDG PET could remain a major functional backbone of precision neurology and psychiatry: not because it answers every biological question, but because it continues to provide a clinically scalable representation of how disease is functionally expressed in the living brain.

CLINICS CARE POINTS

- Future [18F]FDG PET applications should remain driven by clinically defined questions.
- Network-based, metabolic connectivity, and AI-assisted approaches should support expert clinical interpretation, with outputs that remain anatomically explicit, explainable, and actionable.
- Dynamic [18F]FDG PET, functional PET, and total-body PET are promising tools for studying temporal physiology and brain-body interactions.
- Standardization of acquisition, metadata, processing, reporting, and quality control is essential.
- Within multimodal precision neurology, [18F]FDG PET should be positioned as a functional biomarker, complementary to MRI, fluid biomarkers, and pathology-specific PET tracers, particularly when downstream network dysfunction is clinically relevant.

DISCLOSURES

Nothing to disclose.

REFERENCES

1. Guedj E, Varrone A, Boellaard R, et al. EANM procedure guidelines for brain PET imaging using [18F]FDG, version 3. Eur J Nucl Med Mol Imag 2022;49(2):632–51.
2. Arbizu J, Morbelli S, Minoshima S, et al. SNMMI procedure Standard/EANM practice guideline for brain [18F]FDG PET imaging, version 2.0. J Nucl Med 2025;66(Suppl 2):S45–60.
3. Norgaard M, Matheson GJ, Hansen HD, et al. PET-BIDS, an extension to the brain imaging data structure for positron emission tomography. Sci Data 2022;9(1):65.
4. Knudsen GM, Ganz M, Appelhoff S, et al. Guidelines for the content and format of PET brain data in publications and archives: a consensus paper. J Cereb Blood Flow Metab 2020;40(8):1576–85.
5. Naseri M, Ramakrishnapillai S, Carmichael OT. Reproducible brain PET data analysis: easier said than done. Front Neuroinf 2024;18:1420315.
6. Cavaliere C, Galli A, Meneghini C, et al. Molecular connectivity studies of cerebral glucose metabolism and blood flow: a scoping review. Neurosci Biobehav Rev 2026;185:106623.
7. Foster NL, Heidebrink JL, Clark CM, et al. FDG-PET improves accuracy in distinguishing frontotemporal dementia and Alzheimer's disease. Brain 2007;130(Pt 10):2616–35.
8. Meyer PT, Frings L, Rücker G, et al. 18F-FDG PET in Parkinsonism: differential diagnosis and evaluation of cognitive impairment. J Nucl Med 2017;58(12):1888–98.
9. Traub-Weidinger T, Arbizu J, Garibotto V, et al. EANM practice guidelines for an appropriate use of PET and SPECT for patients with epilepsy. Eur J Nucl Med Mol Imag 2024;51(7):1891–908.
10. Jha S, Nagaraj C, Mundlamuri R, et al. FDG-PET in autoimmune encephalitis: utility, pattern of abnormalities, and correlation with autoantibodies. Ann Indian Acad Neurol 2022;25(6):1122–9.
11. Villien M, Wey HY, Mandeville JB, et al. Dynamic functional imaging of brain glucose utilization using fPET-FDG. Neuroimage 2014;100:192–9.
12. Verger A, Guedj E. The renaissance of functional 18F-FDG PET brain activation imaging. Eur J Nucl Med Mol Imag 2018;45(13):2338–41.
13. Hicks RJ, Rahmim A, Lodge MA, et al. Total-body PET/CT: pros and cons. Semin Nucl Med 2025;55(1):11–20.
14. Reed MB, Ponce de León M, Vraka C, et al. Whole-body metabolic connectivity framework with functional PET. Neuroimage 2023;271:120030.
15. Currie GM, Hawk KE. Artificial intelligence augmented cerebral nuclear imaging. Semin Nucl Med 2025;55(4):616–28.
16. Zhou B, Xie H, Liu Q, et al. FedFTN: personalized federated learning with deep feature transformation network for multi-institutional low-count PET denoising. Med Image Anal 2023;90:102993.
17. García-Gutiérrez F, Hernández-Lorenzo L, Cabrera-Martín MN, et al, Alzheimer's Disease Neuroimaging Initiative. Predicting changes in brain metabolism and progression from mild cognitive impairment to dementia using multitask deep learning models and explainable AI. Neuroimage 2024;297:120695.
18. Sohn B, Chung SJ, Lee JR, et al, Harvard Brain Imaging Study, Japanese Alzheimer's Disease Neuroimaging Initiative, Alzheimer's Disease Neuroimaging Initiative. [18F]FDG-PET-based deep learning for predicting cognitive decline in non-demented elderly across the Alzheimer's disease clinical spectrum. Radiol Adv 2024;1(3):umae021.
19. European Parliament and Council of the European Union, Regulation (EU) 2024/1689 of 13 June 2024 laying down harmonised rules on artificial intelligence (Artificial Intelligence Act), *Off J Eur Union*, 2024, OJ L, 2024/1689. Available at: https://eur-lex.europa.eu/eli/reg/2024/1689/oj/eng.

9780443520884